Metallic Foam Bone

Related titles

Bone Response to Dental Biomaterials
(ISBN 978-0-08-100287-2)

Biomaterials Science, 3e
(ISBN 978-0-12-374626-9)

Surface Coating and Modification of Metallic Biomaterials
(ISBN 978-1-78242-303-4)

Woodhead Publishing Series in Biomaterials

Metallic Foam Bone

Processing, Modification and Characterization and Properties

Edited by

Cuie Wen

ELSEVIER

AMSTERDAM • BOSTON • HEIDELBERG • LONDON
NEW YORK • OXFORD • PARIS • SAN DIEGO
SAN FRANCISCO • SINGAPORE • SYDNEY • TOKYO
Woodhead Publishing is an imprint of Elsevier

WP
WOODHEAD PUBLISHING

Woodhead Publishing is an imprint of Elsevier
The Officers' Mess Business Centre, Royston Road, Duxford, CB22 4QH, United Kingdom
50 Hampshire Street, 5th Floor, Cambridge, MA 02139, United States
The Boulevard, Langford Lane, Kidlington, OX5 1GB, United Kingdom

Notices
Knowledge and best practice in this field are constantly changing. As new research and experience broaden our understanding, changes in research methods, professional practices, or medical treatment may become necessary.

Practitioners and researchers must always rely on their own experience and knowledge in evaluating and using any information, methods, compounds, or experiments described herein. In using such information or methods they should be mindful of their own safety and the safety of others, including parties for whom they have a professional responsibility.

To the fullest extent of the law, neither the Publisher nor the authors, contributors, or editors, assume any liability for any injury and/or damage to persons or property as a matter of products liability, negligence or otherwise, or from any use or operation of any methods, products, instructions, or ideas contained in the material herein.

Library of Congress Cataloging-in-Publication Data
A catalog record for this book is available from the Library of Congress

British Library Cataloguing-in-Publication Data
A catalogue record for this book is available from the British Library

ISBN: 978-0-08-101289-5 (print)
ISBN: 978-0-08-101290-1 (online)

Publisher: Matthew Deans
Acquisition Editor: Laura Overend
Editorial Project Manager: Natasha Welford
Production Project Manager: Poulouse Joseph
Designer: Victoria Pearson

Typeset by TNQ Books and Journals

Contents

List of contributors

A. Ataee RMIT University, Melbourne, Victoria, Australia

C.C. Berndt Swinburne University of Technology, Hawthorn, Victoria, Australia; Stony Brook University, Stony Brook, NY, United States

S. Fujibayashi Kyoto University, Kyoto, Japan

P. Hodgson Deakin University, Geelong, Victoria, Australia

T. Kokubo Chubu University, Kasugai, Aichi, Japan

Y. Li RMIT University, Melbourne, Victoria, Australia

J. Lin Zhejiang Industry & Trade Vocational College, Wenzhou, Zhejiang, China; Jilin University, Changchun, Jilin, China

T. Matsushita Chubu University, Kasugai, Aichi, Japan

S. Minagar Swinburne University of Technology, Hawthorn, Victoria, Australia

K.S. Munir RMIT University, Melbourne, Victoria, Australia

A. Nouri University of Toronto, Toronto, ON, Canada

L. Ren Institute of Metal Research, Chinese Academy of Sciences, Shenyang, China

G. Song CSIRO Manufacturing Flagship, Clayton, Victoria, Australia

A. Vahidgolpayegani Deakin University, Geelong, Victoria, Australia

C. Wen Swinburne University of Technology, Hawthorn, Victoria, Australia; RMIT University, Melbourne, Victoria, Australia

S. Yamaguchi Chubu University, Kasugai, Aichi, Japan

K. Yang Institute of Metal Research, Chinese Academy of Sciences, Shenyang, China

Preface

The nine chapters of this book deal with various topics associated with foam bone: materials, processing, surface modification, characterization, and properties.

Chapter 1 provides a review of the development of metallic scaffold implants through selective laser melting (SLM), an emerging additive manufacturing technique for the fabrication of complicated near net shape scaffold implants, which are otherwise difficult or impossible to fabricate with other conventional manufacturing techniques. The influence of the processing parameters and the characteristics of starting materials on the microstructure, mechanical, and biological properties of the fabricated scaffolds are elucidated. The advancements, limitations, challenges, and future potential of SLM in the manufacturing of metallic scaffold implants are also explained.

A variety of fabrication methods for porous magnesium (Mg) and some of its alloys and their characterization for biodegradable implant applications are presented in Chapter 2. The macro- and microstructures, mechanical and corrosion properties, and in vitro and in vivo biocompatibility of different porous Mg and its alloys produced through different methods are highlighted. Furthermore, the manufacturing methods for producing Mg scaffolds that are technologically, scientifically, and technically advanced are reviewed. We also provide an insight into the future research directions in the field of porous Mg alloy biomaterials.

Chapter 3 presents a review of electron beam melting (EBM) as a promising technology for manufacturing complex nonstochastic metal scaffolds in the field of biomedical applications. The processing parameters, mechanical properties, and structural characteristics of the metal scaffolds manufactured by EBM are analyzed. The disadvantages, advantages, and the potentials of this state-of-the-art 3D printing technology are highlighted, and advancements in the area of biomedical devices are elucidated.

Titanium (Ti) foams with different structures for bone tissue engineering are investigated by both powder sintering and SLM in Chapter 4. The advantages and disadvantages of each method, as well as the structural characteristics, mechanical properties, and surface properties of the Ti foams before and after chemical and heat treatments, are comparatively presented. Both the osteoconduction and osteoinduction of the Ti foams after surface modification are highlighted. The Ti foams applied to a lumbar interbody fusion procedure in patients are demonstrated with improved Japanese Orthopedic Association back pain evaluation questionnaire scores.

Chapter 5 focuses on Ti foams for dental applications. Some of the fundamental parameters of porous dental implants that allow enhanced osseointegration, stability, and effective dental rehabilitation, including dimensional considerations, alloy selection, mechanical properties, and porous characteristics, are elucidated. In particular, an attempt has been made to categorize Ti dental implants according to their type and design, including implants with fully porous structures, implants with porous surfaces and a solid core, and implants with a thin porous surface.

A variety of surface modification techniques suitable for Ti foams are presented in Chapter 6, aiming at inducing their bone-bonding ability. Among them, chemical and heat treatments are simple and inexpensive and can be easily applied for coating the Ti foam surfaces uniformly, even the inner surface of the pores of medical devices with complex shapes. Chemical and heat treatments that are effective for inducing bone-bonding as well as osteoconduction and osteoinduction are described.

The bioactivity and biocompatibility of implant materials are influenced by their chemistry and the topography of the implant surfaces at different dimension levels, that is, at macro-, micro-, and nanoscales. The nanotopography and surface chemistry of nanotubular surfaces and their bioactivity and biocompatibility are presented in Chapter 7. The fabrication of metal oxide nanotubes on metallic biomaterials, especially Ti alloys via anodization, can enhance the bioactivity by inducing the formation of hydroxyapatite (HA), in contrast to the anodized surface and the bare metal alone. The wall thickness of the nanotubes, the nanotubular length, the crystallinity of the nanotubes, and the hydrophilicity are demonstrated to strongly influence HA formation. An increase in cell adhesion on the HA-coated nanotubular surface is clearly observed.

Implant-associated bacterial infections have been a serious problem, and many efforts have been devoted to solving this problem. Copper (Cu) is a well-known, broad spectrum antibacterial agent and can be alloyed with many metals. Chapter 8 focuses on the development of a series of Cu-containing antibacterial metals, including stainless steels, Ti and some of its alloys, and cobalt-based alloys. The various aspects in the development of antibacterial metals, including composition design, material fabrication, microstructure and properties characterization, antibacterial performance, biocompatibility, and medical applications in orthopedics and dentistry are elucidated. The development of antibacterial metals will provide new opportunities for the design and manufacturing of metal implants with antibacterial functions.

Chapter 9 deals with the effects of different surface nanopatterns on the bioactivity and cell response of Ti alloys. The $TiO_2-ZrO_2-ZrTiO_4$ nanotubes are fabricated via anodization using aqueous and nonaqueous electrolytes and exhibit different physical and chemical properties. The morphological, thermal, topographical, chemical, and mechanical properties of the nanotubes are comprehensively characterized, and their bioactivity and influence on cellular functions are presented. The highest cell attachment is demonstrated on the nanotubes fabricated in nonaqueous electrolytes with an inner diameter in the range of optimal nanospacing.

Finally, this book is intended to provide knowledge and insights for researchers and engineers from both academia and industries in the field of metallic foam bone: manufacturing, surface modification, and characterization. Ti, Mg, their alloys, and scaffolds for the manufacture of medical devices and clinical applications are highlighted. It is hoped that the materials presented in this book will also inspire further research, leading to contributions toward the development of the next generation of orthopedic and dental implant devices, with improved functions of allowing new bone tissue ingrowth and vascular invasion, osteoconduction, osteoinduction, and osseointegration. Clinical applications of such medical devices will significantly benefit the aging population and individuals adversely affected by bone abnormalities.

Metallic scaffolds manufactured by selective laser melting for biomedical applications

1

K.S. Munir[2], *Y. Li*[2], *C. Wen*[1,2]
[1]Swinburne University of Technology, Hawthorn, Victoria, Australia; [2]RMIT University, Melbourne, Victoria, Australia

1.1 Introduction

Additive manufacturing (AM) has emerged as a promising technique for developing biomedical implants with complicated shapes. A usual approach in AM is the design and development of a computer-generated 3D solid model of the desired implant, which is then manufactured by an addition of material in the form of a series of thin layers. One of the many advantages of using this technology is the development of implants with complicated profiles and shapes, which are difficult to fabricate by adopting conventional manufacturing routes. The conventional manufacturing techniques usually require expensive tools for finishing procedures, leading to reduced efficiency and productivity of the manufacturing setups. On the other hand, AM offers a solution where a complex shape is required for an implant to fit into irregular defected sites in the human body. Extensive research has been carried out to utilize the potential of AM for the development of porous bone scaffolds and dental implants [1,2]. Developments have shown that AM technologies are effective in the development of simpler and more efficient surgical implants where the fabricated porous scaffolds matched and replicated the skeletal anatomy [3,4]. An optimization of the process parameters in AM technologies allows for an intimate control of the microstructures, appearance, and resultant shape of the fabricated implants and scaffolds. These developments in AM technologies imply the success of surgical operations where any part of the human body, eg, the skull, jaw, ear, etc., can be reconstructed by obtaining images from X-ray CT scans of the patients [5–7]. The key steps involved in the development of biomedical implants and scaffolds are illustrated in Fig. 1.1.

1.2 Advanced manufacturing techniques for tissue engineering scaffolds and implants

AM techniques are generally equipped with laser-assisted technologies in which the power of a highly focused laser beam is used for the fusion of metal powders.

Metallic Foam Bone. http://dx.doi.org/10.1016/B978-0-08-101289-5.00001-9

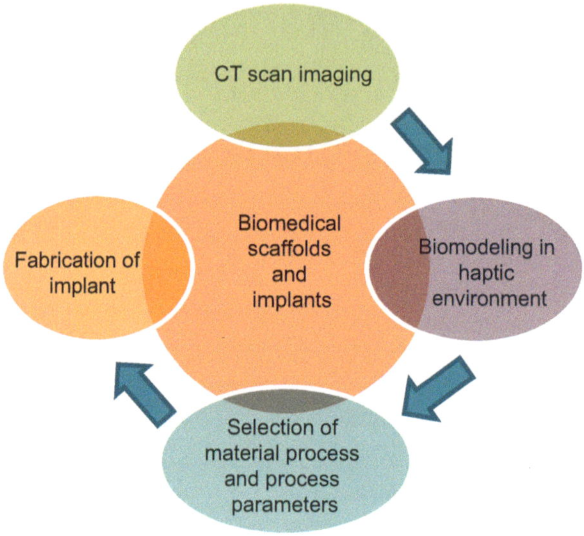

Figure 1.1 Development cycle indicating the key steps involved in the manufacturing of biomedical scaffolds and implants.

Laser-assisted additive manufacturing (LAAM) technologies can use various approaches to fabricate a part, including the following:

- The first approach is to form powder layers in the form of a powder bed from the metal powders fed into the machine. This layer-by-layer fabricated part can be manufactured by using selective laser sintering (SLS) or selective laser melting (SLM) setups.
- The second approach is to directly deposit the fed metal powder onto a substrate that is mounted on a machine table. The movement of the focused laser beam or table can be controlled to obtain a desired part. This technique is used in direct metal deposition technologies.

1.2.1 Selective laser sintering

In SLS a laser is generally employed to build a part using a layer-by-layer method from a fine powder bed. Fig. 1.2 shows a typical configuration of an SLS setup. Recrystallization (sintering) of fine powders takes place once illuminated by a high-power beam of a laser. The scanning laser beam is controlled via a deflection system for building each layer; this deflection and control of the laser beam is governed by a corresponding cross-section calculated from a predesigned CAD model. The next layer is then built up by depositing and spreading powder on the previously processed layer, and this cycle continues to manufacture the whole 3D part [8]. The entire stack of layers is bonded together during the SLS process to generate a specific shape, as described by the predesigned 3D model. The powder deposition system in SLS is generally composed of a roller or a scraper, which enables SLS to deposit successive powder layers with a thickness range of 20−150 μm. The powder deposition is generally carried out under an

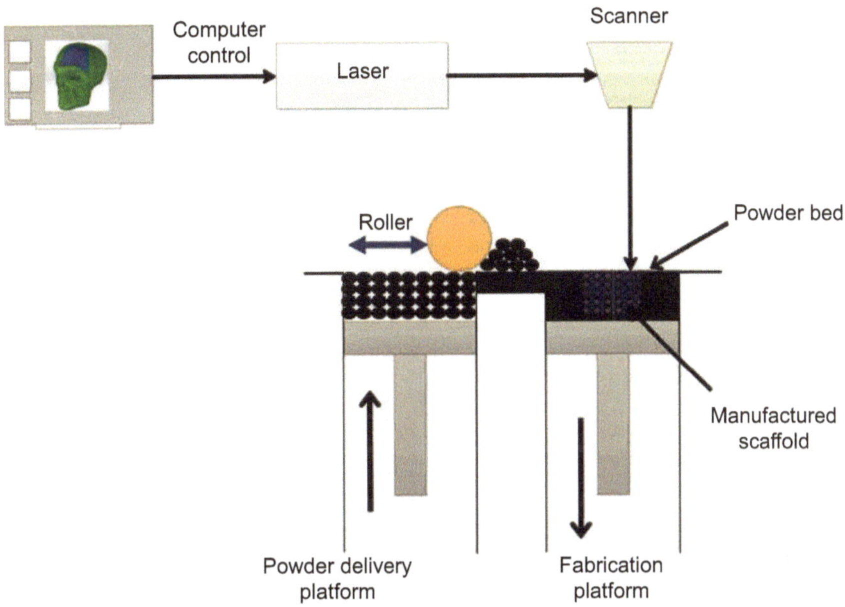

Figure 1.2 Typical configuration of a selective laser sintering setup for manufacturing metal scaffolds.

inert atmosphere (eg, argon, nitrogen) to avoid any environmental contamination and undesired oxidation of powders during the sintering process. SLS printers accommodate a variety of lasers in their setups, eg, CO_2 laser, lamp, or diode pumped Nd:YAG laser, disk or fiber laser, etc. [9]. The unsintered powder bed supports the manufactured part during the SLS process, enabling a support-free production [10]. A promising feature of SLS is the efficient utilization of powder, as the remaining unmelted powder can be recycled. However, previous studies have mentioned a poor surface finish and dimensional inaccuracies of manufactured parts via the SLS process, which require expensive postprocessing treatments such as machining, heat treatments, polishing, etc. [11]. The microstructures of the porous structures and scaffolds can be controlled by optimizing the critical processing parameters of SLS, including laser power, powder bed temperature, laser scan speed, etc. [12].

The layer-by-layer stacking methodology in SLS allows for fabricating scaffolds with complicated geometries. The efficient and productive attributes of SLS have made it a promising technology for the fabrication of tissue engineering scaffolds [7,13]. Kruth et al. [14] adequately described a powder deposition method in SLS in which bonding of powder particles takes place below their melting points. However, pure metallic structures require high sintering temperatures to achieve sufficient metallurgical bonding between metal powders. This constraint makes the SLS process more convenient for polymers. During the early development stages of SLS various materials were fabricated by adopting different processing parameters, including nylon, polycarbonate, nylon–glass composite, ceramics, metal–polymer powders, hydroxyapatite, etc. Later on, efforts were carried out to fabricate high-strength metals using the powder mixtures of Fe–Cu, WC–CO, TiB_2–Ni, TiC–Ni/Co/Mo, Fe_3C–Fe, etc. In those metal-based powder mixtures, powders with low melting points acted as binders for other high melting point powders [15,16].

1.2.1.1 Previous work on tissue engineering scaffolds and implants using selective laser sintering

SLS has been reported as an efficient and productive technology for the development of polymer-based materials for scaffolds and bioimplants. Previous research on SLS has successfully fabricated scaffolds from polycaprolactone (PCL) powders for bone tissue engineering [7]. Fig. 1.3 shows a pig condyle scaffold manufactured by SLS.

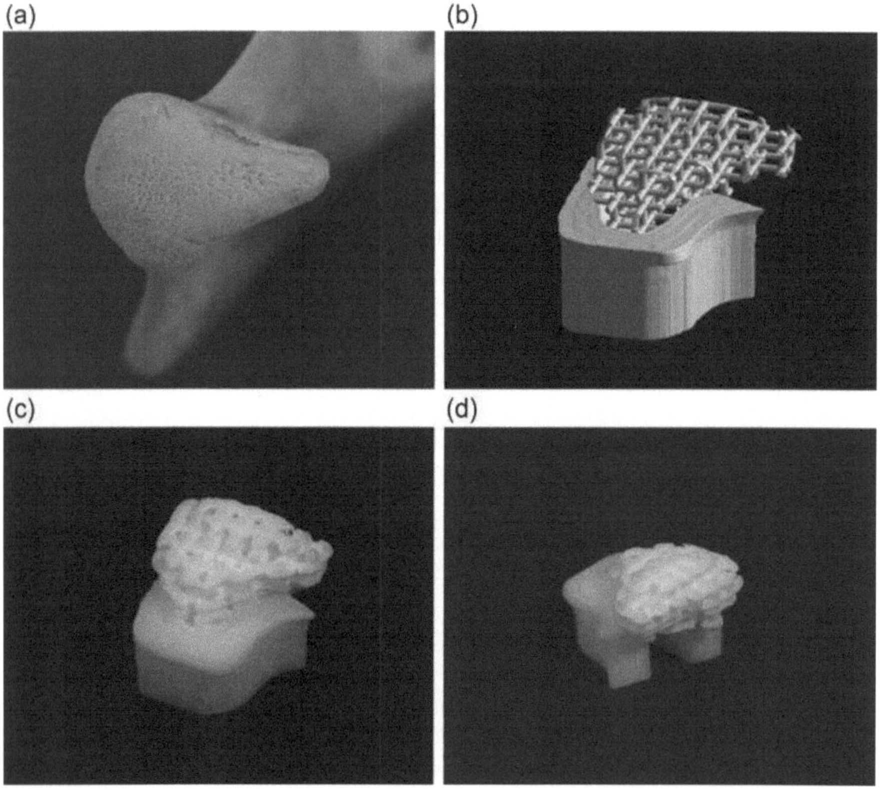

Figure 1.3 (a) An actual pig condyle, (b) surface rendering of STL design file for a pig condyle scaffold, (c) front view, and (d) back view of the pig condyle scaffold fabricated by selective laser sintering.
Reproduced from Williams JM, et al. Bone tissue engineering using polycaprolactone scaffolds fabricated via selective laser sintering. Biomaterials 2005;26(23):4817–27.

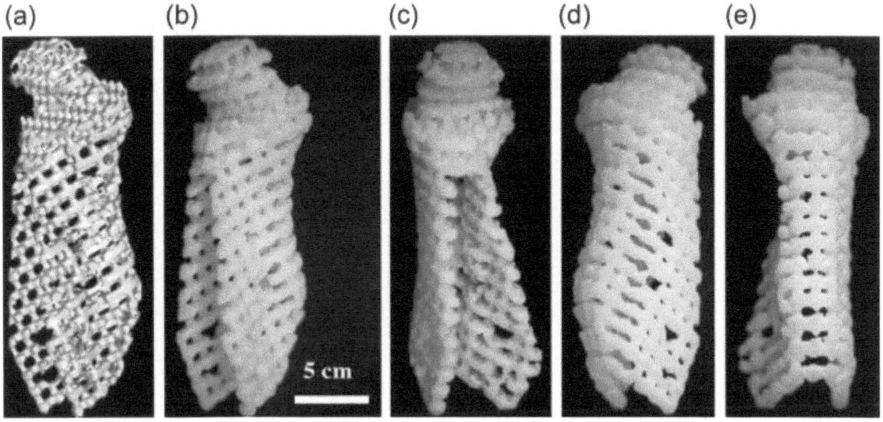

Figure 1.4 Development of an actual human condyle scaffold: (a) 3D rendition of human condyle scaffold, (b–e) polycaprolactone scaffold produced by selective laser sintering. Reproduced from Partee B, Hollister SJ, Das S. Selective laser sintering process optimization for layered manufacturing of CAPA® 6501 polycaprolactone bone tissue engineering scaffolds. J Manuf Sci Eng 2006;128(2):531–40.

Mechanical properties of fabricated scaffolds using SLS have been reported as close to properties of trabecular bone. Partee et al. [17] reported a successful development of tissue engineering human condyle scaffolds prepared from PCL powders by SLS. Fig. 1.4 shows the manufactured human condyle scaffold. In some studies a deviation of actual porosity from designed porosity was reported, which was attributed to the adherence and bonding of excess powders on orthogonal porous channels [18]. Another problem that was observed in the early studies was the insufficient densification of the designed solid regions, as they exhibited 20% microporosity. These problems directly affected the microstructure and eventually the load-bearing capability of the fabricated scaffolds. Later on these issues were addressed by controlling the critical processing parameters of SLS.

The fabrication of the customized passive dynamic response ankle-foot orthoses further enhanced the potential of SLS, which improved the walking abilities of patients with neuromuscular disorders and provided support during various phases of gait [19].

1.2.1.2 Advantages, challenges, and key materials processed by selective laser sintering

One of the major limitations of SLS is the poor surface finishing of the fabricated parts, which requires postprocessing procedures to improve those surfaces. Polymers have been used extensively to be processed by SLS; however, these materials also have some issues, such as shrinkage and warping due to thermal distortion in the fabricated parts. Table 1.1 presents an overview of the advantages, disadvantages, and materials processed by SLS reported in the literature to date.

Table 1.1 Advantages and disadvantages of additive manufacturing using the selective laser sintering technique

Advantages	Disadvantages	Materials used for the fabrication of scaffolds	References
• Fabrication of complicated shapes • Quick processing • Wide range of materials • Self-support of the powder bed	• Not useful for pure metals • Poor surface finish • Defects in the manufactured parts due to large shrinkage rates • Postprocessing treatments are necessary to improve the surface quality	• Polycaprolactone • Calcium phosphates • Carbon-fiber composites • Hydroxylapatite	[7,10,12,13,15,17,19,20]

1.2.2 Selective laser melting

SLM has emerged as a promising AM technique to effectively and efficiently fabricate complicated 3D parts of a wide range of materials [21,22]. SLM was introduced to rectify some of the densification issues in the SLS manufacturing technique by using a focused high-energy laser beam of 0.03 mm diameter [23]. A CAD model is generally used to govern the laser beam, which consolidates a thin layer of supplied metal powders. Fig. 1.5 shows the schematic illustration of the design to surgery road map of a fabricated part via SLM.

During the SLM process, the metal powders are generally spread out mechanically on a metal plate; the powder bed is then scanned by a focused high-temperature laser beam. Fusion of the powder bed occurs with the metallic plate, and a second layer is then built by spreading the powder bed on the consolidated layer by lowering the metallic plate. The laser beam scans the powder bed again and merges with the previously scanned layer. Generally a step of 0.05 mm is placed to build successive layers in the Z direction to fabricate any complex part [14,21]. Fig. 1.6 shows the step-by-step design to production phases involved in the manufacturing of tissue engineering scaffolds using SLM. The fabrication of scaffolds is the most critical step in tissue engineering for a number of reasons: scaffolds not only act as transplant vehicles for the attachment of cells, but they also act as templates for guiding tissue regeneration. Previous studies on the development of tissue engineering scaffolds and implants revealed the importance of 3D porous scaffolds for the attachment of cells and the subsequent regeneration of bone and cartilage [24]. Therefore any AM technique and corresponding process parameters should be selected carefully to achieve the required characteristics of the scaffolds.

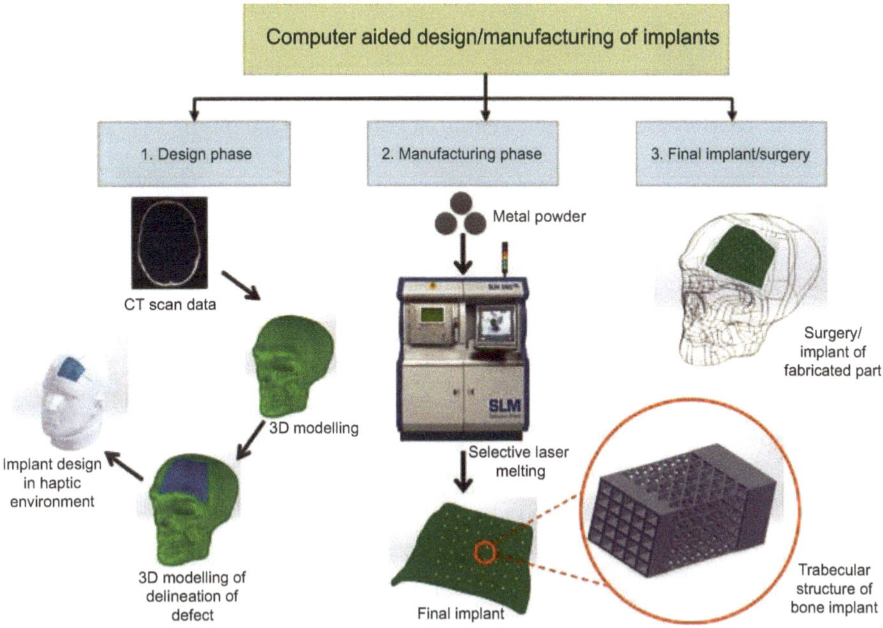

Figure 1.5 Schematic illustration of different phases involved in the design, production, and surgery of a selective laser melting-processed human skull plate.

1.2.2.1 Required characteristics of a tissue engineering scaffold

An ideal scaffold should possess the following characteristics: (1) a 3D porous structure with an interconnected pore network for enhanced cell attachment and growth, (2) compatible mechanical properties matching the tissue or bone of the defected site, (3) biocompatibility to eliminate or minimize adverse tissue reactions, and (4) an appropriate surface roughness to encourage cell attachment and proliferation. Fig. 1.7 shows the illustration of the four important required characteristics that directly influence the properties and performance of a tissue engineering scaffold.

Hollister [24] defined a "4Fs theory" summarizing the required characteristics of a scaffold for a particular defect site, which were given as **f**orm (referring to an appropriate 3D design and geometry of the scaffold to fill the complex defected site); **f**ixation (referring to the fixation requirements of the scaffold to be fixed into the defected site during surgery and to prevent any loosening); **f**unction (referring to the requirement of a scaffold to temporarily perform as a substitute tissue in the defected site); and **f**ormation (referring to the ability of the scaffold to encourage bone tissue ingrowth and regeneration by the controlled release of biowastes, mass transportation, and communication with other organs by providing sufficient signals). Fig. 1.8 shows a typical tissue engineering scaffold designed for a calvarial (skullcap) reconstruction and fabricated by SLM.

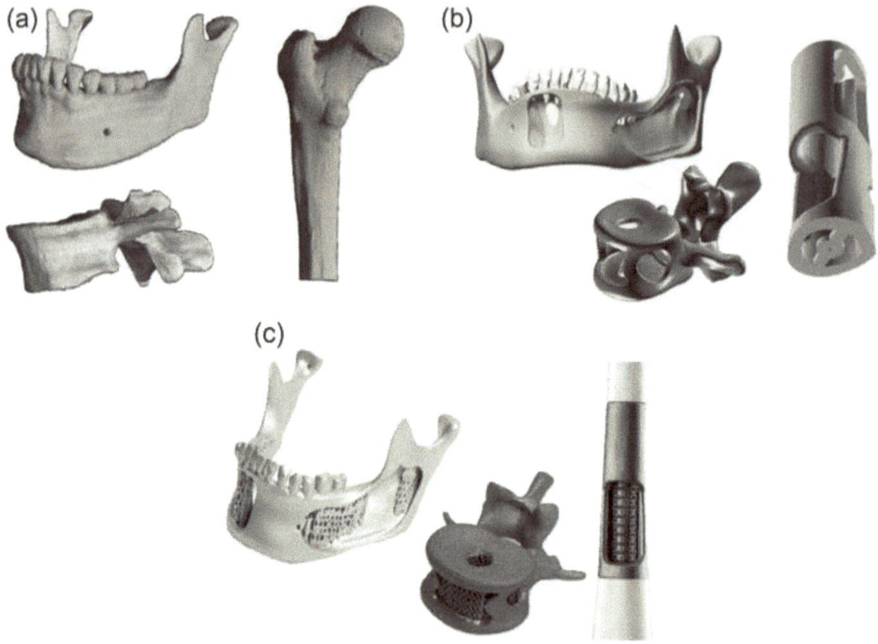

Figure 1.6 Production route of tissue engineering scaffolds by selective laser melting: (a) CT scan images from plastic models, (b) development of CAD anatomic models based on the CT scans, and (c) real parts manufactured by selective laser melting.
Reproduced from Wehmöller M, et al. Implant design and production—a new approach by selective laser melting. In: International congress series. Elsevier; 2005.

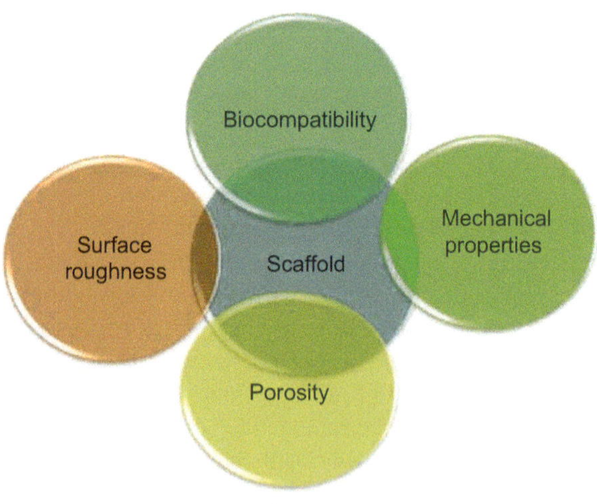

Figure 1.7 Critical characteristics required for a successful tissue engineering scaffold.

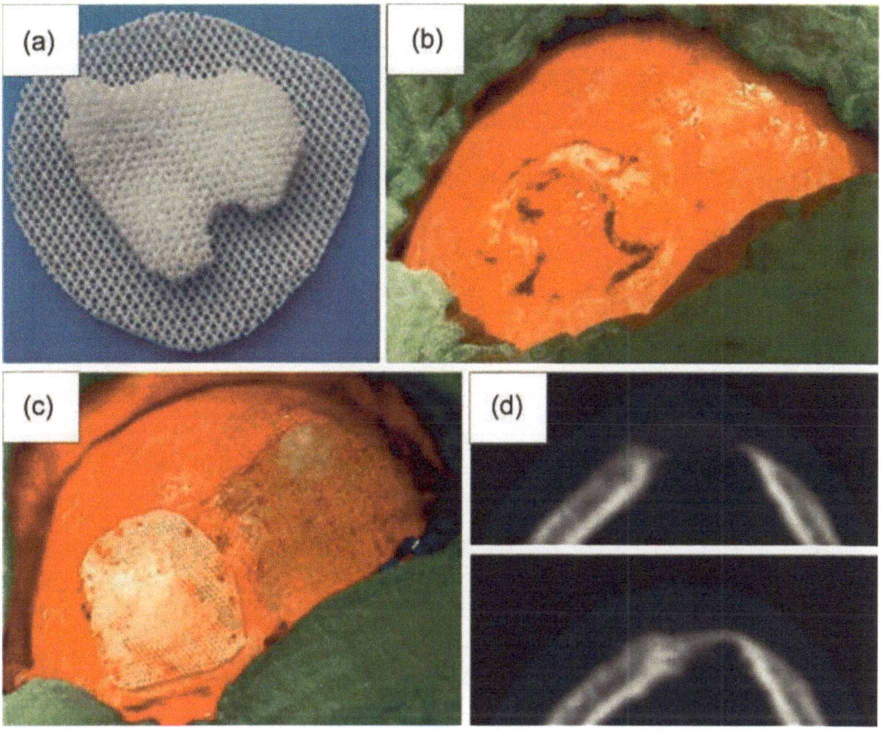

Figure 1.8 Development of tissue engineering for calvarial reconstruction fabricated by selective laser melting: (a) scaffold designed from X-ray CT scan imaging data, (b) clinical surgery showing the calvarial defect site, (c) fixation of the defect after a surgery with calvarial scaffold after a surgery, and (d) CT scan images showing the bony consolidation of the defect after 6 months.
Reproduced from Probst F, et al. [Calvarial reconstruction by customized bioactive implant]. Handchirurgie, Mikrochirurgie, plastische Chirurgie. Organ der Deutschsprachigen Arbeitsgemeinschaft fur Handchirurgie: Organ der Deutschsprachigen Arbeitsgemeinschaft fur Mikrochirurgie der Peripheren Nerven und Gefasse: Organ der V 2010;42(6):369–73.

1.2.2.2 Effect of porous structure on the osteoconductivity of scaffolds

The geometry and shape of a scaffold play an important role in bone regeneration. The bone-implant interface determines the efficiency of tissue and bone ingrowth. Previous studies on SLM-processed scaffolds highlighted the enhanced cell attachment (osteoconductivity) in the scaffolds with a porous structure [27,28]. Such porous structures of the fabricated scaffolds enhance bone ingrowth by migration of the cells to the pores. The migrated cells in the porous structure of scaffolds need quick vascularization to improve the required nutrition. Especially in the case of dental implants, an early vascularization is critical in the large osseous defect sites. In such large defect sites, distances must be bridged to improve the transportation of nutrients, bone

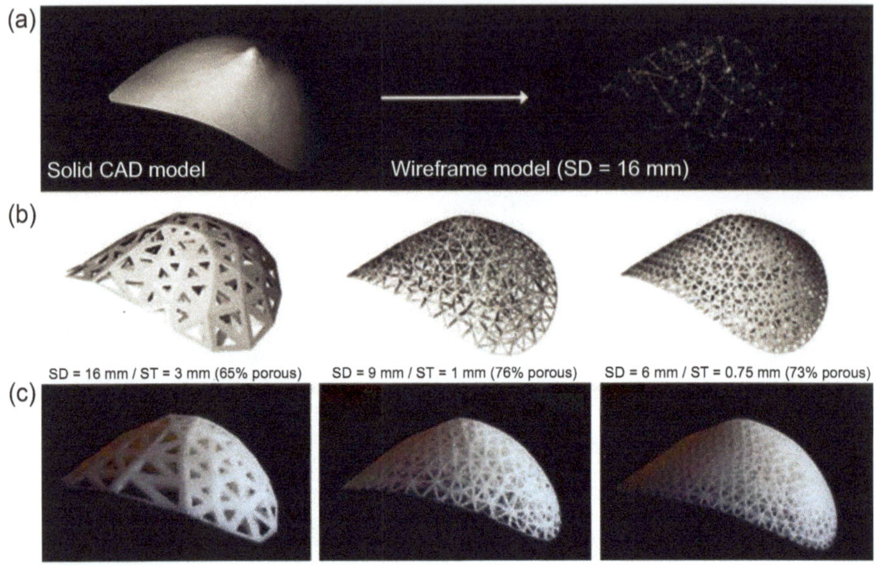

Figure 1.9 Personalized scaffolds for human breast reconstruction showing an effect of seeding points in the meshed model to porous structure of the fabricated scaffold: (a) generation of mesh from a designed CAD 3D model, (b) optimization of seeding distances and strut thicknesses in the CAD model and their effect on the pore sizes and resultant porosity, and (c) actual manufactured scaffolds.
Reproduced from Melchels F, et al. CAD/CAM-assisted breast reconstruction. Biofabrication 2011;3(3):034114.

ingrowth, and metabolic functions [29,30]. Different studies [31] demonstrated the effect of pore size optimization on the development of new blood vessels (angiogenesis). A heterogeneous pore size distribution of 20−1500 μm has been reported for the bone tissue engineering titanium (Ti) scaffolds [31]. In some cases, polymer biocompatible coatings, eg, PCL, are incorporated on the porous scaffolds to enhance the proangiogenic migration factors, which improves the survival of cells attached to the scaffolds and helps in bone regeneration [32−34]. The pore sizes and shapes of the scaffolds can be controlled and tailored by: (1) optimization of the density of seeding points during the creation of tetrahedron mesh in 3D modeling and (2) choosing an appropriate strut thickness. Fig. 1.9 shows the development of a porous scaffold of human breast optimized by controlling the density of seeding points in the meshed model.

Bael et al. [36] studied the role of pore size and shape on the in vitro proliferation and differentiation of 3D human cells (hPDC). Six different Ti-6Al-4V scaffolds were fabricated via SLM with various pore shapes (triangular, hexagonal, and rectangular) and two different pore sizes (500 and 1000 μm). Fig. 1.10 shows the different pore sizes and shapes of the scaffolds used in their study.

In vitro studies revealed a circular cell growth pattern that was independent of the pore size and shape; however, the differentiation of hPDC was dependent on both pore shape and pore size. A higher amount of cell growth was observed on the periphery of

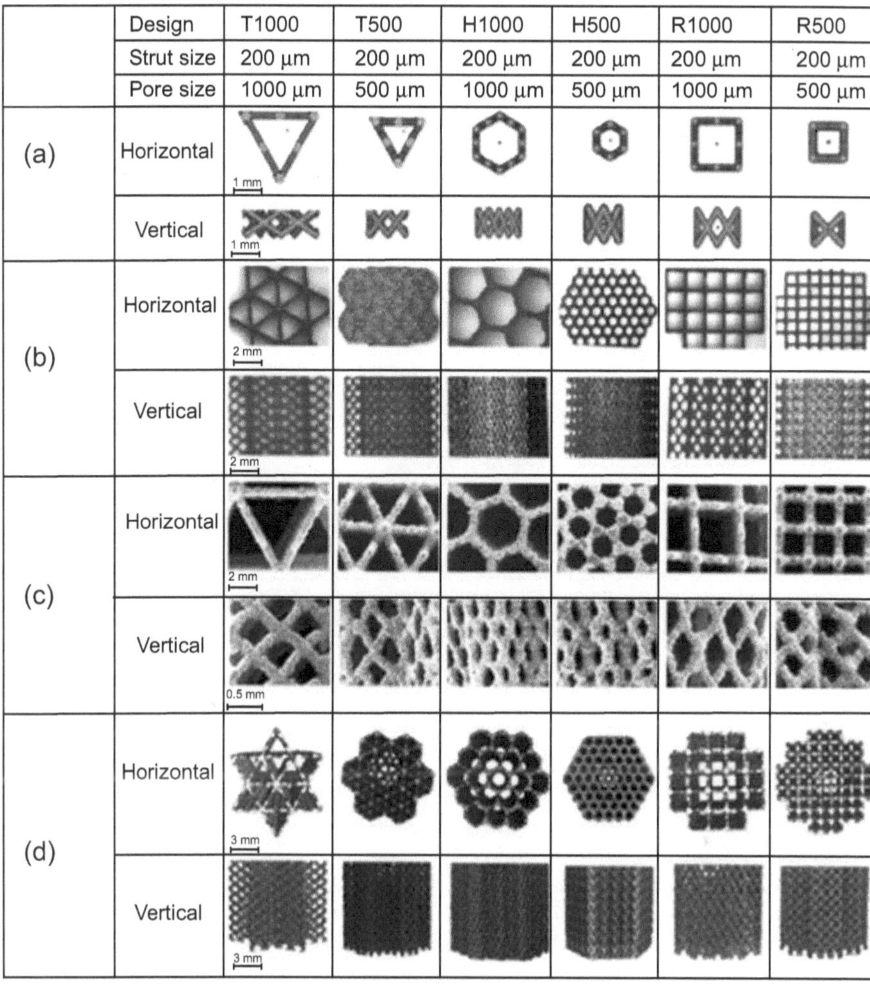

Figure 1.10 Designed scaffolds with different pore sizes, strut thicknesses, and pore shapes: (a) unit cells of the designed Ti-6Al-4V scaffolds, (b) optical microscope images of fabricated scaffolds, (c) scanning electron micrographs of scaffolds, and (d) 3D models generated from X-ray CT scan images from fabricated scaffolds.
Reproduced from Van Bael S, et al. The effect of pore geometry on the in vitro biological behavior of human periosteum-derived cells seeded on selective laser-melted Ti-6Al-4V bone scaffolds. Acta Biomater 2012;8(7):2824–34.

the Ti-6Al-4V bone scaffolds with 500 μm pores, as shown in Fig. 1.11. Their work suggested the development of a functionalized scaffold with a combination of small pores for initial cell attachment and larger noncircular pores to avoid pore occlusion.

Stok et al. [28] conducted in vivo studies to observe the effect of strut size of SLM-fabricated porous Ti-6Al-4V scaffolds, as shown in Fig. 1.12. They developed

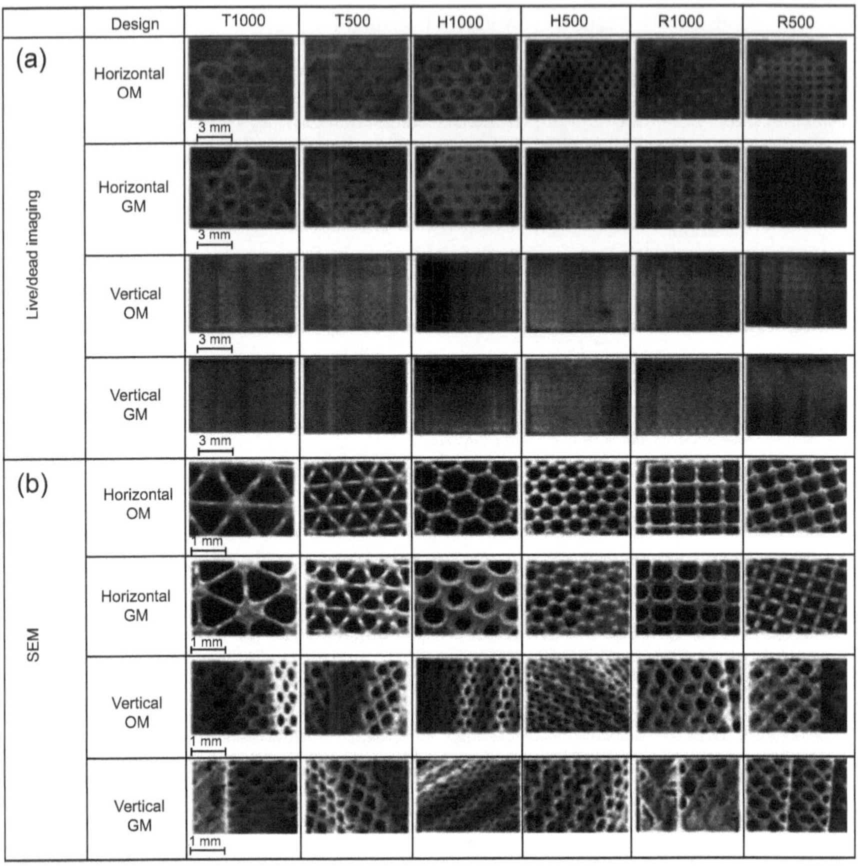

Figure 1.11 In vitro cell proliferation and differentiation analysis within the different designs: (a) live/dead cell staining after cell culturing for 14 days in osteogenic medium and growth medium (green fluorescence indicates the growth of live cells) and (b) scanning electron micrograph images in the horizontal and vertical places of hPDC on various Ti-6Al-4V scaffolds. *GM*, growth medium; *OM*, osteogenic medium.
Reproduced from Van Bael S, et al. The effect of pore geometry on the in vitro biological behavior of human periosteum-derived cells seeded on selective laser-melted Ti-6Al-4V bone scaffolds. Acta Biomater 2012;8(7):2824–34.

two different scaffolds with strut sizes of 120 μm (Ti–20) and 230 μm (Ti–230) for a load-bearing critical femoral bone defect in rats. The reduction of strut sizes provides a positive impact on bone formation but reduces the stiffness.

Their work suggested improved bone fixation with implanted Ti scaffolds. CT scan images of the defect sites revealed the regenerated bones of 18.4 ± 7.1 and $18.7 \pm 8.0\ mm^3$ for Ti–20 and Ti–230 scaffolds, respectively. Biomechanical tests revealed improved bending strength (~62%) of Ti–120 scaffolds as compared to ~45% of Ti–230 scaffolds.

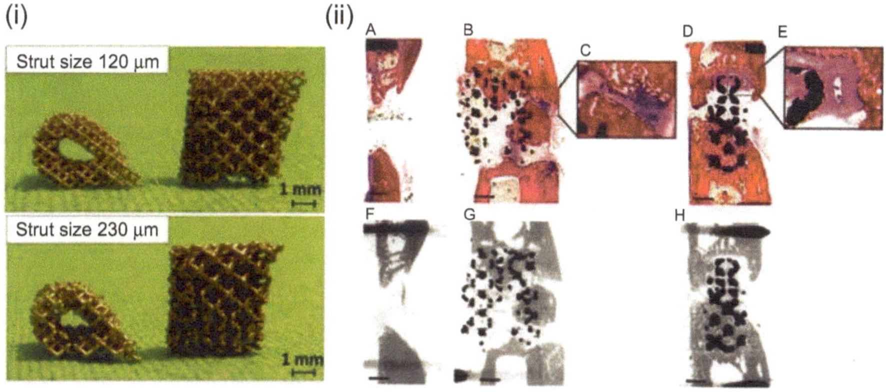

Figure 1.12 Ti-6Al-4V scaffolds fabricated by selective laser melting with different strut sizes and in vitro tests of the defect sites after the implantation: (i) fabricated Ti-6Al-4V scaffolds with strut sizes of 120 and 230 μm and (ii) histological slides with corresponding micro-CT scan images: (A and F) empty defect, (B and G) Ti-120 scaffold, (D and H) Ti-230 scaffold, (C and E) detailed interface view of Ti-120 and Ti-230 scaffolds, respectively.
Reproduced from Van der Stok J, et al. Selective laser melting-produced porous titanium scaffolds regenerate bone in critical size cortical bone defects. J Orthopaedic Res 2013;31(5): 792–9.

1.2.2.3 Role of critical process parameters of selective laser melting

The microstructure, physical, and mechanical properties of the fabricated parts depend upon the selection of process parameters of SLM as well as the properties of the starting materials [37]. Fig. 1.13 shows the key parameters of SLM and the important properties of starting materials, which influence the consolidation mechanism and densification of fabricated complex parts.

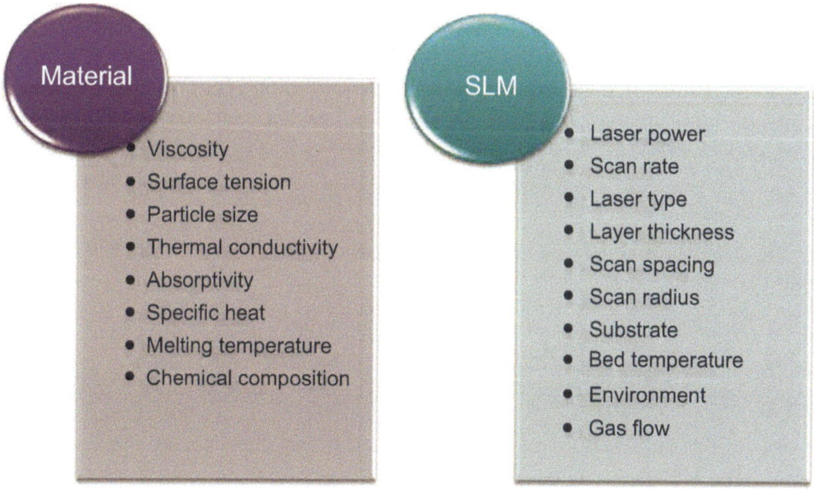

Figure 1.13 List of material and selective laser melting (SLM) variables that influence the densification, microstructure, and resultant properties of the manufactured parts.

The critical parameters of SLM, ie, scanning speed, laser type, laser power, and scanning rate, affect the microstructure of the fabricated parts by controlling the interfacial interactions, reflections, and phase transformations in the processed materials. Therefore it becomes necessary to establish the relationship between the SLM parameters and the resultant thermo-physical and mechanical properties of the manufactured parts [38,39].

Laser energy density used during the SLM process governs the microstructure and properties of as-built parts. This energy density is the measure of the average applied energy from the laser per volume of material during the scanning of an individual layer.

This volume-based energy density, E (J/mm^3), can be defined by the following equation [40]:

$$E = \frac{P}{v \times h \times t} \tag{1.1}$$

where E is the energy density (J/mm^3), P is the laser power (Watt), v is the laser scan speed (m/s), h is the hatch spacing (mm), and t is the layer thickness (m).

Verhaeghe et al. [41] developed a pragmatic model to study the key aspects of the SLM process using an enthalpy formulation and accounting for shrinkage and laser light penetration into the material during the processing stages. Their work took into account the various phase transitions exhibited by the processed material (Ti–6Al–4V) during the SLM process, including the evaporation phenomenon. Their work suggested that inert gas flow over the powder bed (ie, nitrogen or argon) is responsible for absorbing the vapor phases during the melting process in SLM. Extensive research has been carried out to investigate the potential of SLM for the development of near net shaped tissue engineering scaffolds and biomedical implants. Successful examples of dental prosthesis manufactured via SLM from Ti–6Al–4V and Co–Cr–Mo have been reported by Vandenbroucke et al. [42]. They used a diode-pumped Nd:YAG laser with a laser power of 95 W in manufacturing the parts from both materials. Their work suggested that compared to Co–Cr–Mo, Ti-6Al–4V required a higher energy density ($\sim$195 J/mm^3) and a lower build rate of 1.8 cm^3/h, while the energy density required by Co–Cr–Mo was 85 J/mm^3 with a build rate of 4.0 cm^3/h. Theoretically, in the design of the tissue engineering scaffolds, patient-specific issues related to biological, mechanical, and geometrical requirements should be considered and addressed [43,44]. One solution to address these issues is to design a scaffold with a porous structure. The key processing parameters of SLM, which have been discussed above, can then be adjusted or optimized to attain scaffolds with the required porosity, shape, pore size, and intricate interconnectivity for cell migration, bone ingrowth, and the formation of blood vessels [45,46].

1.2.2.4 Previous work on tissue engineering scaffolds and implants using selective laser melting

Previous studies on SLM-processed scaffolds show that an optimal control of pore size and porosity enhances the cellular adhesion, proliferation, and formation of the extracellular matrix. The internal microstructure and architecture of porous implants determine the resultant mechanical properties of the fabricated scaffolds [47,48]. A wide range of materials have been processed by SLM for various applications, generally biomedical implants and tissue engineering scaffolds. Markhoff et al. [49] studied the role of different 3D open porous Ti scaffolds on human osteoblast behavior in static and dynamic cell investigations. Their work suggested that a Ti scaffold with smaller pores (400–620 μm), a high porosity of 75%, and an open-porous pyramidal basic structure provides the highest metabolic cell activity and cell migration. However they did not conduct in vivo tests to further validate the cell response of the fabricated scaffolds. Table 1.2 summarizes some of the studies conducted to explore the key parameters and potential of SLM.

Among various AM techniques, SLM has been widely used in developing complicated shapes of very fine 3D porous structures. Fig. 1.14 shows the porous scaffolds that have been manufactured by SLM.

1.2.2.5 Advantages, challenges, and key materials processed by selective laser melting

Although SLM has emerged as a promising AM technique for tissue engineering scaffolds and implants, studies on SLM-processed scaffolds reveal that the relationship between the starting powder characteristics and key processing parameters still needs to be established. The key research areas in the SLM process are the mass flow rate of the melt pool and heat transfer among the layers and the substrate. Table 1.3 presents an overview of the advantages, challenges, and materials processed by SLM in previous studies.

1.3 Future research directions

The development of metallic tissue engineering scaffolds and implants via LAAM techniques is fascinating; however, processing limitations and challenges do not allow for the full utilization of the potential of these AM techniques. Such unavoidable constraints restrict the fabrication of patient-specific scaffolds and implants. Previous studies on SLS-processed scaffolds report the challenges of wide hatch spacing in the form of the high spatial resolution of laser beams and segmentation, which were attributed to inaccuracies and limitations of the SLS setup [18]. In LAAM techniques, the accumulation of laser energy provided to powder beds has been reported as a major bottleneck. The absorption of thermal energy by the top layer of the powder bed is specifically higher in the materials exhibiting low thermal conductivities, eg, Ti, which act as a heat sink. Wang et al. [56] reported a similar problem in WC–Co powder mixtures in which accumulated energy was absorbed in the powder bed surface; 96% of the energy absorption was accumulated in the powder bed at a depth of 0.4 mm. The lack of laser thermal energy provided to powder particles in certain depths leads to a thermal gradient, which may trigger the warping of the powder bed, voids and cracks in the microstructure, and delamination in the stacked layers. The osteoconductivity of

Table 1.2 Comparison of various materials, selective laser melting parameters, and key findings from previous studies

Starting powder	Selective laser melting model and parameters	Key findings	Applications	References
Ti–6Al–4V	• MCPRealizerSLM • Laser spot size = 30 μm • Layer step size = 50 μm • Build rate = 5 cm^3/h	• Mesh scaffolds with accurate pore sizes were developed. • Scaffolds with a pore width of 0.45 mm showed enhanced compressive strength. • The porosity in the selective laser melting-fabricated scaffold increased with increasing pore width. • Enhanced biocompatibility with 0.45 mm pore width.	Tissue engineering scaffolds	[50]
Ti–TiH_2	• CO_2 laser (λ = 10.60 μm) • Laser spot size = 600 μm • Average laser power = 1 kW • Scan speed = 0.01–0.05 m/s • Scan line spacing = 0.2 mm • Layer step size = 150 μm	• The increase in TiH_2 content lead to increased porosity. • TiH_2–40 wt% Ti samples were fabricated with pore sizes of 200–500 μm. • The porosity increased linearly when the scan speed was raised from 0.01 to 0.03 m/s but decreased at a higher scan speed of 0.05 m/s.	Tissue engineering scaffolds and biomedical implants	[51]
Stainless steel 316L	• SLM PM 100 • YLR-50 CW Ytterbium fiber laser (λ = 1.07 μm) • Laser spot size = 70 μm • Average laser power = 50 W • Scan speed = 0.14 m/s • Layer step size = 20–60 μm	• A 3D filter fabricated via selective laser melting exhibited a regular pore structure. • Square-shaped pores were uniformly distributed with a pore width of 1 mm.	Thin-walled 3D porous baffle filters	[52]
Ti (Grade 1)	• Neodymium-doped yttrium aluminum (Nd: YAG) laser • Laser spot size = 800 μm • Average laser power = 50 W • Scan speed = 0.002–0.016 m/s	• The pore shape changed from crack-like to round as the peak power increased. • Samples fabricated at a high laser power of 1 kW showed less fatigue strength. • High scanning speeds lead to more porosity in the samples.	Biocompatible Ti parts for implants and prostheses	[53]

	• Layer step size = 400 μm	• Scanning speeds of 4, 6, and 8 mm/s resulted in high density, while the evaporation of powder particles occurred at a scan speed of 2 mm/s, which lead to high porosity. • Increased laser power lead to an increase in oxygen content in the fabricated samples. • Postprocessing of fabricated samples, eg, hot isostatic pressing, enhanced the fatigue strength of samples.		
Ti–Nb–Zr–Sn alloy	• MTT SLM 250 HL • Yb:YAG fiber laser • Laser spot size = 80 μm • Average laser power = 200 W • Scan speed = 0.05–0.90 m/s • Layer step size = 100 μm	• High scanning speeds lead to more porosity in the samples. • Low scanning speeds lead to a poor surface finish. • An optimal scan speed of 0.55 m/s was used to fabricate a high-density part with an acceptable surface finish. • Fabricated samples showed improved mechanical properties, ie, a low elastic modulus of ~53 GPa, ultimate tensile strength of 660 MPa, and ductility exceeding 10%. • The density and microhardness of fabricated samples increased with a higher laser energy density.	Low-modulus biomedical beta titanium components and precise acetabular cup	[54]
Carbon nanotubes/AlSi10Mg	• HRPM-II-type SLM • Continuous fiber laser • Laser spot size = 80 μm • Average laser power = 240–360 W • Scan speed = 0.55–0.75 m/s • Layer step size = 30 μm	• High scanning speeds lead to more porosity in the samples. • Increasing laser power resulted in an enhanced densification of the processed samples. • Laser power of 360 W resulted in improved surface quality of the processed samples.	Metal matrix composites with improved thermo-physical and mechanical properties	[55]

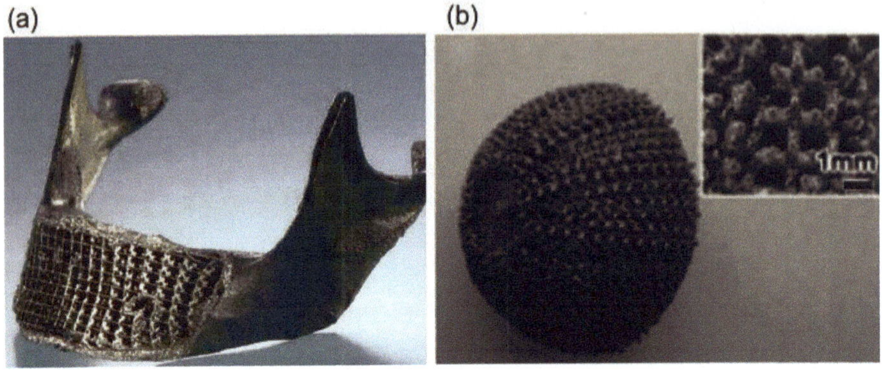

Figure 1.14 Tissue engineering scaffolds manufactured by selective laser melting: (a) a human mandible part produced by selective laser melting with a well-defined porous internal structure and outer dimensions meeting the patient's needs *(Reproduced from Warnke PH, et al. Rapid prototyping: porous titanium alloy scaffolds produced by selective laser melting for bone tissue engineering. Tissue Eng Part C: Methods 2008;15(2):115−24.)* and (b) a precise acetabular cup fabricated by selective laser melting; the inset shows the fine-scale porous structure that had been created in the surface to promote bone ingrowth. *(Reproduced from Zhang L, et al. Manufacture by selective laser melting and mechanical behavior of a biomedical Ti−24Nb−4Zr−8Sn alloy. Scripta Mater 2011;65(1):21−4.)*

Table 1.3 Advantages and disadvantages of additive manufacturing using the selective laser melting technique

Advantages	Disadvantages	Materials used for the fabrication of scaffolds	References
• Fabrication of complicated shapes • Fabrication of high-density metallic implants and scaffolds • Reduced requirements of postprocessing	• Slow part-building rates • Expensive process • High laser power is required • Difficult to remove unprocessed powder from the fabricated part	• Ti−6Al−4V • Pure Ti (Grade 1 and 2) • Ti−TiH_2 • Co−Cr−Mo alloys • Ti−Nb−Zr alloys • Aluminum • Stainless steel 316L • Carbon nanotube reinforced composites	[22,50−55]

porous scaffolds has been reported as better than solid ones, which also facilitates bone ingrowth and tissue regeneration, as discussed in previous sections. However, a relationship is yet to be established between the processing parameters and the pore sizes, and strut sizes and the in vivo osteoconductive behavior are yet to be investigated. This is specifically related to the provision of laser energy density and the physical, thermal, and chemical composition and morphology of starting powders. The establishment of such relationships between the processing parameters and the shape and sizes of pores demands further in-depth research.

The development of porous metallic scaffolds is a hot area of research in which the shape of unit cells and pore and strut sizes play critical roles in the resultant mechanical and biomedical performance of fabricated scaffolds. Previous research on SLM-processed scaffolds highlighted the poor surface roughness and issues of microporosity in the struts of fabricated porous scaffolds [57]. Such residual microporosity in the struts of porous structures may adversely affect the mechanical properties of the scaffold, especially for load-bearing applications, eg, human knee and hip implants, in which high compressive and fatigue strengths are required from the fabricated scaffolds. A high surface roughness in laser-processed Ti and its alloys also demands significant research for improvement. The surface roughness majorly depends upon the characteristics of the starting powder and processing parameters, eg, the type of material, powder particle size distribution, layer thickness, laser scanning parameters, and surface posttreatment methods [38]. Another research area aims to reduce the unprocessed powders left in the fabricated porous structures due to unmelting or partial melting. The unprocessed powder may trigger occlusion or the blockage of pores, resulting in the need for postprocessing operations. Previous research on the fabrication of metallic scaffolds via LAAM technologies highlighted the physics of melt pool in the powder bed, which experiences high thermal and surface tension gradients, resulting in waviness in the top surface of fabricated parts as they gain in vertical height by the progressive stacking of the layers [58]. The complexity of laser processing of metallic scaffolds hinders experimental investigations to develop an understanding of such processes, and the most complicated research area is to take in situ measurements of the localized melt pool formed under the focused laser beam [59]. Various numerical, mathematical, and finite element modeling approaches are needed to establish an adequate understanding of the laser sintering or melting process. This area has not been sufficiently explored and demands focused research for further development and improvements in the fabrication of metallic tissue engineering scaffolds and implants.

1.4 Conclusions

The development of metallic tissue engineering scaffolds and implants is a multidisciplinary research area that needs specialized experience in the fields of material science, biology, medicine, chemical engineering, mechanical engineering, and manufacturing engineering. SLM is an emerging AM technique for the fabrication of complicated near net shape scaffolds and implants, which are not possible to fabricate with other conventional routes of manufacturing. The processing parameters and characteristics of the starting material play a vital role in determining the microstructural, mechanical, and biomedical properties of the fabricated scaffolds. Studies in SLM-processed scaffolds and implants mark a significant breakthrough; however, a certain relationship between the processing parameters and the resultant microstructure is yet to be established. The control of these processing parameters allows for fabricating scaffolds with desired geometrical and structural features. Remarkable advances have been made in establishing an understanding of the effects of the processing parameters on the scaffolds processed with a variety of materials; however, it is expected that the next decade will focus more on bridging the gap between the problems faced by patients in whom these implants have been surgically implanted and desired improvements. A strong collaboration among material scientists, surgeons, and SLM technology experts can bridge the research gaps and improve the existing scaffolds and implants by imparting them with the highly desirable properties described above. All of these efforts in exploring the new manufacturing technologies and new candidate materials for tissue engineering scaffolds and implants give hope to mankind to recover fully from any unfortunate injuries or accidents.

Acknowledgments

This research is financially supported by the National Health and Medical Research Council through grant GNT1087290.

References

[1] Hutmacher DW. Scaffold design and fabrication technologies for engineering tissues—state of the art and future perspectives. J Biomater Sci Polym Ed 2001;12(1):107−24.
[2] Sachlos E, Czernuszka J. Making tissue engineering scaffolds work. Review: the application of solid freeform fabrication technology to the production of tissue engineering scaffolds. Eur Cell Mater 2003;5(29):39−40.
[3] Truscott M, et al. Using RP to promote collaborative design of customised medical implants. Rapid Prototyping J 2007;13(2):107−14.
[4] Sun W, et al. Bio-CAD modeling and its applications in computer-aided tissue engineering. Computer-Aided Des 2005;37(11):1097−114.
[5] Liacouras P, et al. Designing and manufacturing an auricular prosthesis using computed tomography, 3-dimensional photographic imaging, and additive manufacturing: a clinical report. J Prosthet Dent 2011;105(2):78−82.
[6] Werner H, et al. Additive manufacturing models of fetuses built from three-dimensional ultrasound, magnetic resonance imaging and computed tomography scan data. Ultrasound Obstetrics Gynecol 2010;36(3):355−61.
[7] Williams JM, et al. Bone tissue engineering using polycaprolactone scaffolds fabricated via selective laser sintering. Biomaterials 2005;26(23):4817−27.

[8] Olakanmi E. Selective laser sintering/melting (SLS/SLM) of pure Al, Al−Mg, and Al−Si powders: effect of processing conditions and powder properties. J Mater Process Technol 2013;213(8):1387−405.
[9] Gibson I, Shi D. Material properties and fabrication parameters in selective laser sintering process. Rapid Prototyping J 1997;3(4):129−36.
[10] Berry E, et al. Preliminary experience with medical applications of rapid prototyping by selective laser sintering. Med Eng Phys 1997;19(1):90−6.
[11] Wong KV, Hernandez A. A review of additive manufacturing. ISRN Mech Eng 2012; 2012.
[12] Wiria FE, et al. Improved biocomposite development of poly (vinyl alcohol) and hydroxyapatite for tissue engineering scaffold fabrication using selective laser sintering. J Mater Sci Mater Med 2008;19(3):989−96.
[13] Eshraghi S, Das S. Mechanical and microstructural properties of polycaprolactone scaffolds with one-dimensional, two-dimensional, and three-dimensional orthogonally oriented porous architectures produced by selective laser sintering. Acta Biomater 2010; 6(7):2467−76.
[14] Kruth J-P, et al. Binding mechanisms in selective laser sintering and selective laser melting. Rapid Prototyping J 2005;11(1):26−36.
[15] Zhou WY, et al. Selective laser sintering of porous tissue engineering scaffolds from poly (L-lactide)/carbonated hydroxyapatite nanocomposite microspheres. J Mater Sci Mater Med 2008;19(7):2535−40.
[16] Kruth J-P, et al. Lasers and materials in selective laser sintering. Assem Autom 2003;23(4): 357−71.
[17] Partee B, Hollister SJ, Das S. Selective laser sintering process optimization for layered manufacturing of CAPA® 6501 polycaprolactone bone tissue engineering scaffolds. J Manuf Sci Eng 2006;128(2):531−40.
[18] Krishna BV, Bose S, Bandyopadhyay A. Low stiffness porous Ti structures for load-bearing implants. Acta Biomater 2007;3(6):997−1006.
[19] Faustini MC, et al. Manufacture of passive dynamic ankle−foot orthoses using selective laser sintering. Biomedical Engineering. IEEE Trans 2008;55(2):784−90.
[20] Yang S, et al. The design of scaffolds for use in tissue engineering. Part I. Traditional factors. Tissue Eng 2001;7(6):679−89.
[21] Song B, et al. Vacuum heat treatment of iron parts produced by selective laser melting: microstructure, residual stress and tensile behavior. Mater Des 2014;54:727−33.
[22] Olakanmi E, Cochrane R, Dalgarno K. A review on selective laser sintering/melting (SLS/SLM) of aluminium alloy powders: processing, microstructure, and properties. Prog Mater Sci 2015;74:401−77.
[23] Morgan R, et al. High density net shape components by direct laser re-melting of single-phase powders. J Mater Sci 2002;37(15):3093−100.
[24] Hollister SJ. Hierarchical bioactive materials for tissue reconstruction: integrated design and manufacturing challenges. Jom 2011;63(4):56−65.
[25] Wehmöller M, et al. Implant design and production—a new approach by selective laser melting. In: International congress series. Elsevier; 2005.
[26] Probst F, et al. [Calvarial reconstruction by customized bioactive implant]. Organ der Deutschsprachigen Arbeitsgemeinschaft fur Handchirurgie: Organ der Deutschsprachigen Arbeitsgemeinschaft fur Mikrochirurgie der Peripheren Nerven und Gefasse: Organ der V. Handchirurgie, Mikrochirurgie, plastische Chirurgie 2010;42(6):369−73.
[27] Fukuda A, et al. Osteoinduction of porous Ti implants with a channel structure fabricated by selective laser melting. Acta Biomater 2011;7(5):2327−36.

[28] Van der Stok J, et al. Selective laser melting-produced porous titanium scaffolds regenerate bone in critical size cortical bone defects. J Orthopaedic Res 2013;31(5):792–9.

[29] Muller D, et al. Vascular guidance: microstructural scaffold patterning for inductive neovascularization. Stem Cell Int 2010;2011.

[30] Saran U, Piperni SG, Chatterjee S. Role of angiogenesis in bone repair. Arch Biochem Biophys 2014;561:109–17.

[31] Loh QL, Choong C. Three-dimensional scaffolds for tissue engineering applications: role of porosity and pore size. Tissue Eng Part B: Rev 2013;19(6):485–502.

[32] Wulf K, et al. Surface functionalization of poly (ε-caprolactone) improves its biocompatibility as scaffold material for bioartificial vessel prostheses. J Biomed Mater Res Part B: Appl Biomater 2011;98(1):89–100.

[33] Cipitria A, et al. Polycaprolactone scaffold and reduced rhBMP-7 dose for the regeneration of critical-sized defects in sheep tibiae. Biomaterials 2013;34(38):9960–8.

[34] Dash TK, Konkimalla VB. Poly-ε-caprolactone based formulations for drug delivery and tissue engineering: a review. J Controlled Release 2012;158(1):15–33.

[35] Melchels F, et al. CAD/CAM-assisted breast reconstruction. Biofabrication 2011;3(3): 034114.

[36] Van Bael S, et al. The effect of pore geometry on the in vitro biological behavior of human periosteum-derived cells seeded on selective laser-melted Ti6Al4V bone scaffolds. Acta Biomater 2012;8(7):2824–34.

[37] Agarwala M, et al. Direct selective laser sintering of metals. Rapid Prototyping J 1995; 1(1):26–36.

[38] Yadroitsev I, Smurov I. Selective laser melting technology: from the single laser melted track stability to 3D parts of complex shape. Phys Proced 2010;5(Part B):551–60.

[39] Yadroitsev I, Smurov I. Surface morphology in selective laser melting of metal powders. Phys Proced 2011;12(Part A):264–70.

[40] Thijs L, et al. A study of the microstructural evolution during selective laser melting of Ti–6Al–4V. Acta Mater 2010;58(9):3303–12.

[41] Verhaeghe F, et al. A pragmatic model for selective laser melting with evaporation. Acta Mater 2009;57(20):6006–12.

[42] Vandenbroucke B, Kruth J-P. Selective laser melting of biocompatible metals for rapid manufacturing of medical parts. Rapid Prototyping J 2007;13(4):196–203.

[43] Hutmacher DW. Scaffolds in tissue engineering bone and cartilage. Biomaterials 2000; 21(24):2529–43.

[44] Hollister SJ, Maddox R, Taboas JM. Optimal design and fabrication of scaffolds to mimic tissue properties and satisfy biological constraints. Biomaterials 2002;23(20):4095–103.

[45] Taboas J, et al. Indirect solid free form fabrication of local and global porous, biomimetic and composite 3D polymer-ceramic scaffolds. Biomaterials 2003;24(1):181–94.

[46] Chu T-MG, et al. Mechanical and in vivo performance of hydroxyapatite implants with controlled architectures. Biomaterials 2002;23(5):1283–93.

[47] Magan A, Ripamonti U. Geometry of porous hydroxyapatite implants influences osteogenesis in Baboons (Papio ursinus). J Craniofac Surg 1996;7(1):71–8.

[48] Hing K, Best S, Bonfield W. Characterization of porous hydroxyapatite. J Mater Sci Mater Med 1999;10(3):135–45.

[49] Markhoff J, et al. Influence of different three-dimensional open porous titanium scaffold designs on human osteoblasts behavior in static and dynamic cell investigations. Materials 2015;8(8):5490–507.

[50] Warnke PH, et al. Rapid prototyping: porous titanium alloy scaffolds produced by selective laser melting for bone tissue engineering. Tissue Eng Part C: Methods 2008;15(2):115–24.

[51] Wang Y, et al. Development of highly porous titanium scaffolds by selective laser melting. Mater Lett 2010;64(6):674–6.
[52] Yadroitsev I, et al. Manufacturing of fine-structured 3D porous filter elements by selective laser melting. Appl Surf Sci 2009;255(10):5523–7.
[53] Santos E, et al. Microstructure and mechanical properties of pure titanium models fabricated by selective laser melting. Proc Inst Mech Eng Part C: J Mech Eng Sci 2004;218(7): 711–9.
[54] Zhang L, et al. Manufacture by selective laser melting and mechanical behavior of a biomedical Ti–24Nb–4Zr–8Sn alloy. Scripta Mater 2011;65(1):21–4.
[55] Zhao X, et al. Selective laser melting of carbon/AlSi10Mg composites: microstructure, mechanical and electronical properties. J Alloys Compounds 2015.
[56] Wang X, et al. Direct selective laser sintering of hard metal powders: experimental study and simulation. Int J Adv Manuf Technol 2002;19(5):351–7.
[57] Yasa E, Kruth J-P. Microstructural investigation of Selective Laser Melting 316L stainless steel parts exposed to laser re-melting. Proced Eng 2011;19:389–95.
[58] Hayashi T, et al. Selective laser sintering method using titanium powder sheet toward fabrication of porous bone substitutes. JSME Int J Ser A Solid Mech Mater Eng 2005; 48(4):369–75.
[59] Jeong Y-H, et al. Hydroxyapatite thin film coatings on nanotube-formed Ti–35Nb–10Zr alloys after femtosecond laser texturing. Surf Coat Technol 2013;217:13–22.

Production methods and characterization of porous Mg and Mg alloys for biomedical applications

2

A. Vahidgolpayegani [1], *C. Wen* [2,3], *P. Hodgson* [1], *Y. Li* [3]
[1]Deakin University, Geelong, Victoria, Australia; [2]Swinburne University of Technology, Hawthorn, Victoria, Australia; [3]RMIT University, Melbourne, Victoria, Australia

2.1 Introduction

An increase in human and animal body injuries has resulted in a high demand for implant biomaterials. These implants are used to repair the damaged body parts or replace them completely. The application period of the implants inside the body can be classified into two groups: short-term and long-term implants. Long-term implants remain in the body permanently, but short-term implants have to be removed after healing, leading to additional surgery. The most critical problems with postsurgery processes involve the increase in medical costs, time of treatment, and pain for patients. Therefore biomaterials that are soluble in the body environment and absorbable by living tissue, thus eliminating additional surgery processes, are highly desired. This inspired the development of a new generation of biomaterials called biodegradable or bioabsorbable material [1,2]. These biomaterials, which dissolve within the body and produce bioabsorbable products after a complete healing process, have attracted extensive attention in the fields of medical applications such as cardiac stents and orthopedic and trauma surgeries [3,4].

Polymers and natural polymers such as poly-glycolic acid, poly-lactic acid [4], collagen, and chitin [5] as well as ceramics or bioactive glasses [6] have been developed as biodegradable materials, but their low mechanical strength and brittleness as well as transparency to radiation have limited their applications, particularly for bone replacements where load-bearing capacity is necessary. In contrast, biodegradable metals exhibit the required mechanical properties for bone substitutes, such as mechanical strength and fracture toughness for load-bearing applications.

Magnesium (Mg) and its alloys can be gradually dissolved within the body, and their corrosion products are biologically absorbable and nontoxic, unlike other metallic biomaterials such as stainless steel as well as titanium (Ti)-, cobalt (Co)-, and chromium (Cr)-base alloys [7–9]. The low density ($1.74 \sim 2.0\ g/cm^3$) and Young's modulus ($41 \sim 45$ GPa) [10] of Mg and its alloys are close to those of human bone ($1.8 \sim 2.1\ g/cm^3$, $10 \sim 40$ GPa) [11]. Furthermore, the strength of Mg and its alloys

Metallic Foam Bone. http://dx.doi.org/10.1016/B978-0-08-101289-5.00002-0

is greater than that of ceramic and polymeric biomaterials. These characteristics as well as the function of stimulating the growth of new bone tissue [10,12,13] make them highly desirable for bone substitute materials [5].

Mg is necessary for human metabolism with an amount of 375 mg/day, and its cation is ranked as fourth among the other essential cations in the body and approximately half of that stored in bone tissue [3,14]. Excessive Mg is innocuous and can be excreted through urine [15]. However, the low corrosion resistance of Mg and its alloys, which results in a high rate of degradation and decline in mechanical integrity, limits their applications [6,13].

Based on the physical, chemical, and mechanical properties as well as the biological functions of Mg alloys, they appear to be more suitable for use as a bioabsorbable Mg-base implant with a sufficient time frame of degradation for bone cells to settle on and form an extracellular matrix for support prior to complete degradation and dissolution of the implant material. The development of new, high-quality Mg-based implant materials has the potential to meet this demand.

In addition to the base material, allocation of a specific open-cell porous structure for implants would offer bone cell ingrowth capacity and transportation pathways for body fluids. Polymeric and ceramic scaffolds have been used as porous implant materials [16–18], but these materials exhibit low mechanical strength, thus they are not suitable for load-bearing implant applications. This issue leads to the demand for metallic foams such as Ti-based and aluminum (Al)-based foams that display higher mechanical strength [19,20]. However, Ti-based and Al-based scaffolds materials would remain permanently in the body because they are not biodegradable. Therefore porous bioabsorbable Mg and Mg alloys offer new solutions. These materials have great potential for use as bone substitutes with-bone mimicking characteristics. Since the structures of bone tissue and porous Mg materials are similar, host bone cells can grow into the pores of an Mg scaffold and form new bone tissue after implantation for 3–4 months [10,21].

Different production methods have been developed in the fabrication of porous Mg and Mg alloys such as casting, metal–gas eutectic solidification [21], powder metallurgy (PM) with a blowing agent or space holder [1], infiltration, and a negative salt-pattern molding process [22]. Some methods are not economically viable, produce a porous structure that is not suitable for implant applications due to the non-biocompatible residues in the final product, and have inappropriate pore size and porosity. Therefore it is crucial to choose a production method that is suitable for the production of porous Mg and Mg alloys with controlled pore size, shape, and porosity.

In this chapter, various production methods and materials used in the fabrication of porous Mg and Mg alloys are elucidated. The characteristics and properties of the porous Mg structures are analyzed. The effects of the important processing parameters of the porous structures, including the base material, pore type, size, morphology, and porosity, on the biocompatibility of the implant materials are explained. Production methods that produce porous Mg and Mg alloys with the most suitable structure and properties are presented. Future research directions in the field of porous Mg alloy biomaterials are also suggested.

2.2 Production methods for porous Mg and some of its alloys

There is a variety of production methods for manufacturing porous Mg and Mg alloys. These methods can be classified into two categories, melt processing methods and solid processing methods, according to the state of materials that are being processed [23]. The melt processing methods are based on the introduction of a blowing agent into the molten metal followed by stirring, or the infiltration of a bed of hollow spheres, or by introducing a gas or even a vacuum into Mg melt prior to solidification. However, in the solid processing methods, Mg powders, chips, or even strips are mixed with blowing agents or space holder particles to produce gas bubbles or are removed at low or moderate temperatures to create the pores, respectively. A sintering at higher temperatures is followed to assure the bonding of metal particles [24,25]. In the following section, various methods and the specifications of the resultant porous Mg and Mg alloys are introduced.

2.2.1 Melt processing methods

2.2.1.1 Melt processing method with a blowing agent

Mg melts can be foamed by adding blowing agents, which release gas during their decomposition. TiH_2 is one of the most common materials serving as a blowing agent, which releases hydrogen gas in Mg melt [25]. $CaCO_3$ has also been used as a blowing agent in melt foaming processing with a higher decomposition temperature than TiH_2. Hur et al. [26–29] carried out a study on the fabrication of Mg alloy foams by using $CaCO_3$ as a blowing agent. In their process, granular calcium (Ca) is introduced into the melted Mg alloy at 660–750°C by the impeller to raise the viscosity of the melt. $CaCO_3$ powder is dispersed into the melt while stirring, which causes the melt to foam gradually, defined as the stirring foaming stage. Immediately following the foaming stage, the melt is held for 2 min to let the bubbles grow, forming a porous structure. The crucible is then removed from the furnace, and the foamy melt is solidified by air blowing and water spraying. Note that to prevent the melt from ignition, the entire process is performed under a mixed gas of CO_2 and SF6 (Fig. 2.1).

Seo et al. [29] fabricated porous AZ91 and AZ31 Mg with a pore size of 3–5 mm and a porosity of 60–79%, and the ranges of yield strength of their porous Mg alloys were 4.5–10 MPa. Hur et al. [28] attempted to control the porous structure of the specimens by adding zirconium (Zr) to AZ31 Mg alloy. They found that the addition of Zr led to an increase in porosity as well as pore size. The samples with the addition of 1 wt% Zr were not effectively foamed, but a high porosity of 72.9% and a pore size of 0.97 mm were achieved with the addition of 3 wt% Zr. However, any addition of Zr resulted in a decrease in compressive strength, yield strength, and energy absorption as well as an increase in hardness. Yang et al. [26] demonstrated that the blowing agent in this process was not CO_2 but CO, which is the consequence of the reaction between melted Mg and $CaCO_3$. The residue of CaO, MgO, and $Ca(OH)_2$ confirmed the presence of this reaction.

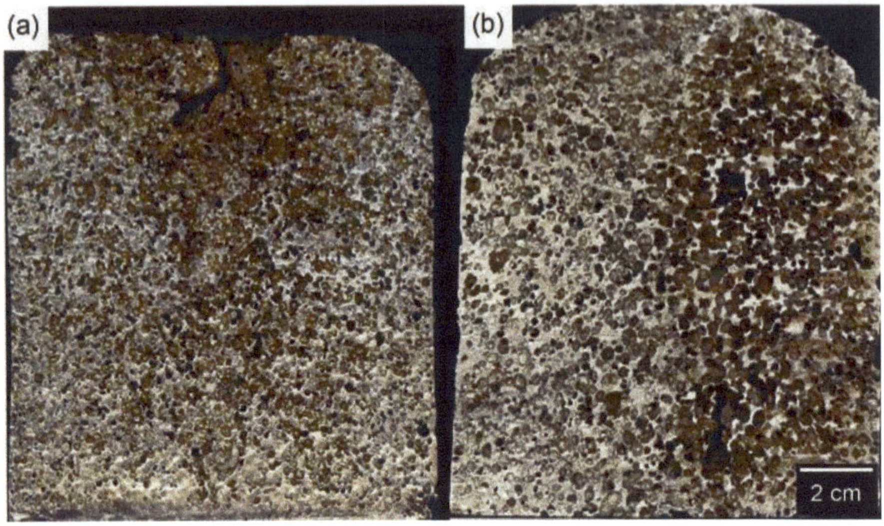

Figure 2.1 (a) Porous AZ91 Mg alloy foamed at 700°C with a porosity of 57.4% and a mean pore size of 1.9 mm and (b) porous AM60 Mg alloy foamed at 700°C with a porosity of 59.1% and a mean pore size of 1.8 mm [26].

In this process, the structure and the type of pores were linked to the melt temperature and the release rate of the blowing gas. The higher temperature led to a higher gas release rate that ultimately resulted in higher porosity, a bigger pore size, and smaller pore numbers. Two porous Mg alloys, namely AZ91 and AM60, have been fabricated so far, and some other porous Mg alloys are expected to be fabricated based on this process. Yang et al. [30] reported that the yield strength of porous Mg increased from 8.69 to 27.11 MPa with decreasing porosity from 71.1% to 53%, respectively, and their specific strength was 33.2 MPa/g cm^3. Both are considered to be superior to Al foams. Zhao et al. [31] also used this process for the fabrication of porous AZ31 and found that the increase in processing temperature resulted in a more homogenous porous structure with better pore distribution and also an increase in compressive strength. The processing temperature exhibited an ambivalent effect on the porosity. An increase in processing temperature from 660 to 720°C led to an increase in the porosity from 41.2% to 73.3%, followed by a decrease to 61.6% when the processing temperature was further increased to 750°C. Xia et al. [32] fabricated a closed-cell AZ31 foam by using this process with a porosity of 55% and a mean pore size of 1.5 mm and investigated the effect of homogenizing heat treatment (HHT) on the compressive strength. The energy dispersive x-ray spectroscopy (EDX) results confirmed the existence of MgO in the matrix due to the reaction between $CaCO_3$ and Mg melt. They also found that HHT increased the yield strength as well as the energy absorption capacity of the porous Mg alloy (Fig. 2.2).

Moreover, Xia et al. [33] reported that an increase in the thickness/width ratio led to a longer stress–strain plateau and an improvement in energy absorption but a

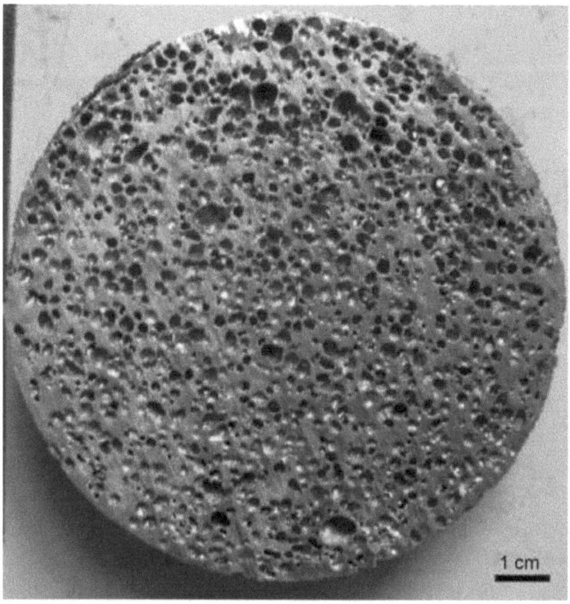

Figure 2.2 Structure of closed-cell AZ31 foam [32].

reduction in yield strength. Porous AZ91 with a porosity of 60–90% and a mean pore size of 0.9–1.6 mm has been fabricated via this method.

Xu et al. [34] used metal Ca and SiC particles to thicken the melt, then added the blowing agent to the melt and stirred. Finally, the melt was cooled in air after foaming. They indicated that the cell edge size decreased with the decrease in cell size. A smaller cell size resulted in more stable deformation and a higher strength of the porous Mg alloy. However, there was an optimum average pore size due to the strength reduction in the porous Mg alloy when the pores became too small, as there was not enough metal in the cell walls. Moreover, some defects could occur. It was indicated that cell shape changed with porosity, as the spherical cells turned to polyhedron when the porosities were more than 70%.

The producibility of Mg–12Al–3Ca alloy foam using the direct foaming method was investigated by Luo et al. [35]. They melted the alloy at 700°C, added SiC particles as a stabilizer at 620°C, and stirred. Some $MgCO_3$ was then added as a foaming agent, and Al_2O_3 particles were used as the dispersant, then stirred for some minutes. The expandable melt was removed to another holding furnace at 590°C and held for a few minutes to foam the bubbles. Finally, the foamed block was chilled by water and cut. They considered the effect of the foaming agent material as well as the amount and size, stabilizer properties, and stirring and foaming parameters on the quality of foam. Their results indicated that adding $MgCO_3$ as a foaming agent led to enhanced quality of the porous Mg alloys compared to the porous Mg alloy foamed by other hydrides and carbonates. Moreover, the porosity of the porous Mg alloy increased from about 58% to 78% when increasing the amount and size of $MgCO_3$ particulates from 1 wt% and 100 mesh to 3 wt% and 200 mesh, respectively. Any further increase in the amount and size of $MgCO_3$ particulates led to a decrease of porosity to ~67% and an increase in the density from ~0.4 to ~0.6 g/cm^3. The porosity and density of the porous Mg alloy were also influenced by the stirring parameters such as stirring velocity, time, and temperature. The apparent density of the porous Mg alloy decreased with an increase in the stirring temperature, which led to more porosity. However, the oxidation of Mg melt became severe at elevated temperatures (above 600°C). The longer stirring time as well as foaming time led to more porosity, but when the stirring time lasted more than 5 min the cell walls could be broken, and a foaming time longer than 4 min could create some defects in the internal porous structures. Therefore according to the maximum expansion ratio achieved by researchers, it was determined that a foaming temperature at 600–620°C is the most efficient foaming state to reduce the foaming time, as a higher foaming temperature resulted in decreased porosity.

Thixocasting processing can also be used to fabricate porous Mg and Mg alloys. Solórzano et al. [36,37] employed this process (called integral foam molding, IFM) in the fabrication of porous AZ91 by injecting the liquid or semisolid alloy at a high velocity into a permanent steel mold. Prior to the casting, the molten Mg alloy was mixed turbulently with MgH_2 as the blowing agent, which was located in a cavity between the injector nozzle and the mold. By using this method they produced a porous AZ91 with porosities ranging from 8% to 39%. It was indicated that the fabrication of intact samples with a homogenous structure and smooth external surface was very difficult, and only a low range of porosities was obtainable (Fig. 2.3).

This process has also been used by Körner et al. [38] for the fabrication of porous AZ91 and AM60, using the same blowing agent. They produced porosity gradient structures (Fig. 2.4) with a porosity of 5% in relatively solid skin, gradually changing to a highly porous core with a porosity of 70%. The compression test results show that the ultimate strength of the samples decreased from 360 to 230 MPa, and elongation at rupture decreased from 52% to 22% when the density decreased from 1.72 to 1.03 g/cm^3. A recognizable stress plateau was observed for the samples with a mean density of lower than 1.2 g/cm^3. The three point bending tests exhibited a rise of bending stiffness while the density decreased. It was demonstrated that there was an increase in the weight-

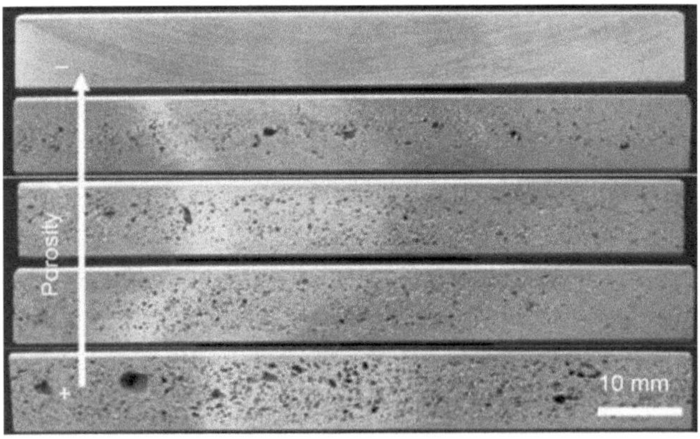

Figure 2.3 Thixocasting processed porous AZ91 with different porosities up to 39% [36].

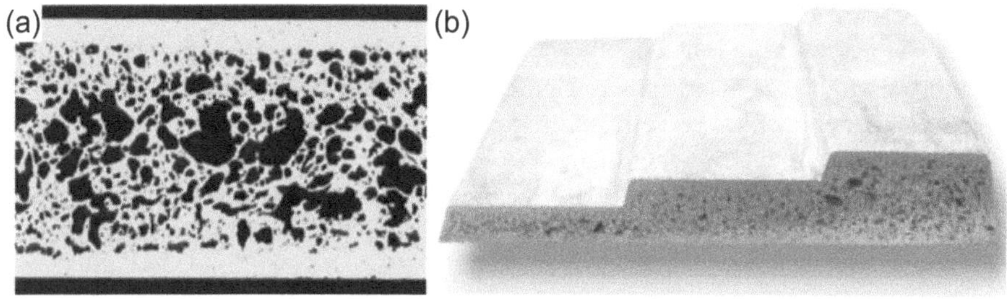

Figure 2.4 (a) Optical micrograph of porous AZ91 with cellular core and relatively dense skin [39] and (b) section of a porous AZ91 Mg door handle with a wall thickness of 30 mm [37].

specific bending stiffness of up to 60% for 6 mm panels when the porosity gradient structures were used [38,39].

2.2.1.2 Melt infiltration in a preform

This process is based on the infiltration of a bed of hollow spheres. In other words, a porous pattern is poured with molten Mg and removed after solidification of the metal. Yamada et al. [40] poured polyurethane foam with plaster slurries and heated the impregnated foam at 480°C to burn the polyurethane. They infiltrated a plaster preform with a porous structure with molten AZ91 while evacuating it at the bottom to facilitate the molten Mg flowing through the narrow routes. Finally, they broke down the plaster mold washing with a water spray. Mg foam with an open-cell structure and a density of 0.05 g/cm^3 was obtained (Fig. 2.5). The Mg foam exhibited column spacing of 4.5 mm and strut thickness of 0.3 mm. They demonstrated that the random cellular structure of the Mg foam was similar to that of the polyurethane foam with no closed-cell structure [40,41].

Wen et al. [42–44] investigated the effect of T6 heat treatment on the mechanical properties of Mg foams and found that as-cast Mg foams have higher relative stress

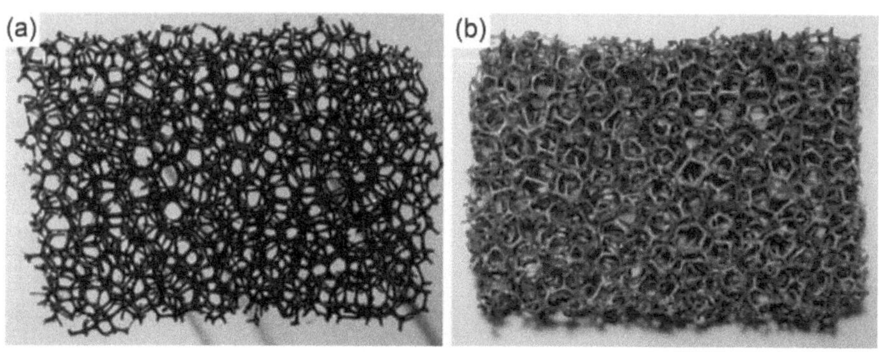

Figure 2.5 Structure of (a) polyurethane form used in infiltrating processing and (b) open-cell porous AZ91 [41].

than T6 heat-treated foams. They suggested that the mechanism of strengthening based on T6 heat treatment in bulk Mg alloy is different from that of cellular alloy.

Yamada et al. [45] also used laser lithography in the fabrication of epoxy foams, which exhibited a controlled cellular structure. Plaster preforms were prepared by using the abovementioned method and were used in the infiltration processing of Mg alloy foams with controlled cellular structures that included square- and diamond-shaped cells. Compressive tests were carried out on the Mg alloy foams with different cell shapes, and the results indicated that the deformation mode of the Mg alloy foams with a random cell structure and a diamond cell structure were the same with a collapsed stress of about 0.1 MPa and a plateau region with a constant flow stress. Moreover, they concluded that the densification strain of the Mg alloy foams during compression depended only on the relative densities.

The collapse stress of the Mg alloy foams with square cells was 0.4 MPa, 4 times higher than those of the Mg alloy foams with a random cell or a diamond cell structure. The Mg alloy foam with a square cell structure also showed a much fluctuating flow stress in the plateau region as compared to the foam with a random cell or diamond cell structure, indicating the anisotropy of the mechanical properties due to the different deformation mode of foam struts.

Yamada et al. [46] produced open cellular SG91A Al alloy foam and compared its compressive properties with the abovementioned porous AZ91 Mg alloys. They indicated that the stress–strain behavior of both cellular materials was almost the same, although solid AZ91 exhibited lower ductility than solid SA91A, indicating that the mechanical properties of metallic foams are independent of the ductility of the matrix materials. In other words, the strain hardening of solid materials does not occur in cellular metals. The cell edge collapses at the yield point of the solid and bends quickly at a low increase in stress.

Kirkland et al. [47] employed a commercial 3D printer to produce a rapid prototyped (RP) polymer template with a periodic lattice structure (1×1 mm struts and channels). The template was infiltrated with NaCl slurries to produce an NaCl-polymer composite, which was heat treated to remove the polymer. The resultant salt template was infiltrated with pure molten Mg at 700°C at a pressure of 1.8 bar. After solidification of Mg, the NaCl was washed and removed, which left a periodic Mg foam with an open lattice-type structure. Kirkland et al. indicated that the infiltration conditions affected the surface topologies of Mg foams. The roughness of the surface increased with an increase in the infiltration pressure. Different topologies actually affected the mechanical properties as well as the cell proliferation, which is a significant consideration in orthopedic implant devices [47,48].

The compressive strength of these periodic porous Mg alloys with a theoretical porosity of 41% is ~13 MPa, higher than that of bulk Mg (~11 MPa) and it is just below that of the random porous Mg (15 MPa) reported by Wen et al. [5] for the same porosity. It has also been reported that the pore size of porous metals affects their strength; a porous Mg with a pore size of 1 mm (the same pore size of the periodic porous Mg) exhibited a compressive strength of less than 9 MPa [47].

Open-cell porous Mg has also been produced by casting using a negative salt-pattern. In this so called "negative salt-pattern molding," moistened sodium chloride

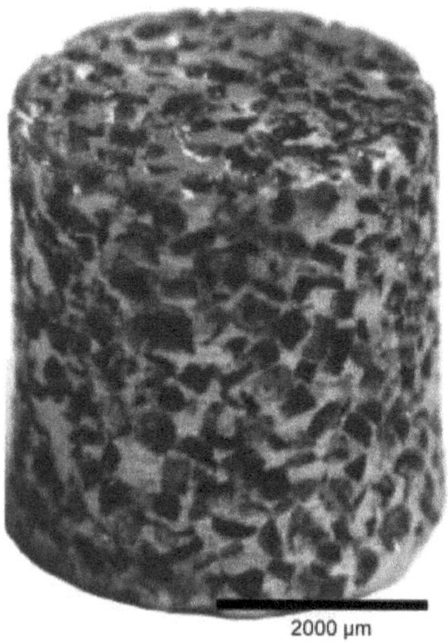

Figure 2.6 AZ91D Mg alloy foam produced via negative salt-pattern molding [22].

grains were poured into a core box and then dehumidified and hardened at 200°C to produce a space holder core. The salt-pattern was then placed into the chill mold, and molten AZ91D was casted using a low-pressure die casting system. Finally, washing out the sodium chloride using a sodium hydroxide solution (to protect Mg from corrosion) resulted in an open-cell porous Mg with a porosity of 72–75% and a pore size of 10–1000 μm [22,49]. The Mg scaffolds produced (Fig. 2.6) were γ-sterilized and implanted into the distal femur condyle of rabbits to investigate the biocompatibility of Mg foam with regard to the inflammatory host response. No serious gas cavities due to slowly corroding Mg were observed, and even slowly produced hydrogen gas diffused into the surrounding tissues [22].

In other research implemented by Lietaert et al. [50], NaCl powder with a particle size of 500 μm was compacted isostatically in a silicon mold to prepare an NaCl preform with a porosity of 75%. AZ63, ZM21, M2, and MZX211 Mg alloys were melted at 690°C, forced into the salt preform under Argon (Ar) gas pressure of 3 bar, and cooled. The composite of Mg/NaCl was machined and leached for 2.5 min in a solution with 0.133 M NaCl and 0.15 M NaF under forced convection to avoid corrosion of the Mg. Fabrication of open-cell porous Mg samples with a porosity of 75% and a pore size of 500 μm is evidence that the "forced flow leaching" process is a reliable route to remove salt preform without a serious corrosion attack on the porous Mg. A hydrogen evolution test of samples for 24 h in simulated body fluid (SBF) at 37°C represented a 3.2–67% weight loss of porous Mg samples, which is too high for biomedical applications.

The weight loss for MZX211 was even higher. The Young's moduli of porous Mg samples with a porosity of 75% varied from 0.6 to 0.8 GPa while their flow stress was in the range of 0.6–3.3 MPa. It has been indicated that the M2 Mg alloy is more suitable than other investigated alloys for orthopedic applications by virtue of its higher mechanical properties before and after a 24 h immersion in SBF [50].

Trinidad et al. [51] used loose NaCl powders with a particle size of 250–500 μm as space holder material in the fabrication of porous Mg. In this process, loose NaCl powders were placed in a steel cylinder, the Mg alloy ingot was placed on the top, and the cylinder was sealed with graphite gasket rings. The cylinder was then located into a resistance furnace under protective gas (CO_2 + 4% SF6) and heated to 740–755°C, according to the Mg alloy composition. When the temperature was homogenized, the molten Mg was infiltrated into the salt grains by increasing the gas pressure to 4–6 bar. Then the cylinder was cooled through a directional solidification to avoid unwanted shrinkages inside the sample. The salt was washed in distilled water with an NaOH solution to reduce corrosion of the Mg. The infiltration pressure was a critical parameter in achieving the porosity of the porous Mg. The highest porosity achieved for this process was 69% at an infiltration pressure of 5 bar for ZWM200, and the lowest porosity was 30% at an infiltration pressure of 6 bar for ZWM200 and ZXM200. However, the porosity of the porous Mg alloy could also be controlled by adjusting other process parameters according to the alloy composition. The highest yield strength of the porous Mg obtained through this process was 12.15 MPa for ZWM200 with 30% porosity at an infiltration pressure of 6 bar. The yield strength decreased to 2.31 MPa with an increase in porosity to 69% at an infiltration pressure of 5 bar for this alloy. The yield strength of the other tested Mg alloys varied from ~3.5 to ~9 MPa with the change of porosity and the alloy composition. For instance, the yield strength of ZXM200 with 44% porosity (8.66 MPa) is 2.5 orders of magnitude greater than that of ZM20 (3.48 MPa) with the same porosity. Moreover, the higher the infiltration pressure used in the process, the greater the yield strength of porous Mg that could be obtained.

Porous pure Mg has also been fabricated through spark plasma sintering (SPS) of Mg/NaCl mixture (Fig. 2.7). In this method, Mg (75–150 μm) and NaCl particles (>170 μm) were mixed together and pressed at 20 MPa in a graphite die. The mixture was placed inside an SPS chamber and sintered at 585°C for 2 h. After sintering, NaCl was washed away by using a 1 M NaOH solution in vacuum while the solution was

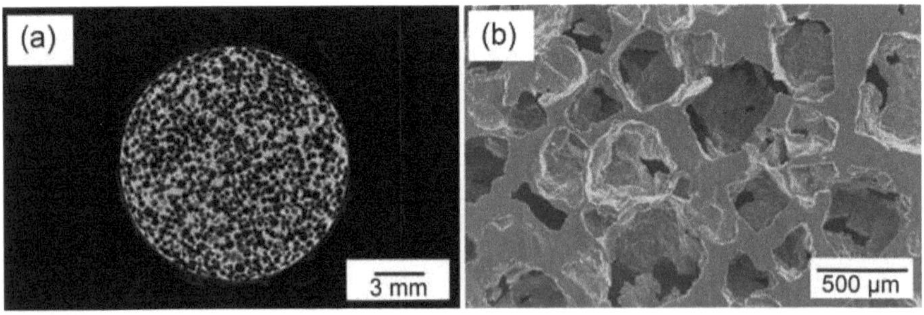

Figure 2.7 (a) Micro-CT image of the cross-section and (b) field emission scanning electron microscope micrograph of noncoated porous Mg fabricated through spark plasma sintering [52].

changed periodically. Porous Mg samples with porosities of 50%, 60%, and 70% were obtained. Then the porous Mg was coated with hydroxyapatite (HA) and tested for biocorrosion in SBF at 37°C. It has been reported that the increase in sintering time from 5 to 120 min doubled the compressive strength of porous Mg samples due to the deterrent effect of nonconductive NaCl particles in the Mg matrix. The highest and lowest compressive strengths measured for the porous samples were 30 and 7 MPa for porosities of 50% and 70%, respectively. The average Young's modulus for the porous samples was reported as 0.23, 0.33, and 0.49 GPa for porosities of 70%, 60%, and 50%, respectively. HA coating showed no serious effect on the mechanical properties of porous samples, but it affected the biodegradation rate due to pH changes in the SBF [52].

Staiger, Nguyen, and coresearchers [53–55] developed an open-cell Mg with periodic architectures (Fig. 2.8). Polymeric templates with different square struts and pore sizes were printed using a 3D modeler. The templates were then impregnated with NaCl slurries and finally removed by heating. The negative NaCl preform was infiltrated with pure melted Mg under pressure of 1.4–1.8 bar. After solidification, the composite structure was washed with an NaOH solution, and a topologically ordered open-cell porous Mg was left.

The removal of the NaCl residues from the surface of the porous Mg and the infiltration of NaCl paste into the polymer template for higher resolution structures are the main challenges of this process. Although the removal of the NaCl template is more feasible than the removal of the plaster preform, which was used in the infiltration processing of porous AZ91 by Yamada et al. [40], some minor residual NaCl was still detected on the surface of the porous Mg [55]. Staiger et al. [55] produced a porous Mg with pore sizes as small as 1 mm and an infiltration distance of 17–18 mm with errors less than 10% (Fig. 2.9). Their results indicated that a pore size less than

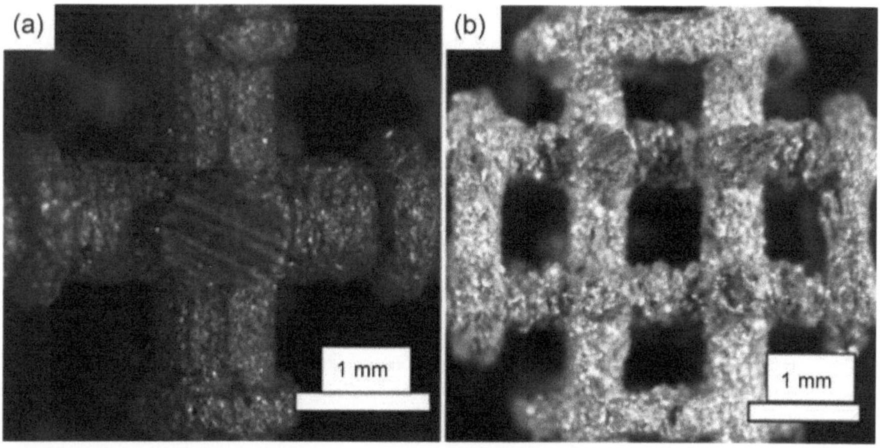

Figure 2.8 Topologically ordered porous magnesium with different architecture structures: (a) fire hydrant, strut, and interface diameter of 0.93 and 1.33 mm, respectively, and (b) crossbar, strut diameter of 0.63 mm [53].

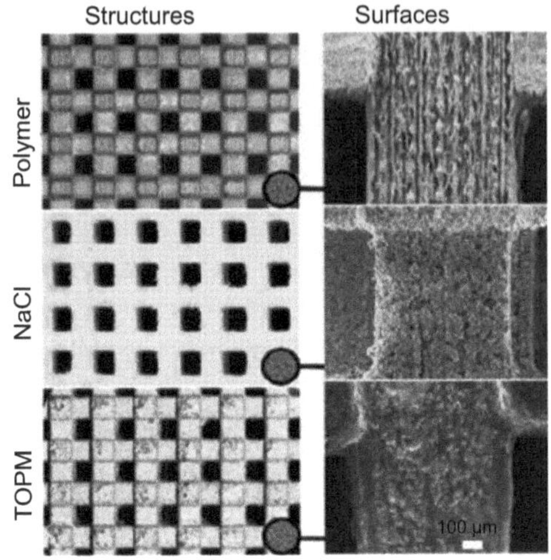

Figure 2.9 Structures of polymer, NaCl, and fabricated porous Mg [55]. *TOPM*, topologically ordered porous magnesium.

1 mm and/or a strut thickness less than 0.8 mm led to difficulties in the infiltration of NaCl paste into polymer and liquid Mg into the NaCl template.

In another method classified in this category, Ti wire was used as the preform or space holder. The principle of this process, which is called the Ti wire space holder (TWSH) method, is similar to melt infiltration, except that no polymeric preform is utilized in the TWSH method. In this process, Ti wires with a diameter of 0.27 mm were entangled to form a cylinder preform with dimensions of Φ10 mm × 20 mm. Mg ingot was melted at 700°C and infiltrated into the entangled Ti wire preform assisted by supersonic vibration. All of the processes were implemented using a mixture of SF6 and CO_2 gases. After solidification the composite sample, consisting of Ti wires in Mg matrix, was immersed in a 40 wt% hydrofluoric acid solution to etch away the Ti wires, then supersonic vibration was again applied. The etching time was about 72 h for a Φ10 mm × 20 mm composite sample. As the Ti wires were removed from the composite completely, a porous Mg with a porosity of 51% and pipe-like shape pores with a diameter of 270 μm were achieved (Fig. 2.10). A comparison of the mechanical properties of porous Mg manufactured using various methods with different porosities is listed in Table 2.1. The mechanical properties of porous Mg are comparable to those of cancellous bone [56].

It should be mentioned that EDS analysis of the inner surface of the pipe-like pores of the porous Mg showed an MgF_2 layer on the Mg surface. This film, which is about 2 μm in thickness, is a passive layer on Mg formed during the etching process in HF solution [56]. Although the effect of this layer on the mechanical properties of the porous Mg is negligible, its biocompatibility still has not been tested.

Wang et al. [57] also fabricated a porous Mg via a melt infiltration technique by using a salt–flour mixture as the space holder. Crude salt was fine-ground and mixed with flour. The mixture was processed into spherical salt–flour mixture particles with

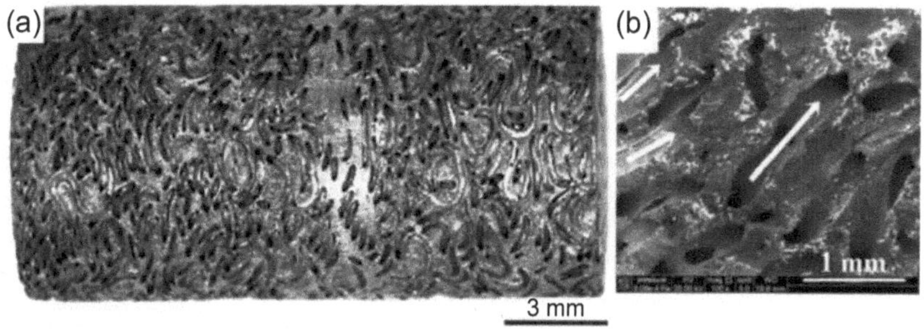

Figure 2.10 (a) Macroscopic structure of porous Mg fabricated via titanium wire space holder method and (b) scanning electron microscope micrograph of the axial section [56].

Table 2.1 **Mechanical properties of the Mg foams with different porosities fabricated using the titanium wire space holder method [56]**

	Porosity (%)		
Mechanical property	**43.5**	**51**	**54.2**
Yield strength (MPa)	6.2	4.6	4.3
Young's modulus (GPa)	1	0.6	0.5

an average size of 1.6 mm by using a pan-type pelletizer. The particles were then heated to 680°C for 2 h to remove the water and flour. The final preform was acquired by pressing the particles into a cylindrical mold. The infiltration process was fulfilled by placing the Mg ingot on the top of the mold and heating the system to 680°C for 1 h under Ar gas. After solidification and machining the ingot acquired the desired dimensions, and the salt particles were dissolved and removed in a 0.001 M NaOH water solution. The salt–flour particles were nearly spherical, and their size could be optimized by adjusting the granulation parameters. The porous Mg exhibited a porous structure with a pore size of 0.6–1.5 mm. The yield strength and Young's modulus of the porous Mg varied from 3.57 to 8.65 MPa and 0.0206 to 0.050 GPa when the porosity increased from 54.4% to 70.4%, respectively. No harmful residues of Cl or other elements were detected on the surface of the porous Mg, indicating no chemical reaction during the infiltration process.

2.2.1.3 Melt/gas eutectic solidification process

In this method, high-pressure hydrogen is introduced into the Mg melt to produce a hydrogen-saturated Mg melt. Then the temperature is lowered, causing the melt to undergo a eutectic transition and decompose to solid and gas. As the Mg melt is solidified, hydrogen bubbles form and are entrapped in the solidified Mg. The pore morphologies largely depend on the chemical composition of the Mg melt, hydrogen

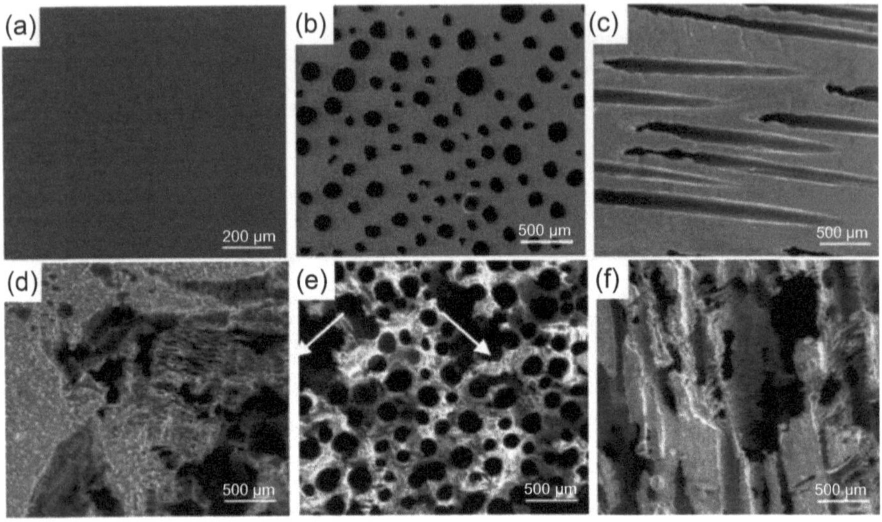

Figure 2.11 Scanning electron microscope images of (a) dense pure Mg, (b) cross-section and (c) longitudinal section of porous pure Mg fabricated via the melt-gas eutectic solidification process, and (d–f) the structures of (a–c) after 7 days immersion in simulated body fluid at 37°C [21].

content, and the pressure and conditions of heat removal during the solidification [25,58,59].

Gu et al. [21] fabricated lotus-type porous pure Mg with a purity of 99.9 wt% (Fig. 2.11). They melted the Mg in a vacuum and then saturated it with hydrogen under 1 MPa pressure. Then the melt was poured into the water-cooled copper (Cu) mold and solidified unidirectionally upward, which resulted in long cylindrical pores in the solidified pure Mg. The average pore size and porosity were about 170 ± 19 μm and $28 \pm 1.3\%$, respectively. They also compared the degradation and cytotoxicity of lotus-type porous Mg with dense pure Mg in SBF and declared that porous pure Mg exhibited a higher corrosion resistance, a slower mass loss rate, and a slower decrease of compressive yield strength during the immersion period than dense pure Mg. Despite a higher Mg concentration in the extract, caused by the larger exposed surface area than that of the dense pure Mg, it was indicated to be still biologically safe in accordance with the Grade I relative growth rate value [21].

Wan et al. [60] also produced lotus-type porous Mg via unidirectional solidification. Their research results indicated that the increase in hydrogen gas pressure led to more uniform pore size and an increase in porosity. Moreover, solidification at the eutectic point at a constant hydrogen pressure resulted in the most uniform distribution of pore size and porosity. Hyun et al. [61] fabricated lotus-type porous Mg via continuous casting and found that the increase in transference velocity led to an increase in pore number as well as the angle between the transference direction and pore growth direction. The pore diameter decreased with increasing transference velocity, but the porosity did not vary much when changing this parameter. Porous

AZ31B and AZ91D with a maximum porosity of 53% were also fabricated under pressurized hydrogen through continuous zone melting and casting. With the casting technique, the trend of pores to be extended in the solidification direction was affected by the amount of alloying elements. However, with the continuous zone melting technique, pores were elongated in the transference direction, and their alignment was independent of the concentration of alloying elements [62].

Liu et al. [63] employed a safe, highly efficient process in which the in-situ reaction combined with unidirectional solidification in the fabrication of a lotus-type porous Mg. They mixed sodium silicate and alumina powder together and spread them on the inner surface of a ceramic mold that was fixed on a Cu cooling crystallizer. The Mg was then melted and cast into the ceramic mold. The liquid metal solidified unidirectionally and entrapped the generated hydrogen, which was the in situ reaction product between the molten Mg with the coating material. By using this process, porous Mg with cylindrical pores and various porosities of 2.5% to ~54% was obtained (Fig. 2.12). Liu et al. reported that the increase in sodium silicate, alumina powder, and solidification rate led to an increase in porosity. However, the increase in temperature resulted in an increase in porosity, which is continued by a decrease.

The lotus-type porous Mg can also be produced through casting molten Mg into a mold containing MgH_2 as a blowing agent and unidirectional solidification. Tane et al. [64,65] indicated that this method was simpler than those processes using pressurized hydrogen. The porosity and pore size could be controlled by adjusting the amount of MgH_2 and by adjusting the solidification process. Zahrani and coresearchers also fabricated lotus-type porous Mg by introducing some pine wood pellets into Mg melt followed by casting into a water-cooled mold. The thermal decomposition of the wood

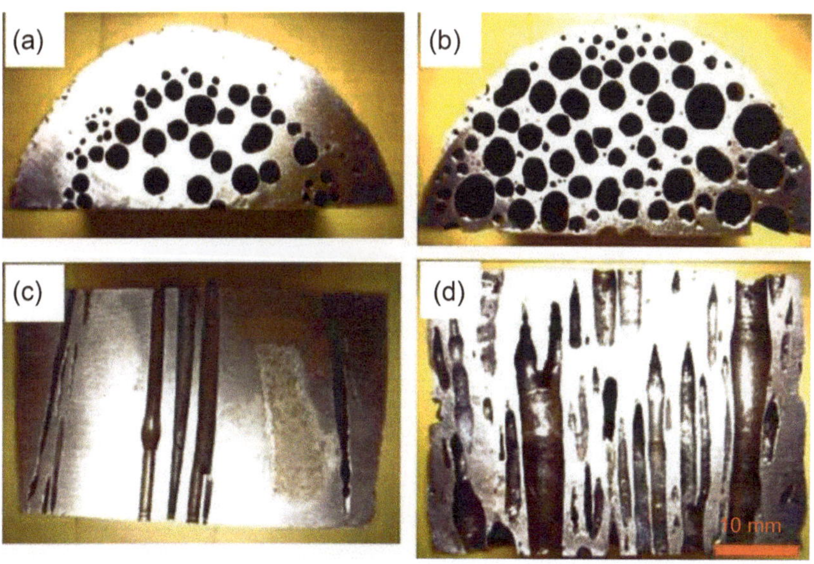

Figure 2.12 The morphology of lotus-type porous Mg with various amounts of sodium silicate binder: (a and c) 5 mL and (b and d) 9 mL [63].

resulted in hydrogen bubbles in the Mg melt, and the unidirectional solidification fulfilled the process by entrapment of the hydrogen in the matrix. Although the porosity and pore size varied by changes in the wood content, other gases such as CO, CO_2, and CH_4 as well as residuals such as tar and char can be formed, which established some impurities in the final product [66].

2.2.1.4 Melt vacuum solidification foaming: vacuum foaming technique

In 2005, Renger and Kaufmann [67] introduced the vacuum foaming technique (VFT) for the fabrication of porous Mg as a cost-efficient foaming process, based on the reduced pressure test. The principle for this process is that gas inclusions in the molten Mg expand when the surrounding pressure is reduced sufficiency. Therefore they used thin-walled, high-pressure die casting Mg scraps as the precursor, since these are a good source of oxides stemming from the high-turbulence casting process. The precursor material was melted quickly, poured into a die, and cooled to form a semisolid state, which resulted in an increase in melt viscosity. The addition of machining chips can be considered as an alternative method to increase the melt viscosity. When the temperature reached the intended foaming temperature, the semisolid metal and die were placed into an autoclave at a reduced pressure of about 0.1 bar. Similar to the reduced pressure test process, the melt expanded, and bubbles formed during solidification (Fig. 2.13). The pore diameter produced by using this process was normally 4–5 mm and 10 mm in low-density foams.

2.2.2 Powder metallurgy

In this method, pure Mg or Mg alloy powder is mixed with a foaming agent. The mixture is pressed and heated at moderate temperatures to produce the foam structure.

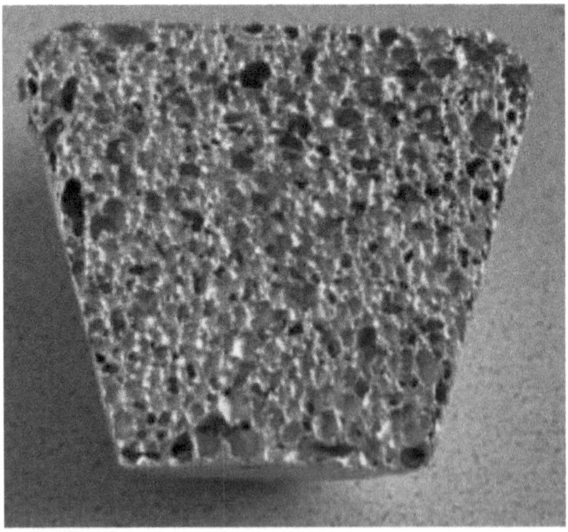

Figure 2.13 Cross-section of porous AZ91 prepared by using a melt/vacuum solidification foaming method at 600°C [67].

Then, a sintering process at elevated temperatures is carried out, so a strong foam structure can be achieved. The foaming agent can be considered as either a blowing agent (to generate gas in an Mg matrix) or as spacer material (to be removed from the Mg matrix prior to sintering). Therefore there are two major PM-based processes for Mg foam [24]. However, Mg foam fabrication without a foaming agent and spacer is also feasible, although rare. For instance, Kaya [68] used no blowing agent or space holder but rather different compaction pressures to control the porosity. The researcher just mixed the Mg and Al powders and used compaction pressures of 400 and 600 MPa, sintering the samples at 465°C for 4 h under Ar atmosphere. Kaya reported that the increase of compaction pressure leads to a decrease of porosity and encourages the Mg phase to transform to the Mg17Al12 phase.

2.2.2.1 Blowing agent-based powder metallurgy

In this process, porosity is created by entrapping gas that is commonly released from the hydride foaming agent into the Mg powder [25]. TiH_2 is the most powerful blowing agent in powder-based routes. However, $CaCO_3$ is considered as a substitute for TiH_2 due to the fact that carbonates are safer and fabricate finer and more homogenous cell structures in PM processing [69,70].

In addition to the size, morphology, and quality of initial powders, some supplementary elements can influence the foaming quality. For instance, Plorin et al. [71] suggested that adding zinc (Zn) powder to the mixture of Mg and TiH_2 powders and a heat treatment following the injection process can improve the foaming behavior. They explained that Zn diffuses into the Mg matrix through the heat treatment and consequently halts the Mg diffusion. Therefore some voids form in place of previous Zn spots in the matrix and actually result in the formation of pores prior to the start of the foaming process. These pores cause the hydrogen to be separated at temperatures lower than the Mg melting point and can also decrease the pressure of the hydrogen gas released by TiH_2 decomposition. Moreover, these pores lead to slower crack formation during the initial stages of foaming, which finally results in more homogenous pore distribution in the final foam. They also mentioned that the finer powder sizes can produce higher quality foams with more homogenous cell wall thicknesses.

The extrusion method as well as Al powders can be considered as an alternative method and supplementary element, respectively, to facilitate the consolidation process of Mg powders in this method. Experiments carried out by Neu and coworkers [72] revealed qualified results. They mixed Mg and Al powders (as a precursor) with a blowing agent, consolidated into green compact, and finally heated above the solidus temperature. They prepared the precursors with and without TiH_2 and employed uniaxial pressing as well as extrusion methods to consolidate the powders. Two foaming processes were utilized. The ambient pressure process was performed by heating the precursors to about 100°C above the melting point of the alloy and holding them isothermally at 150 s followed by natural cooling, all under a 1.2 bar Ar atmosphere. In the pressure-induced foaming (PIF) process, the furnace was filled by Ar to 10 bar, which caused the precursor to be melted. Cooling followed the gas release to 1 bar. Based on their results, both pure Mg and Mg–Al alloy foams, with reasonable foam structures and 60–70% porosity, can be produced only via the PIF process and extruded precursors containing TiH_2. In extruded samples, the shear stresses break the oxide layers on the powder surface and lead to better metallurgical bonding and superior foams. However, in uniaxial compacted precursors, part of the generated gas during heating is lost, which results in crack-like pores and an unstable foam structure with low density. The researchers reported that Al increases the expansion as well as the pore size. Al acts as a plasticizer and improves the consolidation, which produces high-density precursors. Moreover, it decreases the melting point of the alloy and facilitates the formation of a liquid phase. Therefore generated gas entrapped in the sample leads to expansion and then crack formation. They also stated that PIF is essential for foaming of blowing agent-free precursors. In such samples without TiH_2, absorbed MgH_2 on powder surfaces generates some gas during heating, which can be preserved only when the external pressure is high enough to slow down gas losses. In samples with TiH_2, the gas losses during melting can also be compensated by these additional gas sources [72].

2.2.2.2 Space holder-based powder metallurgy

The foaming stage, in this process, is the removal of the space holder material from the Mg matrix, which creates hollow spaces between Mg particles prior to joining. A heat treatment process is then used to join the Mg powders and obtain a suitable strength.

So far, Mg powders with various specifications, different spacer materials, and several production parameters have been investigated, which resulted in Mg foam with various characteristics.

Wen et al. [1] fabricated open cellular Mg foam with a pore size in the range of 200–600 μm by using ammonium hydrogen carbonate particles or carbamide particles as space holder materials with the same range of size. They stated that the control of porosity, pore size, and morphology of the porous Mg foams via the space holder-based powder metallurgy (SHPM) process is feasible. The production of Mg foam with a specific pore size range appropriate to the pore size range of bone tissue could be both useful and commercially viable. Furthermore, these produced foams have sufficient strength to make them feasible for handling and implantation. The researchers measured the compressive strength and Young's modulus as 2.33 MPa and 0.35 GPa, respectively, for 50% porosity.

Wen et al. [5,73] also utilized different carbamide particle sizes, ie, 45–100, 100–200, 200–300, and 300–500 μm to fabricate various pore sizes (73, 168, 251, and 412 μm) and a range of porosities (35–55%) of Mg foams (Fig. 2.14). They reported that the pore size of porous Mg can be controlled by the particle size and volume of carbamide particles. Specimens with a porosity of 35% (pore size ~250 μm) revealed a high Young's modulus of 1.8 GPa and a high peak stress of 17 MPa, whereas specimens with a porosity of 45% (pore size ~73 μm) showed a Young's modulus of 1.3 GPa and a high peak stress of 16 MPa. Moreover, they showed that the number of isolated pores, which are not interconnected, as well as the Young's modulus of Mg foams decrease with increasing porosity and pore size. With respect to the ductility and modulus of bone tissue [11], it has been suggested that porous

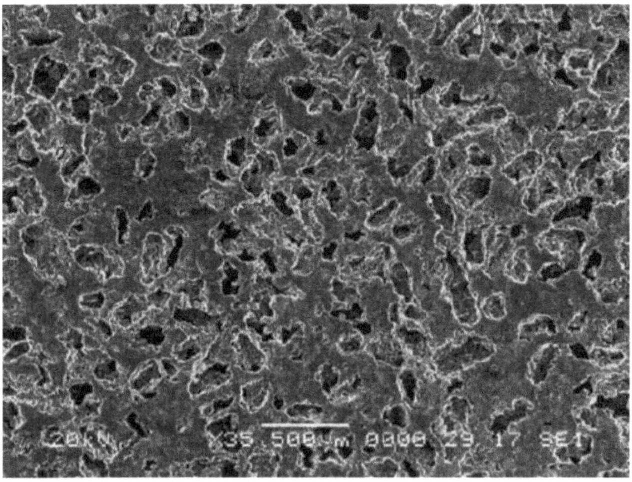

Figure 2.14 Microstructure of open cellular Mg foam fabricated by the space holder-based powder metallurgy method with a porosity of 45% and a pore size of 168 μm [5].

Mg can be used for bone implant material. However, in terms of residual materials through the production process, they reported that no nitrogen and very little carbon was observed on the cell wall surfaces, which means that Mg and carbamide reacted during the sintering, and further investigation is needed on the bioproperties of the residual materials.

Carbamide particles with a size range of 200–400 μm were also used by Zhuang and coworkers [74]. Open-cellular Mg foams with a pore size and porosity range of 200–400 μm and 36–55%, respectively, were fabricated. Isolated microporosities were also observed within the wall of macropores. They mentioned that the compressive strength and the Young's modulus of foam increase from 15 to 100 MPa and 3.6 to 44 GPa, respectively, by decreasing the porosity from 55% to 0%. They also investigated the effect of porosity on the biodegradation of specimens in physiological saline solution (0.9% NaCl solution) after 144 h. They observed that the weight loss of the specimens with a porosity of 55% and 36% is 60% and 15%, respectively. Moreover, the degradation rate of specimens with a porosity of 55% is more than specimens with a porosity of 36% due to more connecting areas that facilitate the transportation of the solution and accelerate the rate of chemical reactions. Therefore these results reveal that porous Mg samples have "changeable in vitro degradable rates" that are boosted by increasing the porosity.

Open-cellular Mg foams (Fig. 2.15) with a porosity range of 40–80% and pore size range of 0.5–2 mm have also been fabricated by Hao and coresearchers [75–78] using different volume fractions and particle sizes of carbamide as the space holder. They investigated the manufacturing parameters and found the optimized parameters, according to compression properties, that can be achieved when the compacting pressure is 200–300 MPa and the sintering temperature is 610–630°C. Their Mg foams showed a long plateau region with a small plateau stress, where both the peak elastic

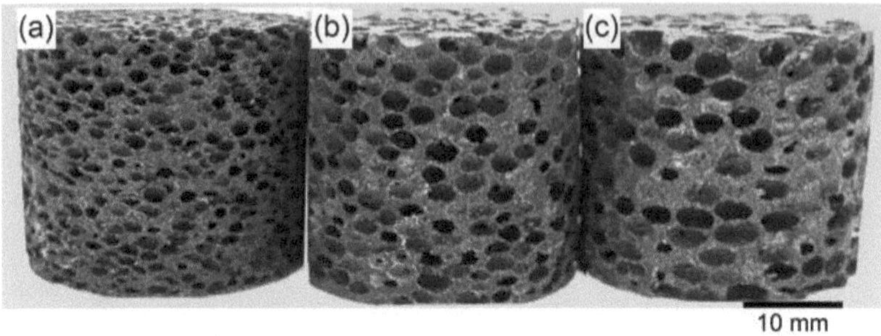

Figure 2.15 Porous Mg samples manufactured using the space holder-based powder metallurgy method with a porosity of 70% and pore sizes of (a) 0.75 mm, (b) 1.25 mm, and (c) 1.75 mm [75].

stress and the plateau height increase with an increase in the relative density. Moreover, increasing porosity or decreasing pore size will increase the damping properties of the foam.

Aghion and coresearchers [79] employed a PM process to fabricate Mg alloy foam as a biodegradable drug delivery platform. They milled Mg alloy powder mixed with ammonium hydrogen carbonate and pressed at a pressure of 100 MPa. The green compact was heated under a low vacuum (0.1 Torr) to enable the evaporation of the space holder and then sintered at a temperature range between 450 to 630°C under high vacuum (10^{-5} Torr). They produced Mg foams with 10% and 25% porosity with an average pore size of 40 and 140 μm, respectively (Fig. 2.16). They stated that the increase of time and temperature of sintering decreases the number and size of pores. The 25% spacer has more porosity and interconnected open pores than the 10% spacer, which makes it superior for absorbing, carrying, and releasing a larger amount of drug. Therefore the amount of delivered drug, as well as the time for delivery, can be controlled by the porosity, which is determined by the amount of space holder material. They also expressed that the corrosion resistance of Mg foams, in

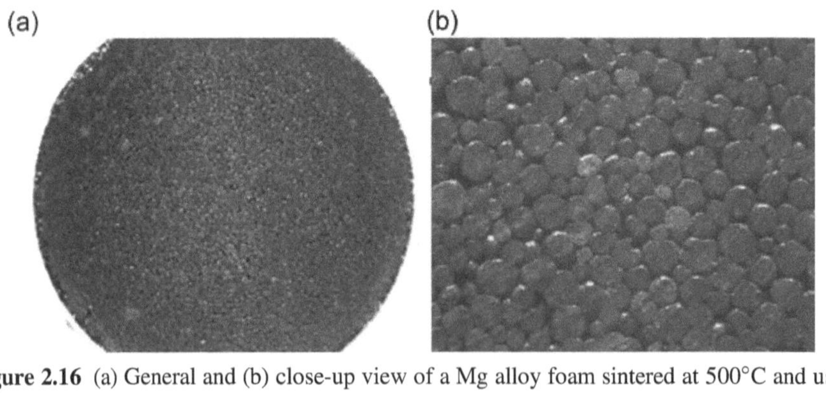

Figure 2.16 (a) General and (b) close-up view of a Mg alloy foam sintered at 500°C and used for drug delivery [79].

phosphate buffer saline (PBS) solution, increases by decreasing the spacer content, which results in lower porosity. Mg foams with 25% spacer expose more surface area to the corrosive solution.

0 to 20 vol% of ammonium bicarbonate powder (250–500 μm) has also been used as space holder material by Čapek and Vojtěh [80]. They manually mixed this powder with Mg powder as well as 30 vol% liquid hexane (to avoid segregation) for 30 min. Then the mixture was uniaxially cold pressed (at 265 MPa) and heat treated in two steps: 130°C for 4 h and 550°C for 6 h under Ar atmosphere. Porous Mg samples were prepared with the porosity of 12–38 vol%. The experiments showed that the flexural strength of samples decreases from 38 to 4.4 MPa by increasing the porosity from 12 to 38 vol% [81]. The shape of Mg powders is also an effective parameter on the quality of foams, as the flexural strength of samples prepared with spherical powders is interestingly higher than samples that have been prepared with irregularly shaped Mg powders, such as Mg chips [82]. They also mentioned that a longer sintering time and the purity of the Ar atmosphere improve the flexural strength of Mg foams. Their results suggest that sintering for longer than 6 h should be carried out under a shielded Ar atmosphere. Sintering under a technical Ar atmosphere results in oxidation of the powder surface and decreases the mechanical properties [80,81].

In addition to Mg and spacer powder, some alloying elements can be added to Mg foams to modify the properties and allocate the foams to specific applications. Hao et al. [83] have increased the damping capacity of porous AZ91 Mg alloy by adding Cu particles, as reinforcement, to AZ91 alloy powder. They mixed Mg and Cu powders with a size of 50 and 4 μm, respectively, and then carbamide particles with a size of 1.25 mm were added. The mixture was compacted under 300 MPa pressure for 2 min. The green compact was put in an $NaHCO_3$ water solution to remove the majority of the space holder materials and then heated at 250°C for 3 h and sintered at 610°C for 2.5 h. They stated that the produced samples with a porosity of 40–80% and different pore sizes have a higher damping capacity in comparison with a porous AZ91 alloy with the same porosity and pore size but unreinforced. Porous Mg/Alumina composites (with porosity of 10–38% and pore size of 25–100 μm) have also been fabricated by Cay and coworkers [84]. They mixed the Mg powder with alumina powder (with the size of 0.5 μm) and carbamide, as a space holder, in a planetary ball mill. The mixture was pressed at a pressure of 120 MPa, heated at 250°C for 4 h, and sintered at 630°C for 2 h. Results show that the yield strengths of porous composites are higher than both cast bulk Mg and porous pure Mg with the same porosity and pore size. Moreover, the pore size of porous samples increases with an increase in porosity [84].

Zn powder has also been added to Mg powder to produce an Mg–Zn alloy foam. The Mg–Zn powder was mixed with carbamide particles, uniaxially pressed at 100 MPa, heat treated at 250°C to remove the space holder, and finally heated up to different temperatures ranging from 500–580°C. Three classes of samples with porosity volume fractions of 21, 29, and 36 vol% and a pore size of 200, 100–300, and 200–400 μm, respectively, were obtained. Results show that Zn refines the Mg grain size and so improves the mechanical properties of porous Mg–Zn alloy foams. Both the Young's modulus and the compressive strength of the porous samples increase when the Zn content is increased. The highest compressive strength and Young's modulus obtained for porous Mg-6%wt Zn with a porosity of ~15% and a pore size of 200–400 μm (sintered at 550°C) are ~60 MPa and ~7.3 GPa, respectively. Experiments also show that an increase in sintering temperature results in the reduction of Young's modulus as well as compressive strength [85].

Zhang et al. [86] also produced Mg foams using an SHPM process. However, unlike other studies, they used ground salt as the space holder material. They ground salt and sieved it to three different particle sizes, 250–350, 350–500, and 500–700 μm, and then dried it at 200°C for 24 h. Then 30 wt% of salt and 70 wt% of spherical Mg powder were layered alternately and hot pressed under a pressure of 40 MPa for 20 min at 640–650°C. The composite of salt/Mg was cut and immersed into a solution of glycerine and ethanol for 48 h. The salt particles were removed, leaving a porous structure on the surface of the samples, with a porosity of 8%, 10%, and 6% respectively achieved, while the inner compact structure was reinforced by salt particles. Macro- and micropores were observed on the outer surface in the Mg foams that formed due to the dissolving out of salt particles and the sintering process of Mg powders, respectively. Two types of pores, interconnected and isolated pores, can be seen in Mg foam structures, favoring bone ingrowth (Fig. 2.17).

X-ray diffraction and energy dispersive spectroscopy (EDS) analysis results exhibit no salt residue on the surface of the specimen or the cell walls. However, small amounts of carbon and oxygen were detected on the cell walls. The compressive yield strength and Young's modulus of Mg foams increased with an increase in the size of salt particles to 55–79 MPa and 2.5–3.1 GPa, respectively, when the salt particle size changed from 250 to 700 μm.

Table 2.2 summarizes the parameters used by various researchers to produce Mg alloy foams through SHPM process.

2.2.3 Other processes

In addition to the abovementioned processes, there are other methods that are a mixture of some former methods and actually have been invented and investigated by some researchers. The main foundation of these routes is the use of a blowing agent and the generation of a gas or the utilization of free spaces between consolidated particulates. In the following two new methods for Mg foam have been introduced.

2.2.3.1 Forming and blowing agent-based process

In this process, which has been done for three Mg alloys by Kitazono and coworkers [87], 1.0 mass% of TiH_2 particles, used as the blowing agent, are dispersed on Mg alloy strips. Then the strips are stacked and diffusion-bonded by hot pressing in air. The stacked strips are heated at elevated temperatures according to the alloy composition and then uniaxially pressed to achieve a 50% strain. The flat plate is cut and plates are stacked again, and after a second diffusion bonding, preforms with a 10 mm thickness are obtained. The preforms are heated in Ar by a high-frequency induction coil to form closed-cell foams. The researchers showed that the specimens expanded to the axis of the hot pressing direction. They also stated that the porosity and the average pore size increase with increasing temperature. However, heating at

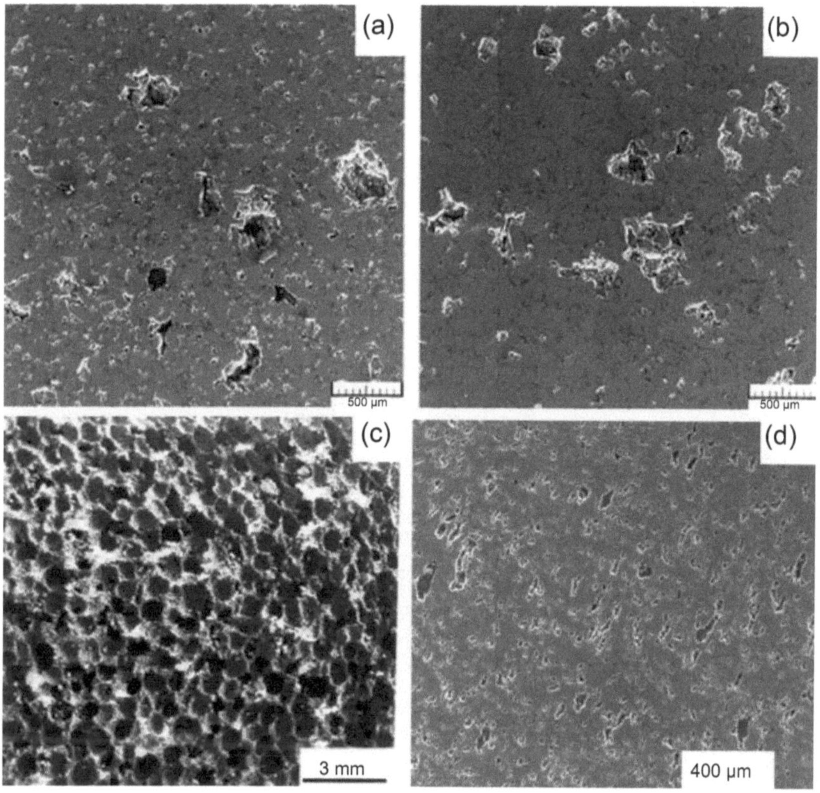

Figure 2.17 Microstructure of Mg foams produced via the space holder-based powder metallurgy method: (a and b) Mg foam with porosities of 28% and 33%, respectively, (c) AZ91 foam with a porosity of 71% and a pore size of 0.75 mm, and (d) Mg/1%alumina composite foam with a porosity of 10% [77,81,84].

higher temperature ranges causes shrinking of the Mg matrix and decreasing porosity. The cell morphology depends on the chemical composition of the Mg alloy, so that ZA146 alloy with a low solidus temperature produces fine cell morphology. They claim that this process has an advantage over the PM process because there is no need for flammable and expensive Mg powder. However, more investigations are necessary to optimize the cell morphology, porosity, and pore size. Various porous Mg alloys, such as AZ31, AZ91, and ZA146, with maximum porosities of 46%, 55%, and 60%, respectively, were achieved in this study. Kikuchi and coworkers [88] used the same process and space holder material, but of 0.5 and 2.0 mass%, for AZ31 Mg alloy. The samples containing 2.0 mass% TiH_2 represented more porosity than those of 0.5 mass%.

Mehara and coworkers [89] have also produced closed-cell Mg foams based on this process. Machined chips of AZ91D Mg alloy were mixed with TiH_2 as the blowing agent. Three production methods, hot extrusion, compressive torsion, and compressive torsion followed by hot extrusion, were used to prepare precursors

Table 2.2 **The production parameters of pure Mg or Mg alloy foams produced using the space holder-based powder metallurgy method**

Mg alloy	Metal powder particle size (μm)	SH material	SH particle size (μm) [amount (vol%)]	Compacting pressure (MPa) and compacting period (min)	Burning temperature (°C) and burning period (h) of SH material	Sintering temperature (°C) and sintering period (h)	Pore size (μm)	Porosity (%)	Residual material formed during fabrication	References
Pure Mg	≤180	Ammonium hydrogen carbonate	200–600	100	200 [5]	500 [2]	200–500	50	–	[1]
Mg	≤180	Carbamide	45–100; 100–200; 200–300; 300–500	100	200 [5]	500 [2]	70–400	35–55	Carbon	[5]
Pure Mg	≤40	Carbamide	200–400	100	250 [4]	500 [2]	200–400	7, 36 and 55	Carbon, oxygen	[74]
Pure Mg	100	Carbamide	0.5–1.0, 1.0–1.5 and 1.5–2.0 mm	300 [2]	Immersion in NaOH water solution for 0.5–5 h followed by heat treatment at 250°C for 3 h	630 [2.5]	0.5–2.0 mm	40–80	–	[75]

Mg-10Al	45	–	–	400 and 600	–	465 [4]	–	9.2–9.7	–	[68]
AZ91	50	Carbamide	1.25 mm	300 [2]	250 [3]	610 [2.5]	Hundreds micro-meter to several millimeters	40–80	–	[77,83]
Mg–Zn	<100	Carbamide	200–400 [15,25,35]	100	250 [4]	500, 550, 565, 580 [2]	150–400	21–36	MgO $Mg7Zn_3$ MgZn	[85]
Mg + 3.1 wt% Nd, 0.46 wt% Zr, 0.01 wt% Si, 0.004 wt% Fe, 0.001 wt% Cu, and 0.001 wt% Ni	100–150	Ammonium hydrogen carbonate	50–200 [10,25]	100	150 Under 10^{-1} Torr vacuum	450–630 [48] Under 10^{-5} Torr vacuum	40–140	10, 25	MgO, Si	[79]
Mg	75–150	Ammonium hydrogen carbonate	250–500 [0,5,10,15,20]	265	130 [4]	550 [6]	>200	12–38	MgO	[81]
Mg/alumina	45	Carbamide	–	120	250 [4]	630 [2]	25–100	10–38	–	[84]

SH, space holder.

from the mixture. The consolidated precursors were heated in an induction furnace under Ar gas protection, and the expansion was evaluated with a video camera. After the maximum level of expansion, the specimens were cooled by helium gas. The results show that the compressive torsion process, regardless of being followed by extrusion, is more effective than other processes to break thin oxide films on the machined chips. It also consolidates them firmly and disperses the blowing agent homogeneously. Moreover, the porosity and the number of pores were higher in the specimens processed by the compressive torsion process in comparison to specimens prepared by hot extrusion.

2.2.3.2 Pulse electric current sintering process

Okumura and coworkers [90,91] used electric current to sinter and join the AZ91D, AZ31, and AM60B Mg alloy chips for Mg foam fabrication. The chips of the alloy, as the raw material, were provided by a lathe machine, poured into a graphite mold, and put between electrodes in a hydraulic press apparatus. Sintering was carried out by current flowing through the chips under Ar gas atmosphere, which led to surface melting of the chips. The samples were held at different sintering temperatures for 10 min. The low sintering temperature, the small amount of low melting compounds in the alloy, and the narrow semisolid temperature range of the alloy lead to weak joints between the chips. Moreover, an increase in the amount of chips causes a decrease of porosity due to the low intensity of the pulse current that passes thorough chip contacts. The plateau stresses obtained for AZ91D Mg alloy by these researchers range from 1.3 to 37 MPa for porosities of 76% to 50%, respectively. They also indicated that the porosity is the most effective parameter on the plateau stress.

2.2.3.3 Fiber sintering process

New results show that porous Mg can also be made through liquid phase sintering of Mg short fibers. Morgenthal et al. [92] used melt-extracted MgY4 and WZ21 Mg alloy fibers (with an average length of 6–7 mm and a mean diameter of 180 μm) as the initial material. Homogeneously deposited fibers on the sinter substrate were heat treated at 630 and 610°C for MgY4 and WZ21 alloys, respectively, under high-purity Ar gas. Porous Mg alloy samples with a porosity of 65–75% and a fine-grained microstructure were achieved (Fig. 2.18). Compression test results confirm the anisotropic mechanical properties of produced porous Mg. Moreover, mechanical properties depend on alloy composition and the direction of loading. Loading samples perpendicularly to the direction of fiber deposition results in a higher compressive strength and stiffness. The average compressive strength and stiffness of porous samples, loaded in the former direction, are reported as ~14 MPa and 1.7 GPa, respectively, for WZ21 alloy and as ~22 MPa and 2.8 GPa for MgY4 alloy. The researchers also tested the corrosion rate of porous samples through hydrogen evolution in Dulbecco's Modified Eagle Medium solution at 37°C, which is lower than that of the initial material.

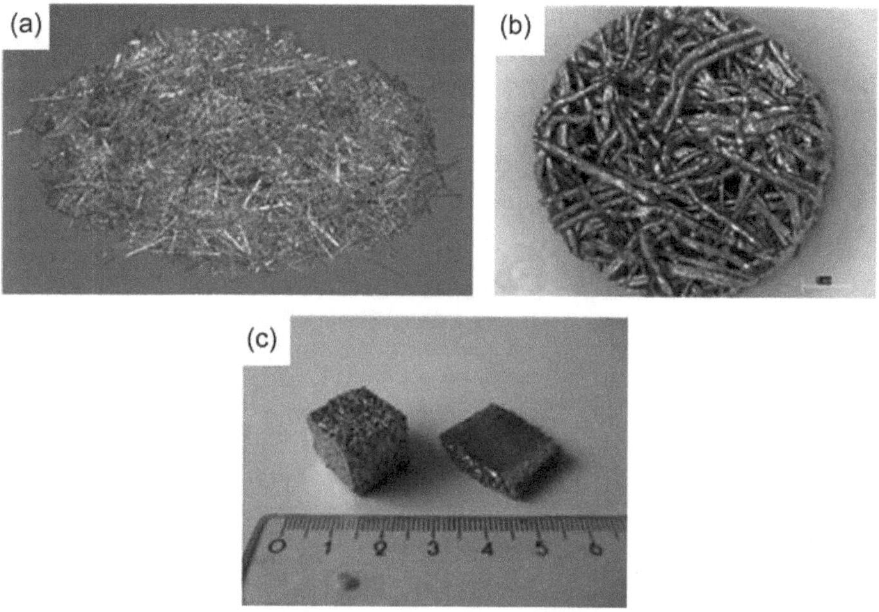

Figure 2.18 (a) MgY4 fibers, (b) laser-beam cut of MgY4 (W4) foam sample, sintered at 630°C, porosity ~70%, and (c) sample before and after compression test [92].

2.2.3.4 Fiber deposition hot pressing technology

In this process, in contrast to the previously explained method (fiber sintering (FS)), Mg fibers are lined up regularly to a network structure unit of Mg fibers to be formed. The fibers of each layer are perpendicular to the neighboring fiber layers, and the space between each fiber layer is about 0.5 mm. Then 15 network units are layered in graphite die and hot pressed under a pressure of 55 MPa at 640°C for 20 min to fabricate a porous Mg scaffold with a porosity of 33–54%. The shape of the pores is rectangular, and the distribution of the pores is almost even. The pore size is controlled by the fiber spacing and fiber size (height) as well as the hot pressing temperature or pressure. Mechanical properties of fiber deposition hot pressing (FDHP)-manufactured Mg foams (Table 2.3) are anisotropic, as their axial compression flow stress is higher than that of lateral flow stress and much higher than those porous scaffolds produced via other techniques [93].

2.2.3.5 Mechanical perforation technique

Tan and coworkers [94] fabricated a predesigned porous Mg by utilizing a pulsed laser power supply and a machine tool. They controlled equipment using software to prepare an Mg scaffold with different pore arrangements (Fig. 2.19). Researchers stated that the compression behavior of fabricated porous Mg via the mechanical perforation

Table 2.3 Mechanical properties of Mg foams fabricated using the fiber deposition hot pressing method [93]

		Porosity (%)	
		33	**54**
Young's modulus (GPa)	Axial	0.37	0.10
	Lateral	0.67	0.19
Compressive strength (MPa)	Axial	30.3	11.1
	Lateral	15.1	7.8

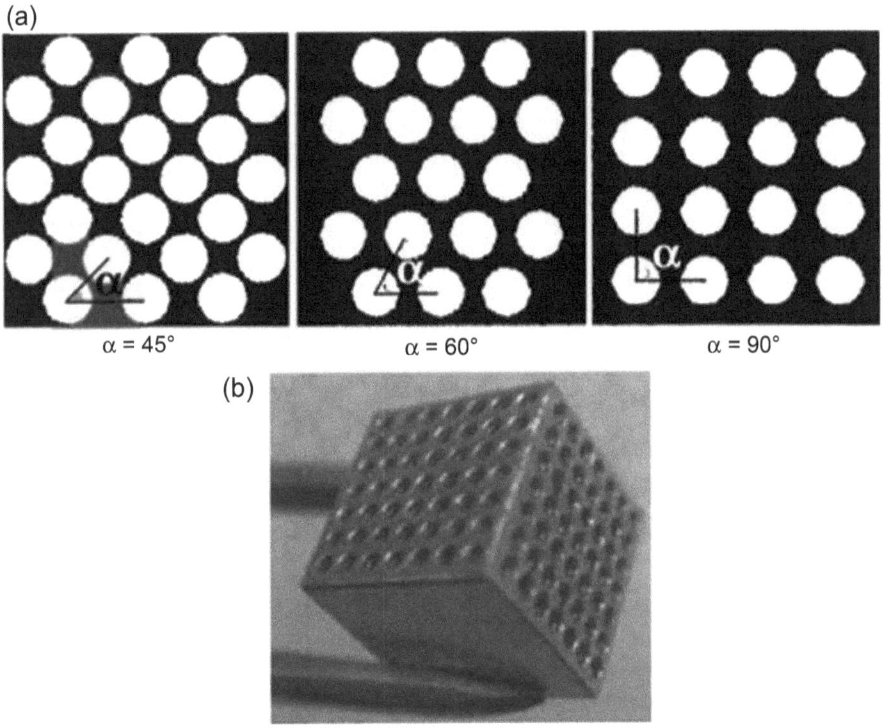

Figure 2.19 (a) Different pore arrangements of Mg scaffold and (b) porous Mg scaffold produced by the mechanical perforation technique with a pore arrangement of $\alpha = 90$ degrees [94].

(MP) method is anisotropic. So, the compressive strength of samples in the direction of pore growth is the highest, and perpendicular to the pore growth direction is the lowest. Moreover, compressive properties of prepared Mg scaffolds can be affected mainly by the pore arrangements [94].

2.3 Discussion

As can be seen in the previous section, there are various procedures that can be used to produce Mg foams with a wide variety of properties and characteristics. However, some methods are limited due to their affiliation to various and/or accurate production parameters. Moreover, properties of Mg foams produced by some methods are not admissible specifically in biomedical applications. Some advantages and disadvantages, as well as critical factors and parameters for the production and application of biodegradable Mg and Mg alloy foams for biomedical applications, will therefore be discussed below.

2.3.1 Effect of alloy composition

The composition of an Mg matrix, in biocompatible and biodegradable Mg foams, influences both the porous structure and the biocompatibility of the porous structure, so the effects of composition should be investigated mutually. The effect of the composition of an Mg matrix on the porous structure itself can be considered from two points of view: the effect of the alloying elements on either the intrinsic properties of the Mg alloy or on the foaming behavior, which both consequently change the properties of Mg foam [95].

The alloying elements, which change the initial properties of Mg and consequently improve the properties of Mg foam, can be categorized as common alloying elements such as those that serve in solid alloys [51] (structural modifiers [85] and reinforcements [83,84], for example). However, some other alloying elements alter the foaming behavior of Mg alloys through changes in size or the morphology of pores, porosity, or pore orientation. They change the properties of Mg melt [27], casting properties [22,36,67], solidification characteristics of Mg melt [60,62], solidus temperature [87], and structural properties [71,85,87] of the Mg alloy and influence the foaming characteristics. For instance, the cell morphology of Mg foams fabricated via the forming and blowing agent-based process (FBA) is influenced by the chemical composition of the Mg alloy, so that finer cell morphology can be observed in ZA146 alloy foams than that of AZ31 and AZ91 alloy foams due to its low solidus temperature [87].

As can be seen in Table 2.4, various chemical elements have been used for porous Mg structures. However, the effects of some elements on foam characteristics such as foam expansion behavior, cell structure, and consequent physical and mechanical properties have not yet been established.

Most of the Mg alloys considered for use in porous Mg structures are existing commercial Mg alloys originally designed for industrial applications, and Al and Zn are the most common alloying elements [96,97]. Although these alloys exhibit excellent mechanical properties and corrosion resistance and are well developed for their applications, particularly in the transportation industry [98–100], their biocompatibility and biodegradability should be given serious attention. The performance of biomaterials is governed by biofunctionality as well as biocompatibility. Biofunctionality refers to the mechanical properties of the biomaterial, whereas biocompatibility is defined as the compatibility of material with surrounding tissues [101].

Table 2.4 Different Mg alloy foams fabricated using various foaming techniques

	Pure Mg	MgZn3	MgZn6	MgSn3	MgZnSn alloys, gZnSi,	Mg-Al alloy	Mg-Zn alloy	AZ31	AZ31+1,2,3,%Zr	AZ31B	AZ91	AZ91D	AZ91E	AZ63	AZ181	Mg-12Al-3Ca	AM60	AM60B	M2	MZX211	WE43	WZ21	ZA146	ZM21	ZM20	ZWM200	ZXM200	MgNdZrSiFeCuNi	MgY4
MBA	×							×	×		×					×	×							×	×	×	×		
MIP	×										×		×	×					×	×	×								
GASAR	×									×		×																	
MVS											×				×														
BAPM	×	×	×	×	×	×																							
SHPM	×						×	×			×												×					×	
FBA												×																	
PECS								×				×						×											
FS																						×							×
MP	×																												

In other words, elements that are advantageous for mechanical properties and acceptable for the design of industrial Mg alloys may be detrimental to bioabsorbable Mg-based alloys. Implanted biomaterials interact with cells and release metal ions into the surrounding tissues, exhibiting specific biological responses. Thus the cytotoxicity of metallic biomaterials is controlled by their composition and the cytotoxicity of component elements [97,102]. The effects of the various elements that have been used widely in Mg foam fabrication, such as Al, Zn, manganese (Mn), Si, Zr, Ca, Cu, nickel (Ni), iron (Fe), Li, Y, and Nd, on biofunctionality and biocompatibility of Mg in vivo and in vitro have been extensively investigated. The amount of impurities and additional elements should be strictly controlled, even at very low concentrations, and some of them, such as Ni, should be avoided [14,97,103–109].

Al- and Zn-containing Mg alloys are the most common alloys to have been investigated as bio-Mg-foams. Although these alloys are stable from the mechanical and corrosion points of view [110], and there are no negative records about the affected surrounding tissues, implants by porous AZ91 alloy in rabbits have been reported [49], and Al-free Mg alloys are recommended for implant into humans [6].

Al has a more favorable effect on Mg than any other element. It is commonly used in Mg for grain refining, modifying mechanical properties, and hardness and corrosion resistance. Moreover, it facilitates the casting process of Mg by widening the solidus liquidus range [96,111,112]. It is therefore preferable that Al be utilized as an alloying element for stronger Mg foams that are fabricated via casting processes such as melt foaming methods [29]. Al powders have also been added to Mg powder, using the blowing agent-based powder metallurgy (BAPM) method, as a plasticizer for greater consolidation of the Mg powders, and as a melting point reducer for greater gas entrapment and expansion [72]. However, a high concentration of Al in the human body, especially in the brain, may damage intelligence and neurons and impair osteoblasts. It also raises the risk of developing Alzheimer's disease [113]. Although in some studies Al has been revealed to have no negative effects on human-derived cells cultured on AZ91D alloy, osteoblast activity has been enhanced on guinea pig femora [110]. The safe daily intake of Al from medications has been reported to be as high as 12–71 mg/kg [114], but higher doses may have detrimental effects on humans [103]. Al accelerates the corrosion of Mg alloys in SBFs, which is not appropriate from a degradation point of view [115]. Thus the amount of Al that is used in and released from Mg alloys should be attentively controlled. It is therefore advised that the Al content for bio-Mg foams be kept as low as possible and that other alloying elements or methods be employed to improve the mechanical properties of porous structures.

Zn and Al are pretty close in effectiveness as an alloying element in Mg. Zn is often employed in combination with Al to improve the strength of Mg [96] and form fine grains [112]. Mechanical property testing of an Mg–Al–Zn alloy indicated that the yield tensile strength is enhanced as the contents of Al and Zn are increased and reaches a maximum value at a total element content of 10 wt% [116]. Al- and Zn-containing Mg alloys are used in porous structures, as their mechanical properties are close to those of human bone tissues [92]. Seyedraoufi and Mirdamadi [85] reported that an increase of Zn from 4 to 6 wt% in Mg–Zn alloy foam refined the grain size of Mg and improved the compression strength of the porous structure. Some heat treatments can also improve the mechanical properties of Al- and Zn-containing Mg foams. The HHT of AZ31 foams exhibited an increase in both yield strength and the energy absorption capacity of Mg alloy foams [32]. In contrast, T6 heat treatment of AZ91 Mg foams showed lower relative stress than cast foams [43].

Zn also reduces the harmful effects of impurities, such as Fe and Ni, on the corrosion properties of Mg by transforming such impurities into harmless intermetallic compounds [117]. The corrosion resistance of Mg–Zn–X (X: Ca, Si, Zr) alloys has been enhanced by the addition of Zn [107]. However, an excessive addition of Zn in Mg–Zn alloys has been detrimental to corrosion resistance in NaCl solution. So, the effect of Zn on the corrosion resistance depends on the composition as well as the situation of the Mg alloys, due to various and different amounts of Zn-containing phases formed in Mg alloys [103,118–120]. Zn is a biologically benign element, and Zn-containing Mg alloys are considered to be suitable candidates for biodegradable implants [7,121]. Zn is also a cofactor for enzymes in bone and cartilage and is effective for health and growth. It acts on taste, smell, DNA, RNA, and hormonal mediation [122]. However, the introduction of a large amount of Zn into the body will impair the immune function and lead to neurological disorders and eventually cell death [123]. Zn, as powder, has been added to Mg powder in the BAPM process to improve the foaming behavior and form a more homogenous pore distribution in Mg foams [71].

Mn is the third most abundant element used in combination with Mg for bioporous structures. Mn decreases the grain size of Mg alloys [96,124] and improves the tensile strength as well as the fatigue life of AZ61, AZ31, and AZ21 alloys [125,126]. The role of Mn in corrosion resistance of Mg alloys is similar to Zn. Mn transforms impurities into harmless intermetallic compounds and improves the corrosion resistance of Mg–Zn alloys; however, a high concentration of Mn declines the corrosion resistance of Mg alloys [117]. Biologically, Mn is essential for a healthy immune system and for different enzymes [127]. Mn is toxic when a high level of the element is exposed to the body. Therefore in order to utilize Mn effectively and reduce its drawbacks, it is often included in Al- and Zn-containing Mg alloys [128]. Accordingly, not only has no toxicity been reported by using Mg–Al–Mn alloys, but osseous callous formation on periosteal tissue has also been observed. The addition of Mn plus other alloying elements (such as rare earth elements (RRE), Ca, Al, and Zr) to Mg alloy slows the corrosion rate of pins in vivo [2]. Lietaert et al. [50] stated that because of the high mechanical properties before and after an immersion test, M2 Mg alloy foams with 2 wt% Mn are more appropriate for orthopedic applications than other Mg alloys containing Al, Zn, and Ca.

Ca, which is used in small amounts (0.3–0.5 wt%) in Mg, reduces oxidation in the casting processes, shows a significant grain-refining effect as well as grain-boundary strengthening and hardness increments in Mg alloys, and improves the formability of Mg sheets [13,14,96,129,130]. The higher yield strength of ZXM200 foam (with 0.2% Ca) than ZM20 foam (with 0.00124% Ca) with the same porosity (44%) confirms the effective improvement of Ca in the mechanical properties of Mg foams [51].

Ca is also added to Mg to modify corrosion resistance [131,132]. However, a high concentration of Ca results in the formation of a high-volume fraction of the Mg_2Ca phase, which causes deterioration of the corrosion resistance of the Mg alloy [12,130]. Wan et al. tested various amounts of Ca content in Mg–Ca alloys and reported that 0.6 wt% of Ca can enhance the compressive strength, modulus, and corrosion resistance of an Mg alloy [133]. From a biological perspective, Ca is the most abundant ingredient in the human body, especially in the skeleton as mineral HA [103]. Good cell adhesion on Mg–Ca and Mg–Zn–Ca has also improved the biocompatibility of Ca in Mg alloys [13]. The results of both in vivo and in vitro studies revealed that Mg-1Ca alloy is a promising biocompatible and biodegradable implant material [130]. Histological examination in rats, conducted by Park et al. [134], also confirmed good biocompatibility and a controllable absorption rate of Mg-35Zn-3Ca alloy in vivo. Using the MBA foam production method, 2 wt% Ca is added to pure Mg melt to raise the viscosity and reduce the surface tension of the melt. So the gas bubbles are entrapped and stabilized during the production process and form a more uniform cell structure [26,135]. Metal Ca and SiC particles are also added to AZ91 Mg alloy for melt thickening [34]. Ca compounds are also being used in Mg foam fabrication processes. Calcium carbonate is a better substitution for TiH_2 in the PM process due to safety issues as well as its ability to form a more homogenous and finer porous structure [70]. Moreover, the mismatch of decomposition temperature of TiH_2 and melting temperature of Mg alloys can be overcome [69].

Zr effectively improves the strength and grain refinement of Mg alloys, and it is suggested for Mg alloys, including Zn, RRE, and thorium, but not for Al- and Mn-containing Mg alloys [96,136]. Controlling the pore structure of AZ91 and AZ31 Mg alloys with the addition of Zr has also been investigated. Zr increased the porosity and pore size of such foams. The addition of Zr to AZ31 Mg foams enhanced the energy absorption as well as the hardness of the cellular structures when compared to AZ31 foams without Zr. However, increasing the Zr from 1 to 3 wt% leads to a decrease of energy absorption [28]. The noteworthy effect of Zr on Mg−Zr alloys is the oxide film that forms on such alloys after immersion in a borate buffer solution, which inhibits the corrosion of Mg−Zr alloys [137]. However, Zr addition results in a higher corrosion rate of Mg alloys in 0.1 M NaCl solution, compared to pure and Mn-containing samples, as investigated by Gandel et al. [136]. The biocompatibility of Zr as an alloying element in different Mg alloys, such as Mg−Zr [138,139], Mg−Zn−Zr, Mg−Y−RE−Zr [108], Mg−Zr−Sr [9], and Mg−Zr−Ca [140], has been approved. Low cytotoxicity of Zr^{4+} ions in murine fibroblasts and osteoblast cells have been reported by Yamamoto et al. [141]. The results of these trials suggest a very promising proof of concept, as Zr can be utilized as a biocompatible ingredient in Mg alloys. However, more investigations are still vital since its biocompatibility depends on the amount and the Zr ions formed and absorbed in the usage [103].

As mentioned above, reinforcements can also be added to an Mg foam matrix to improve its properties and allocate it for specific applications. The SHPM method can be considered as a promising route for composite foam production due to its potential for mixing different powders as well as reinforcements. For instance, Cu particles have been added to AZ91 Mg alloy foams to increase the damping capacity of foams [83]. A composite of porous Mg reinforced with alumina particles also exhibited a higher yield strength than bulk and porous pure Mg with the same pore size and porosity [84]. Reinforcements can be used easily via this method, but, importantly, they must be biocompatible in biomaterial applications. Trace elements such as Cu exist in the human body in low concentrations [103] and are utilized in biomaterials [142]. The amount of Cu in the human body is at a level of about 1−3 mg/kg and its daily intake is about 1 mg [143]. The role of Cu as a biological cofactor and in neurodegenerative diseases is crucial [144]. The toxicity class of micro-sized Cu particles is class 5, which is particularly nontoxic. However, nano and ionic Cu particles are moderately toxic (class 3) [145]. Alumina is a bioinert material that has excellent biocompatibility, corrosion, and wear resistance, making it suitable for load-bearing applications [146−148]. However, scrutiny is still vital since the biocompatibility of such materials is affected by particle size, morphology, and content as well as the matrix material [145].

As mentioned above, to date the majority of Mg alloys that have been used for porous structures are commercial Mg alloys designed for engineering, and they are not appropriate for use as biocompatible and biodegradable implant materials. The effects of elements combined with Mg to produce porous implant material should be considered from two perspectives: the effects on the porous structure of Mg and the consequences on the biocompatibility and biodegradability of Mg foams. The effects of some of the elements used as alloying ingredients or process facilitators in foam fabrication processes have not been assessed for use as biocompatible materials. For instance, in the MBA method, some process facilitators such as stabilizer, foaming agent, and dispersant should also be added to Mg melt [26,35] in addition to the alloying elements. This issue restricts the application of such processes in bio-Mg foam fabrication. Moreover, some materials have been investigated just in vitro, and they may behave differently in vivo. Thus scrutiny is still vital, and more research on the exact ingredient of Mg foams to approach a suitable porous structure with proper biocompatibility for implant usage is essential.

2.3.2 Effect of porosity

The porosity of biomaterial implants plays a crucial role in osteogenesis in vivo and in vitro. Lower porosity in vitro results in osteogenesis stimulation, whereas higher porosity in vivo yields more significant bone formation. So, more porosity is preferred in vivo for greater osteogenesis and bone ingrowth, but this propensity deteriorates mechanical properties and has an effect on the degradation rate of scaffolds. Thus it is essential to maintain a balance between the porosity and mechanical properties as well as the rate of bone remodeling and the degradation rate of the implant material [23,149]. In this section, the capability of different methods of Mg foam fabrication to produce a various range of porosities and effects on the biocompatibility of Mg foams will be discussed.

Porosity can be controlled by the fabrication method as well as process variables. Fig. 2.20 represents the range of porosities that can be produced by various methods of Mg foam fabrication. As reported by researchers, some methods, such as using a melt/blowing agent [150], melt infiltration [41], and space holder-based PM [1], are able to produce a wide range of porosities while others, such as melt/vacuum

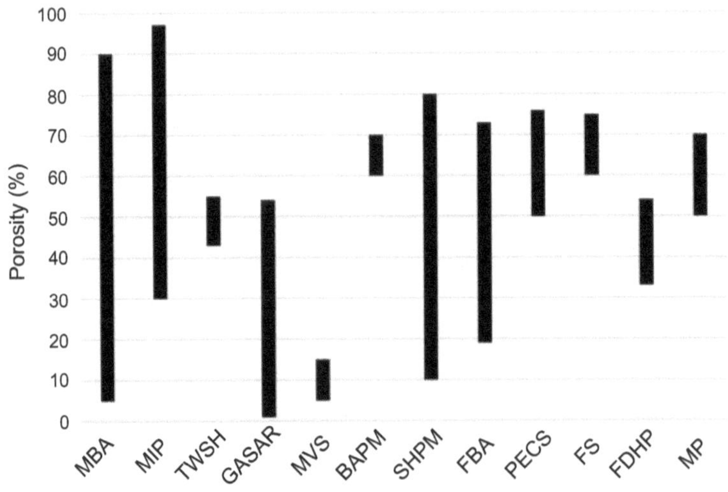

Figure 2.20 Range of porosities produced via different methods.

solidification [67], blowing agent-based PM [72], and pulse electric current [91] methods, have been tested for a limited range of porosities. Thus the method and characteristics of Mg foams can be selected based on the application and required specifications.

Porosity, which is a morphological property of the material, defined as the fraction of void space in a solid material [151], is beneficial for bone tissue formation. Pores allow the bone tissue to creep into the voids and facilitate the migration and proliferation of appropriate cells as well as the transport of nutrients [152,153]. Further, faster and deeper bone ingrowth has been reported for porous scaffolds as compared to solid implants [18,154–157]. Furthermore, the superior attachment of a porous structure to the surrounding bone tissue has received great attention because of the significant benefits of such structures as bone repair materials. The adhesion of tissues to the implanted material can be promoted by the growth of osteoblastic cells to the void space of the biomaterial [158]. Methods using a melt/blowing agent, melt infiltration, and PM-based processes, which are able to produce high porosities, are of great interest for bone ingrowth.

The degradation rate of biomaterials should also be considered as another crucial parameter when porosity is assessed. High porosity exposes a higher surface area to interact with the surrounding tissue, and it increases the oxidation and macrophage function that eventually accelerates the degradation of the implant. Moreover, high-porous implants, such as Mg biomaterials with a high degradation rate, are depleted before substitution by new bone, resulting in implantation failure [149,159]. Zhuang et al. [74] showed that there was a 50% increase of weight loss of Mg foams with a 20% increase of porosity. Aghion et al. [79] also expressed the corrosion resistance increment of Mg foams when porosity increases from 10% to 25%.

The number and connectivity of pores also have a remarkable effect on the yield strength, Young's modulus, and plateau stress of Mg foams [5,91]. Porosity can be beneficial not only through an increase of biological integrity but also advantageously by adjusting the mechanical properties of implanted material to match that of natural bone [2]. This valuable property of porous implants can reduce the stress shielding of bone as well as implant loosening [160]. For instance, in Mg foams fabricated through the SHPM method, when a porosity of 55% is added to a bulk structure, the compressive strength and the Young's modulus decrease from 100 to 15 MPa and 44 to 3.6 GPa, respectively [74], which is close to that of natural bone [93,161]. However, too much porosity will cause a decline in the mechanical properties and make it unsuitable for load-bearing applications. The mechanical properties of various Mg foams fabricated via different methods are presented in Table 2.5. For instance, Mg foams fabricated through melt infiltration in a preform by Yamada et al. [40] with a porosity of 97.3% and a pore size of 4.5 mm, which render a low compressive yield strength of 0.1 MPa, would be inappropriate for orthopedic applications. Such highly porous structures may serve as suitable platforms for drug delivery applications. More porosity can provide more interconnected open pores that can absorb and consequently release a larger quantity of drug. As reported by Aghion et al. [79], porosity plays an important role in controlling the amount and time of drug released from porous structures. The cell shape of Mg foams can also be influenced by porosity. The change of

Table 2.5 Porous characteristics and mechanical properties of various Mg and Mg alloy foams fabricated using different methods

Mg alloy	Cell type	Pore size	Porosity (%)	Density (g/cm^3)	Yield (MPa)	Strength (MPa)	Peak stress (MPa)	Elongation at peak stress (%)	Plateau stress (MPa)	Stress drop ratio (%)	Densification (%)	Hardness (HV)	Energy absorption (MJ/m^3) at densification strain of	References
Melt/blowing agent foaming														
AZ31	Closed	–	–		–		–	–				48.3	–	[28]
AZ31 + 1% Zr		0.43 mm	48.7				12.5	4	15		45	68.8	16.26 [78%]	
AZ31 + 2% Zr		0.71 mm	53.6				9	3	7.5		62	73.1	7.81	
AZ31 + 3% Zr		0.97 mm	72.9				5	4	5		80	81.8	4.37	
AZ91, AZ31	Closed	3–5 mm	60–79	–	–	–	–	–	–	–	–	–	–	[29]
Pure Mg	Closed	0.8–2 mm	53–71		8.69–27.11	Specific strength: 33–18 MPa/g cm^3	~8–28	5	8–24		65	–	4.24–53 [60%]	[30]
AZ31	Closed	0.38–1.52 mm	41–73				5–15	~5	5–16		52–76	37–66	4.5–15.5	[31]
AZ31	Closed	1.5 mm	55		18		17	9	21	26.5	52	51	9 [52]	[32]
AZ31 Homogenized heat treated	Closed	1.5 mm	55		19–28		17–27	8	18–32	3.5–17	54–58	60–80	10 [54]–19 [58]	[32]
AZ91	Closed	0.9–1.6 mm	60–90	0.2–0.8			1.75–2.6	1	1.1–2.3	26–56	65–70	–	–	[34]
Mg-12Al-3Ca	Closed	–	58–81	0.34–0.8	–	–	–	–	–	–	–	–	–	[35]
AZ91 Thixo-casted	Closed	–	8–39	–	–	–	–	–	–	–	–	–	–	[36]
AZ91 and AM60	Closed	<550 μm	5–71	Lowest relative density: 0.3–0.5	–	–	Same as UCS: 230–360	22–53	–	–	–	–	–	[38]

Melt infiltration in a preform														
AZ91	Open	3.8–5.7 mm	97	0.05	0.07–0.13	Relative stress: 9.2×10^{-4}	0.1–0.13	0.1–0.15	0.11	–	56	–	–	[41,46,162]
AZ91 As cast at dynamic strain rate	Open	3.8–5.7 mm	97	0.05	–	–	50–62*	3–6	36–41*	–	35	60–70	–	[43,44]
At quasi-static strain rate					–	–	15–25*	6–14	19–25* 0.11†	–	55		–	
T4 Heat treated at dynamic strain rate					–	–	10–25*	2–5	9–19*	–	40	–	–	
At quasi-static strain rate					–	–	5–14*	2–4	9–11*	–	60	–	–	
T6 Heat treated at dynamic strain rate					–	–	11–40*	2.5–4.5	10–20*	–	35–42	62–118	–	
At quasi-static strain rate					–	–	13–20*	2–4	12–20* 0.12†	–	60		–	
Pure Mg	Open	1 mm	41	–	–	UCS: 13	–	–	–	–	–	–		[47]
AZ63, ZM21, M2, and MZX211	Open	500 μm	75	–	0.6–3.3	Elastic modulus: 0.6–0.8 GPa	–	–	0.6–3.3	–	–	–	–	[50]
AZ91E, WE43, ZM20, ZWM200, ZXM200	Open	–	30–69	–	2.31–12.15	–	2.5–10	1–6	6–8	–	4–35	–	–	[51]
Pure Mg	Open	Av. 242 μm	50,60,70	–		Compressive strength: 7–30 Elastic modulus: 0.23–0.49 GPa	7–34	5–13	8–37	–	39–64	–	–	[52]
Pure Mg	Open	0.8–2.1 mm	35–80			–	–	–	–	–	–	–	–	[53,55]

Continued

Table 2.5 Continued

Mg alloy	Cell type	Pore size	Porosity (%)	Density (g/cm^3)	Yield (MPa)	Strength (MPa)	Peak stress (MPa)	Elongation at peak stress (%)	Plateau stress (MPa)	Stress drop ratio (%)	Densi-fication (%)	Hardness (HV)	Energy absorption (MJ/m^3) at densification strain of	References
Titanium wire space holder														
Pure Mg	Open	270 μm	43.5–54.2	–	4.3–6.2	Young's modulus: 0.5–1 GPa	–	–	–	–	–	–	–	[56]
Melt/gas eutectic solidification foaming														
Pure Mg	Closed	170 μm	28	–	23.9 ± 4.9	–	–	–	–	–	–	–	–	[21]
AZ31B and AZ91D	Closed	–	<53	–	–	–	–	–	–	–	–	–	–	[62]
Pure Mg	Closed	–	2.5–54	0.797–1.696	–	–	–	–	–	–	–	–	–	[63]
Pure Mg	Closed	Diameter: 550–1300 μm	5–40	–	–	–	–	–	–	–	–	–	–	[64,65]
Pure Mg	Closed	1100 μm	1–44	–	65–130	–	60–83	11–17	10–40	–	58–68	–	–	[66]
Melt/vacuum solidification foaming														
AZ91, AZ181	Closed	4–10 mm	5–15	0.4	–	–	7	5	7	–	25	–	–	[67]
Blowing agent-based powder metallurgy														
Pure Mg, MgZn3, MgZn6, MgSn3, MgZn3Sn1.5, MgZn3Sn3, MgZn3Si3, MgZn3SiC5	Closed	0.1–4 mm	–	0.5	–	–	8	7	9	–	52	–	Energy: 9 J	[71]
Reinforced Mg foam				0.55–0.62			10	6	7	–	45	–	Energy: 105–131	
Pure Mg and Mg–Al alloy	Closed	<5 mm	60–70	Relative density: 98.6–99.4%	–	–	–	–	–	–	–	–	–	[72]

Space holder-based powder metallurgy														
Pure Mg	Open	200–500 μm	50	0.87		Young's modulus: 0.35 GPa	7	3.5	2.33	–	50	–	–	[1]
Pure Mg	Open	73–412 μm	35–55	–	–	Young's modulus: 0.75–1.8	11–17.5	2	1–4	–	55–71	–	–	[5,73]
Pure Mg	Open	200–400 μm	36–55	–	–	Compressive strength: 15–100 Young's modulus: 3.6–44 GPa	–	–	–	–	–	–	–	[74]
Pure Mg	Open	0.5–2 mm	40–80	Relative density: >0.55	1–20	–	2.45–3.4	2.5	2.5–3.5	–	60–65	–	–	[75]
AZ91	Open	0.75–1.75 mm	40–80	Relative density: 0.1–0.5	Relative yield: 0.025–0.15	–	2–18	2–4	1–13	–	60–75	–	Damping capacity: 0.0025–0.0325	[77,78]
MgNdZrSi FeCuNi alloy	Closed	40–140 μm	10–25	–		–	–	–	–	–	–	–	–	[79]
Pure Mg	Open	250–500 μm	24–31	–	13–53	Ultimate flexural strength: 3–15, UCS: 20–70	20–70	5–17	25–52	–	50	17–27	–	[80]
Pure Mg	Open	–	11–44	–	–	Ultimate flexural strength: 1.8–38	–	–	–	–	–	–	–	[82]
Pure Mg	Open	–	12–38	–	–	Ultimate flexural strength: 4.4–38	–	–	–	–	–	–	–	[81]
Pure Mg	Open	25–100 μm	10–38	1.08–1.57	43–112	Young's modulus: 3–4.9 GPa	25–140	7	25	–	50	–	–	[84]
Mg–Zn	Open	100–400 μm	21–36	–	–	Compressive strength: 10–60 Young's modulus: 1.5–7.4 GPa	–	–	–	–	–	–	–	[85]
AZ31, AZ91, ZA146	Closed	–	46–60	–	–	–	–	–	–	–	–	–	–	[87]

Continued

Table 2.5 Continued

Mg alloy	Cell type	Pore size	Porosity (%)	Density (g/cm³)	Yield (MPa)	Strength (MPa)	Peak stress (MPa)	Elongation at peak stress (%)	Plateau stress (MPa)	Stress drop ratio (%)	Densi-fication (%)	Hardness (HV)	Energy absorption (MJ/m³) at densification strain of	References
AZ31	Closed	–	10–77	0.41	–	–	–	–	–	–	–	–	–	[88]
Forming and blowing agent-based process														
AZ91D	Closed	<5 mm	19–73	–	–	–	–	–	–	–	–	–	–	[89]
Pulse electric current sintering process														
AZ91D, AZ31, AM60B	Open	–	50–76	0.46–0.91	–	–	–	–	1.3–37	–	–	–	–	[90,91]
Fiber sintering process														
WZ21	Open	–	60–75	–	–	Compressive strength: 8.5–14 MPa Stiffness: 1.7 GPa	–	–	–	–	–	–	–	[92]
MgY4	Open					compressive strength: 15–22 MPa Stiffness: 2.8 GPa								[92]
Fiber deposition hot pressing technology														
Pure Mg ribbon	Open	110–300 μm	33–54	–	–	Compressive strength: 7.8–30.3 MPa Young's modulus: 0.1–0.67 GPa	8–15	5	1–2.5	–	40–45	–	–	[93]
Mechanical perforation technique														
Pure Mg	Open	300–400 μm	50–70	–	–	Compressive strength: 11.75–18.2	–	–	34–56	–	–	–	–	[94]

∗ (Nominal Stress)/(Relative Density)$^{\frac{3}{2}}$(MPa)

† Nominal Stress (MPa)

spherical cells of AZ91 Mg alloy foams to polyhedron cells in porosities larger than 70% has been reported by Xu et al. [34].

2.3.3 Effect of pore size

Pore size is another crucial alternative affecting the properties of Mg foams, especially for biomaterial applications. This characteristic can also be controlled by the fabrication method and process variables. As can be seen in Fig. 2.21, just the melt/vacuum solidification foaming process [67] has been exposed to produce large sizes of pores, ranging from 4–10 mm. So far, the pore sizes that have been produced via other methods range from a few microns [79] to a few millimeters (<5 mm) [41].

Materials used as an implant should mimic organ morphology, function, and structure in order to optimize integration into the surrounding tissue. For instance, the properties of scaffolds that are utilized as bone implant should be suitable for bone remodeling, and materials implanted in soft tissues should imitate the surrounding soft tissues [163,164]. Bone, composed of HA ($Ca_{10}(PO_4)_6(OH)_2$) crystals, is formed from a trabecular core with cortical bone surrounding it. Trabecular bone has a porous structure with a porosity of 50–90% and a pore size of 1 mm, and cortical bone has an almost solid structure with a haversian canal with an approximate diameter of 100–200 μm and 3–12% porosity [161,165].

In a study conducted by Hulbert et al. [166], significant bone deposits were observed in large pores with a pore range of 100–200 μm, while only fibrous and soft tissues penetrated in the smaller pore range of 10–75 μm, and no mineralized tissues were detected. Pore sizes of 25 and 200 μm porous Ti implants, cultured by human fetal osteoblastic cells, represented better results in vitro, and no toxicity was observed in comparison to pore sizes of 50, 300, 400, and 500 μm [167].

On the other hand, bone ingrowth has been observed in all pore sizes of Ti plates implanted in rabbit femurs under non-load-bearing conditions. Based on research

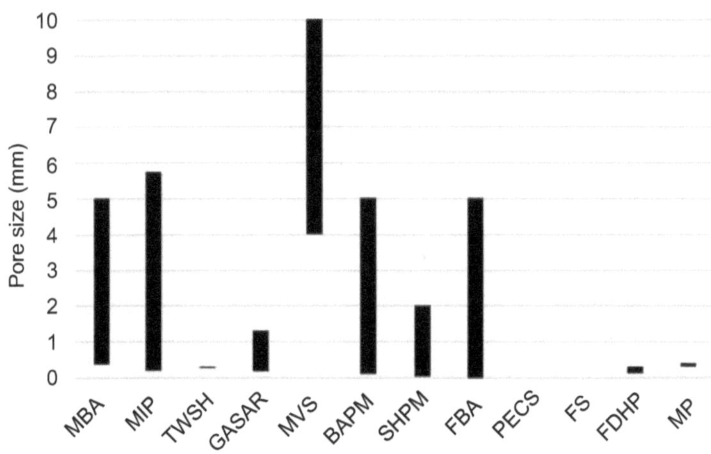

Figure 2.21 Range of pore sizes produced via different methods.

in vivo and in vitro on various biomaterials, in some cases pore size affected the cell migration rate and extent. However, in other cases no significant or statistical difference could be found in the bone formation and cell penetration depth for different pore sizes [149,166]. Thus the effect of pore size can be considered as dependent on the biomaterial, application and its condition, substituted organ, and proliferated cell type. Nevertheless, generally the minimum pore size required for new bone to be deposited in porous implants has been reported as ~100 μm to facilitate vascularization as well as nutrition, which assist direct osteogenesis [17,168,169].

In this regard, almost all of the Mg foam fabrication methods are capable of producing Mg foam with an appropriate pore size for bone implants. In the MBA methods, various parameters such as melt temperature, foaming time and temperature, and stirring time and velocity influence the pore size and porosity of fabricated foams. For instance, longer stirring and foaming times lead to more porosity. However, holding the Mg melt in the stirring and foaming steps for more than the short required periods (just 5 and 4 min, respectively) leads to some defects in the foam structure [26,27,35,170]. Moreover, blowing agent material also influences the size of pores. Some blowing agent materials, such as TiH_2, produce extremely coarse pore structures, while others, such as $CaCO_3$, can form small pore structures. $CaCO_3$ powder reacts with Mg melt involving CO gas as the blowing agent, which is released at a temperature lower than the decomposition temperature of $CaCO_3$. Thus a low foaming temperature of melted Mg leads to a fine pore structure. On the other hand, the high foaming temperature of other blowing agents results in a high Mg melt-blowing agent reaction rate and consequently a high gas releasing rate, which enlarges the bubbles more quickly in the melt and forms coarse pores [26,135].

The control of pore size in some other methods such as the melt infiltration in a preform (MIP), SHPM, and FDHP processes is easier. The pore size can be changed by manipulating the preform pore size and space holder particle size in the MIP and SHPM processes, respectively [5,40,57]. The thickness of the fibers and the spacing between fibers, as well as pressing temperature and pressure, can control the size of pores in the FDHP process [93]. A narrow range of pore sizes can be obtained via some methods, such as SHPM and the melt-gas eutectic solidification process (GASAR). Gradients in pore sizes and porosity are attractive and are recommended for the reproduction of multiple tissues [149]. Foams with various ranges of pore size, such as Mg foams fabricated via the MIP and melt vacuum solidification foaming (MVS) processes, can promote direct osteogenesis and osteoid tissue (correlating to large pore sizes) as well as fibrous and soft tissues (correlating to small pores) [41,67,149]. Fabrication of two-layer-structured Mg foams, having an inner compact structure and porous structure on the outer surface, via the SHPM process, is of interest to biomedicine. The interconnected pores of the outer porous surface present better biocompatibility and allow more bone ingrowth and integration. The interior structure, reinforced with salt particles, can induce and boost the mechanical compatibility of Mg scaffolds [86]. However, the influence and cytotoxicity of the salt reinforcements should be evaluated. An increase in pore size influences the mechanical properties of Mg foams as well. Xu et al. [34] demonstrated that instability in compressive deformation for bigger cell sizes (>1 mm) was more than for smaller cells in AZ91 foams, which can be related to inhomogeneity of density in larger cell sizes.

2.3.4 Effect of pore type

A major classification of porous metals is between open cells and closed cells, which in terms of biomaterial is considerable. In closed-cell foams, an individual cell is isolated from other cells by a thin wall of metal. In open-cell foams, cells are joined together, which results in a structure of interconnected voids [24,25,171].

Closed-cell Mg foams are usually fabricated via random foaming processes in which Mg melt or powder is foamed using a gas and solidified or cooled down, respectively [69]. Gas-containing voids are created with an injection of gas (GASAR process) [59], and decomposition of a blowing agent in melt [26] or powder [71]. In addition to the gas or blowing agent, nonmetallic particles such as ceramics are also employed as a stabilizer to avoid the rupture and merging of gas bubbles [69]. Moreover, since fabrication of closed-cell foams is based on random practices, remarkable variations in porosity and pore size, as well as pore shape and location, can often be observed [160,172]. It is therefore hard to control such processes and obtain specific structures. In addition to closed cells, some methods such as thixocasting (IFM) form a solid skin (0.5−1 mm thickness) on the outer surface of foam. Although this process is a low-cost manufacturing route in which foams can be formed with an adequate surface quality where such a solid layer increases the mechanical properties of Mg foams, it hinders the bone ingrowth and vascularization [36,37].

Open-cell Mg foams are of particular importance in biomaterials, due to their penetration capability. Nutrients as well as vasculature and tissues can infiltrate interconnected pores, which consequently establish an interlocked composite of metal foam and live tissues [23,173,174].

Therefore those methods in which open-cell porosities are created in an Mg matrix, such as MIP, SHPM, FS, and MP techniques, are more suitable and applicable for biomaterials. Although such processes can produce open-cell Mg foams, the control of pore size and shape in some methods such as FS is not completely feasible [92]. Thus in cases with specific porosity, pore size, and pore shape, the MIP, SHPM, and MP methods are more practical. Moreover, to take advantage of the open-cell foams and easy production features of the die-casting process, negative salt-patter molding [22] can also be employed.

2.3.5 Effect of pore shape (pore morphology)

Geometrical and morphological characteristics of pores, in addition to the pore type, mechanical properties, and biocompatibility of Mg foam implants, are also among the critically important parameters of foam materials that must be considered in scaffold fabrication. Geometry and shape change of the pores as well as those of the whole scaffold may influence the flow of body fluids, gases, nutrients, and blood vessels as well as the removal of metabolites through the scaffold [168,175−179]. Moreover, various pore shapes result in different mechanical properties [171,180,181].

For instance, stainless-steel foams with irregularly shaped pores showed less compressive strength and elastic modulus than the same foams with spherical pores [182]. This has been reported for Mg as well as Ti, Al, and polymeric foams [56,183–185]. Van Bael et al. [186] reported that pore occlusion in obtuse-angled pores, such as honeycomb pores, is higher than acute-angled pores, such as triangular pores. They mentioned that human osteoblasts can bridge the corners of a pore. Thus more pore areas can be bridged on hexagonal pores due to a higher number of corners on such pores, in comparison to triangular and rectangular pores. Moreover, they stated that the size of irregularly shaped pores should be less than 200 μm to be bridged by cells. So, if the larger pores were utilized in foams, cells can spread only on the surface of struts. Their experiments showed that in triangular pores, with small sizes and sharp angles, cells attach to several struts, thus making such pores useful for cell proliferation as well as differentiation. Chu et al. [187] showed that the orthogonal-shaped channel of HA scaffolds, implanted in Yucatan mini pigs, resulted in a porous matrix of HA and new bone, while the radial architecture formed a solid bone at the center of the scaffold. In other words, newly formed bone mimics the architecture of the voids of the implant. Jin et al. [188] attributed the occurrence of osteochondral ossification, as the initial phase, in honeycomb-shaped HA to low oxygen conditions in such pore shapes, while in porous block implants, boosted vascularization resulted in direct bone formation.

According to the effects mentioned above, namely pore shape on vascularization and osteogenesis, it would appear to be crucial to fabricate porous structures with predicted pore shapes. Thus it would be possible to control the architecture of newly formed bone as well as the type and quantity of cells generated on the implant. In this regard, some Mg foam processes are advisable, such as MIP- and SHPM-based methods. In the MIP process, the desired architecture of the implant can be made using a preform (initial preform) that is filled with plaster or salt (second preform). After removal of the preform and pouring the porous plaster (or salt) with molten Mg, which is followed by solidification, the required architecture of preform is replicated in the solidified Mg. Therefore an Mg implant with the required pores and channels will be fabricated. Moreover, the mechanical properties of such implants in predetermined directions are also controllable, which is suitable for specified load-bearing applications. As Yamada et al. [45] presented, the collapse stress of AZ91 Mg alloy foam with a controlled-cell structure is 4 times higher than that of random-cell-structured foam. However, the mechanical properties of the former foams are more anisotropic than the latter, which results in more fluctuation of flow stress in the plateau region. Researchers reported a higher compressive strength for periodic pure Mg foams than for random porous pure Mg foams with the same pore size and porosity [5,47].

The size and surface quality of pores also depend on the properties of the template and plaster (or salt) as well as infiltration conditions, which are all controllable [45,47]. Such specifications, as well as the open pore producibility of implants via this process, are heavily desired by the biomedical industry. However, some issues, such as limited infiltration pressures of plaster (or salt) in the preform, molten Mg in the plaster, and poor wetting between Mg and the template at lower temperatures restrict the process. Moreover, the corrosive effect of the removal of plaster or salt from the solidified Mg matrix and limited available materials as an initial and second preform to be inert against the second preform and molten Mg, respectively, confine this process, and further research is required. It should be mentioned that NaCl or plaster residue is the main restriction in this process. Although minor NaCl residue on the surface of the cells in Mg foams fabricated by Staiger et al. [55] is biologically safe, overmuch residue of NaCl, or even a small amount of plaster residue, is not biologically allowed. Thus the size of MIP-fabricated porous implants, which implies an amount of consumed NaCl as preform, is restricted.

SHPM can also be considered as an alternative for the fabrication of controllable porous architectures. In this process, space holder material can be selected and mixed with Mg powder. Subsequent heating and sintering steps remove space holders and join Mg particles, respectively. Thus the size of the space holder material determines the dimension of the created pores and the shape the spacers form in the architecture of voids in the Mg matrix. A wide range of particle sizes has been used for Mg foams [1,5] but only with spherical and irregular shapes of space holder materials. An increase of pore size results in a decrease of Young's modulus and peak stress of Mg foams [5]. The shape of the pores also influences the mechanical properties of porous Mg [181]. Mg foams fabricated with spherical particles using infiltration technology are not brittle, unlike other Mg foams produced using the PM method, and show a typical elastic–plastic deformation characteristic. Wang et al. [57] attributed this to the superior metallurgical bonding obtained from Mg infiltration in spherical particles as well as the cell edge bending of pores during the deformation procedure.

The cost and convenience of this approach have shown this method to be promising for competent Mg foam production. However, this process is more limited than MIP for topologically ordered purposes. The main restriction of the space holder process is the lack of control regarding the distribution of pores in the Mg matrix. Since the spacer particles are thoroughly mixed with Mg powder, and the regular sorting and fixing of particles is impossible, the fabrication of well-distributed, topologically ordered structures is not feasible.

A mechanical perforation technique is also capable of establishing a controllable porous structure. This technique provides reliable process controls and repeatability as well as an excellent surface finish. Thus not only is it possible to obtain more accurate pore sizes and porosities, but also precision can be continued for all the pores throughout the whole scaffold. However, this technique is more restricted than the two previously mentioned methods, since the shape of the pores that can be fabricated is more limited, and the equipment is more costly. The design of intricate architecture and pores with complex shapes such as blind profiles and draft angles are also impossible.

The TWSH method is also capable of replicating porous structures, according to Jiang and He [56]. The porous structure of fabricated Mg foams reflects the shape and size of Ti wires and is thoroughly interconnected, which is favorable for the fabrication of refracted structures for implant applications. However, long and curved pipe-like pores and MgF_2 film on the inner surface of pores may restrict the application of this method in biomaterials. As stated by Jin et al. [188], curved and longer pores in HA porous blocks delay penetration of mesenchymal cells, as well as vascularization, which causes the bone to form only on the outer surface of the porous blocks. On the other hand, in HA porous particles, bone is formed deeply in the particles. Thus the effect of curved and relatively long pores in TWSH-fabricated porous Mg in vivo and in vitro is crucial. Moreover, the biocompatibility of the MgF_2 layer on the Mg surface requires serious attention. It should also be mentioned that the increase of porosity, as well as the size of porous implants, need a greater structure of Ti wire as the space holder. The more Ti wire consumed, the longer the required immersion time in HF solution, which results in a greater and thicker MgF_2 layer on the Mg surface.

Other Mg foam production methods, in which a blowing agent produces gas inside the Mg melt or powder, generate pores with random shapes and sizes. Although the pore size of such Mg foams can be governed by fabrication parameters such as the blowing agent material and the amount and the temperature at which the gas is released, the control of the pore size and its shape are more feasible and precise using the MIP, SHPM, and MP methods.

2.4 Challenges and directions of future research

Although it is feasible to fabricate Mg foams using different methods with various properties and specifications, not all of the foams are suitable and applicable specifically for biomedical applications. Some methods are inefficient, while others are sensitive to working parameters. Some routes are not capable of producing foams with desirable medical properties, and others produce foams that do not qualify mechanically or have some residuals that limit their medical applications.

Novel technological advances have led to increased accessibility to production processes, and consequently a wide range of porous Mg and Mg alloys can be developed. Open- and closed-cell structures of Mg/Mg alloy foams with various physical and mechanical properties can be achieved, which establishes them for a wide range of applications. Such applications, which include biomedical implants, as well as current production processes, are being investigated regarding higher quality, further reliability, and better reproducibility as well as the predictability of properties.

"Higher quality and reliability" for the biomedical application of porous Mg-based materials refers to the homogeneity of morphology and structure, the proximity of mechanical properties to that of surrounding living tissues, and the suitability of surface morphology. Biocompatibility and appropriate biodegradability, which consist of biocompatibility of residual products and excreted compounds as well as an appropriate degradability rate, also influence the mechanical and cell proliferation properties of Mg foams and should be considered charily. Moreover, cost reduction, which can be achieved by utilizing cheaper materials, reducing scraps, and omitting some manufacturing steps, is a crucial issue that needs to be considered. However, it should be noted that all these proceedings must be compatible with biostrategies and bioproperties of produced cellular Mg materials.

According to the discussion above, by using the MBA, GASAR, MVS, BAPM, and FBA processes, various porosities and pore sizes can be achieved. However, pores are closed, and some gases or blowing agent residues remain inside the porous structure, which is not biocompatible. The Mg melt that is used in melt foaming methods is prone to ignition, so special protective gases like CO_2, SF6, and Ar are needed to prevent oxidation. Furthermore, some processes, such as stabilizing, foaming, and dispersing, are employed in such methods. Thus they are very sensitive to working parameters such as melt temperature, foaming time and temperature, and stirring time and velocity. This causes the foam procedure to be too complicated and susceptible. The increase in temperature in both the foaming and stirring steps influences the porosity, pore size, and pore structure and therefore promotes oxidation of Mg material as well. In GASAR processed- and vacuum solidified-Mg foams, residual materials such as H_2 gas and oxides, respectively, are limiting factors for medical applications. Moreover, it is difficult to control the pore properties. The pressure of hydrogen or the amount of oxide precursors can be increased to increase the porosity, but tiny cracks due to gas pressure have been detected near the pores in transmission electron microscopy (TEM) observations by Park et al. [189]. Although reasonable degradation and cytotoxicity tests of lotus-type Mg foams with a pore size and porosity of 170 μm and 28%, respectively, were obtained in SBF [21], more studies are needed to consider their biological and mechanical properties with regard to their various pore sizes and porosities and even in vivo tests. The MVS (VFT) process is a cost-effective technique for pore sizes larger than 4–5 mm. However, control of the process for small pore sizes is difficult.

Other methods such as MIP, SHPM, and MP processes are more reliable for biomedical applications due to the open cellular structures that can be achieved using these methods. Moreover, such processes are more controllable and adjustable than former methods. These processes will allow superior control over parameters and features of porous structures, such as pore geometry, shape, size, and distribution. It is possible to imitate the structure of the preform with minor errors using the MIP method. The SHPM, FS, and MIP processes are more efficient and easier in operation than the MP process. In PM methods, the equipment that is used for working with Mg powders, such as ball milling, mixing, pressing, and extrusion, are more economical because of operating in lower temperatures. Flexibility in alloy choice and the ability to add various additives, even ceramics and fibers, to produce porous composite structures is another advantage of this method. In the SHPM process, pore size and distribution can be controlled by manipulating the shape and size of the space holder material as well as by changing the process parameters, such as compacting pressure, sintering temperature, and time. The SHPM and MIP methods are suitable for producing complex architectures where other manufacturing processes are too costly and time-consuming.

Fabrication of a controlled-cell structure with a required cell wall thickness, porosities of more than 90%, and desirable mechanical properties is feasible by using a periodic-architecture preform via the MIP route. However, there are still some problems. For instance, SHPM-processed foams with low porosities have more residue in the matrix. From a biological perspective, residual material generated from the space holder or by removing the polymer is inappropriate. Mg powders are explosive hazards and have to be protected under an Ar atmosphere to prevent oxidation. PM methods have a lower risk than melt foaming methods due to working in a solid state. In other words, the ability to work in the solid state, which is crucial for active molten metals such as Mg, would be one of the most important and beneficial aspects of PM methods.

Little information is available regarding the MIP method, and so far few materials such as polyurethane, epoxy foam and RP polymer as preform, and NaCl as spacer have been used with pure Mg and AZ91 Mg alloy. Although other water-based solutions, such as NaOH and NaF, have been used to wash and remove the NaCl, the corrosive effect of water, which is commonly used as a solvent in these solutions, should be considered. The investigation of other solutions with lower corrosive effects seems to be effective. The limited size of fabricated Mg foams is the main restriction of the MIP process, and this is related to limited penetration of Mg melt in the preform. Infiltration of molten Mg into an NaCl preform under vacuum, or by using an inert gas or a low-pressure die-casting system, has been carried out to overcome this issue. However, there is an optimum infiltration pressure for both steps. The melt cannot infiltrate the pores of either the polymer or the NaCl preform at a low pressure. High pressure also results in some dimensional changes in the preforms. Therefore optimum tolerances should be considered, which means limited pore sizes and porosities are achievable. Moreover, the infiltration pressure of molten Mg increases the surface roughness of the Mg foam, which consequently influences the maturation of the osteoblast cells. Furthermore, the SHPM and MIP methods are not environmentally clean because of the space holder or polymer removal stage.

From a mechanical properties point of view, the highest Young's modulus and compression strength reported for pure Mg foam fabricated via the SHPM method, with the highest porosity of 55% (pore size: 200–400 μm), are stated as 3.6 GPa and 15 MPa, respectively [74]. Other researchers also have reported on the mechanical properties of pure Mg and Mg-alloy foams, but since these properties depend on several parameters, such as the size and shape of pores, porosity, the shape and size of the initial Mg powder, the compacting method, and the pressure and sintering parameters, the exact comparison of these data is not feasible.

In conclusion, Mg foams are promising new biomaterials that can be used as implant materials, particularly for load-bearing applications. Although significant advancement has been achieved in the fabrication and application of such porous materials, still further research is necessary to determine the relationships between the structural characteristics and the mechanical properties, the in vitro and in vivo biocompatibility, and the biodegradability of porous Mg biomaterials.

References

[1] Wen C, Mabuchi M, Yamada Y, Shimojima K, Chino Y, Asahina T. Processing of biocompatible porous Ti and Mg. Scr Mater 2001;45:1147–53.

[2] Staiger MP, Pietak AM, Huadmai J, Dias G. Magnesium and its alloys as orthopedic biomaterials: a review. Biomaterials 2006;27:1728–34.

[3] Song G, Song S. A possible biodegradable magnesium implant material. Adv Eng Mater 2007;9:298–302.
[4] Brar HS, Platt MO, Sarntinoranont M, Martin PI, Manuel MV. Magnesium as a biodegradable and bioabsorbable material for medical implants. JOM 2009;61:31–4.
[5] Wen C, Yamada Y, Shimojima K, Chino Y, Hosokawa H, Mabuchi M. Compressibility of porous magnesium foam: dependency on porosity and pore size. Mater Lett 2004;58:357.
[6] Witte F, Hort N, Vogt C, Cohen S, Kainer KU, Willumeit R, et al. Degradable biomaterials based on magnesium corrosion. Curr Opin Solid State Mater Sci 2008;12: 63–72.
[7] Zhou Y, Li Y, Luo D-M, Wen C, Hodgson P. Microstructures, mechanical properties and in vitro corrosion behaviour of biodegradable Mg–Zr–Ca alloys. J Mater Sci 2013;48: 1632–9.
[8] Geng F, Tan L, He Y, Yang J, Zhang B, Yang K. Preparation and cytocompatibility of bioactive β-TCP coatings on porous magnesium scaffold surface. Rare Metal Mater Eng 2009;38:318–22.
[9] Li Y, Wen C, Mushahary D, Sravanthi R, Harishankar N, Pande G, et al. Mg-Zr-Sr alloys as biodegradable implant materials. Acta Biomater 2012;8:3177–88.
[10] Gu X-N, Zheng Y-F. A review on magnesium alloys as biodegradable materials. Front Mater Sci China 2010;4:111–5.
[11] Zhou YL, Luo DM, Hu WY, Li Y, Hodgson P, Wen C. Compressive properties of hot-rolled Mg-Zr-Ca alloys for biomedical applications. Adv Mater Res 2011:56–9.
[12] Li Y, Hodgson P, Wen C. The effects of calcium and yttrium additions on the microstructure, mechanical properties and biocompatibility of biodegradable magnesium alloys. J Mater Sci 2011;46:365–71.
[13] Xin Y, Hu T, Chu PK. In vitro studies of biomedical magnesium alloys in a simulated physiological environment: a review. Acta Biomater 2011;7:1452–9.
[14] Li Y, Li M, Hu W, Hodgson P, Wen C. Biodegradable Mg-Ca and Mg-Ca-Y alloys for regenerative medicine. In: 7th Pacific Rim International Conference on advanced materials and processing, PRICM-7. Cairns, QLD, Australia: Materials Science Forum; 2010. p. 2192–5.
[15] Song Y, Shan D, Chen R, Zhang F, Han E-H. Biodegradable behaviors of AZ31 magnesium alloy in simulated body fluid. Mater Sci Eng C 2009;29:1039–45.
[16] Lewandrowski KU, Gresser JD, Bondre SP, Silva AE, Wise DL, Trantolo DJ. Developing porosity of poly(propylene glycol-co-fumaric acid) bone graft substitutes and the effect on osteointegration: a preliminary histology study in rats. J Biomater Sci Polym Ed 2000; 11:879–89.
[17] Yeung HY, Qin L, Lee KM, Leung KS, Cheng JCY. Quantification of porosity, connectivity and material density of calcium phosphate ceramic implants using microcomputed tomography. In: Advanced bioimaging technologies in assessment of the quality of bone and scaffold materials: techniques and applications; 2007. p. 289–305.
[18] Luyten J, Thijs I, Ravelingien M, Mullens S. Bone engineering with porous ceramics and metals. Adv Eng Mater 2011;13:1002–7.
[19] Henriques VAR, Galvani ET, Cairo CAA, Taddei EB. Ti-13Nb-13Zr foams for surgical implants. In: 6th International Latin American Conference on powder technology, PTECH 2007. Buzios - Rio de Janeiro, Brazil: Materials Science Forum; 2008. p. 24–9.
[20] Freyman TM, Yannas IV, Gibson LJ. Cellular materials as porous scaffolds for tissue engineering. Prog Mater Sci 2001;46:273–82.

[21] Gu XN, Zhou WR, Zheng YF, Liu Y, Li YX. Degradation and cytotoxicity of lotus-type porous pure magnesium as potential tissue engineering scaffold material. Mater Lett 2010;64:1871−4.
[22] Witte F, Ulrich H, Rudert M, Willbold E. Biodegradable magnesium scaffolds: part I: appropriate inflammatory response. J Biomed Mater Res A 2007;81:748−56.
[23] Guden M, Celik E, Cetiner S, Aydin A. Metals foams for biomedical applications: processing and mechanical properties. Adv Exp Med Biol 2004:257−66.
[24] Banhart J. Manufacture, characterisation and application of cellular metals and metal foams. Prog Mater Sci 2001;46:559−632.
[25] Banhart J. Manufacturing routes for metallic foams. JOM 2000;52:22−7.
[26] Yang D-H, Hur B-Y, Yang S-R. Study on fabrication and foaming mechanism of Mg foam using $CaCO_3$ as blowing agent. J Alloys Compounds 2008;461:221−7.
[27] Yang D, Seo C, Hur BY. Mg alloy foam fabrication via melt foaming method. J Mater Sci Technol 2008;24:302−4.
[28] Hur BY, Zhao R. Correlation between zirconium addition and compressive properties of AZ31 Mg alloy foams. In: 2nd International Conference on frontiers of manufacturing and design science, ICFMD 2011. Taichung, Taiwan; 2012. p. 75−9.
[29] Seo CH, Seong HG, Song YH, Hur BY. Compressive properties of AZ91 and AZ31 Mg alloy foams at different foaming conditions. In: 68th World Foundry Congress 2008. WFC; 2008. p. 415−7.
[30] Yang D-H, Shang-Run Y, Hui W, Ai-Bin M, Jing-Hua J, Jian-Qing C, et al. Compressive properties of cellular Mg foams fabricated by melt-foaming method. Mater Sci Eng A 2010;527:5405−9.
[31] Zhao R, Li Y, Jeong SR, Yue X, Hur BY. Fabrication, microstructure and compression properties of AZ31 Mg foams. Korean J Mater Res 2011;21:314−9.
[32] Xia X, Zhao W, Feng X, Feng H, Zhang X. Effect of homogenizing heat treatment on the compressive properties of closed-cell Mg alloy foams. Mater Design 2013;49:19−24.
[33] Xia X, Zhao W, Wei Z, Wang Z. Effects of specimen aspect ratio on the compressive properties of Mg alloy foam. Mater Design 2012;42:32−6.
[34] Xu ZG, Fu JW, Luo TJ, Yang YS. Effects of cell size on quasi-static compressive properties of Mg alloy foams. Mater Design 2012;34:40−4.
[35] Luo H, Zhang L, Xu Z, Yang Y. Effect of technological parameters on preparation of Mg-based foam materials. Mater Sci Forum 2013:356−60.
[36] Solórzano E, Hirschmann M, Rodriguez-Perez MA, Körner C, de Saja JA. Thermal conductivity of AZ91 magnesium integral foams measured by the Transient Plane Source method. Mater Lett 2008;62:3960−2.
[37] Hirschmann M, Körner C, Singer RF. Integral foam molding a new process for foamed magnesium castings. Mater Sci Forum 2007:1827−32.
[38] Körner C, Hirschmann M, Bräutigam V, Singer RF. Endogenous particle stabilization during magnesium integral foam production. Adv Eng Mater 2004;6:385−90.
[39] Körner C, Hirschmann M, Wiehler H. Integral foam moulding of light metals. Mater Trans 2006;47:2188−94.
[40] Yamada Y, Shimojima K, Sakaguchi Y, Mabuchi M, Nakamura M, Asahina T, et al. Processing of cellular magnesium materials. Adv Eng Mater 2000;2:184−7.
[41] Yamada Y, Shimojima K, Sakaguchi Y, Mabuchi M, Nakamura M, Asahina T, et al. Processing of an open-cellular AZ91 magnesium alloy with a low density of 0.05 g/cm^3. J Mater Sci Lett 1999;18:1477−80.
[42] Wen C, Yamada Y, Shimojima K, Mabuchi M, Nakamura M, Asahina T. Mechanical properties of cellular magnesium materials. Mater Sci Forum 2000;350:359−64.

[43] Wen C, Yamada Y, Shimojima K, Mabuchi M, Nakamura M, Asahina T, et al. Effects of heat treatment on the compressive properties of AZ91 Mg foam. Mater Trans JIM 2000; 41:1192–5.
[44] Kanahashi H, Mukai T, Yamada Y, Shimojima K, Mabuchi M, Aizawa T, et al. Experimental study for the improvement of crashworthiness in AZ91 magnesium foam controlling its microstructure. Mater Sci Eng A 2001;308:283–7.
[45] Yamada Y, Wen C, Shimojima K, Hosokawa H, Chino Y, Mabuchi M. Compressive deformation characteristics of open-cell Mg alloys with controlled cell structure. Mater Trans 2002;43:1298–305.
[46] Yamada Y, Shimojima K, Sakaguchi Y, Mabuchi M, Nakamura M, Asahina T, et al. Compressive properties of open-cellular SG91A Al and AZ91 Mg. Mater Sci Eng A 1999;272:455–8.
[47] Kirkland NT, Kolbeinsson I, Woodfield TIM, Dias G, Staiger MP. Processing-property relationships of As-Cast magnesium foams with controllable architecture. Int J Mod Phys B 2009;23:1002–8.
[48] Kasemo B, Gold J. Implant surfaces and interface processes. Adv Dental Res 1999;13: 8–20.
[49] Witte F, Reifenrath J, Müller PP, Crostack HA, Nellesen J, Bach FW, et al. Cartilage repair on magnesium scaffolds used as a subchondral bone replacement. Materialwiss Werkstofftech 2006;37:504–8.
[50] Lietaert K, Weber L, Van Humbeeck J, Mortensen A, Luyten J, Schrooten J. Open cellular magnesium alloys for biodegradable orthopaedic implants. J Magnesium Alloys 2013;1:303–11.
[51] Trinidad J, Marco I, Arruebarrena G, Wendt J, Letzig D, Sáenz De Argandoña E, et al. Processing of magnesium porous structures by infiltration casting for biomedical applications. Adv Eng Mater 2014;16:241–7.
[52] Kang MH, Jung HD, Kim SW, Lee SM, Kim HE, Estrin Y, et al. Production and biocorrosion resistance of porous magnesium with hydroxyapatite coating for biomedical applications. Mater Lett 2013;108:122–4.
[53] Nguyen TL, Staiger MP, Dias GJ, Woodfield TBF. A novel manufacturing route for fabrication of topologically-ordered porous magnesium scaffolds. Adv Eng Mater 2011; 13:872–81.
[54] Staiger MP, Kirkland NT, Kolbeinsson I, Woodfield T. Processing of magnesium foams with periodic, controllable architectures. In: ICCM International Conferences on Composite Materials; 2009.
[55] Staiger MP, Kolbeinsson I, Kirkland NT, Nguyen T, Dias G, Woodfield TBF. Synthesis of topologically-ordered open-cell porous magnesium. Mater Lett 2010;64:2572–4.
[56] Jiang G, He G. A new approach to the fabrication of porous magnesium with well-controlled 3D pore structure for orthopedic applications. Mater Sci Eng C 2014;43: 317–20.
[57] Wang X, Li Z, Huang Y, Wang K, Wang X, Han F. Processing of magnesium foams by weakly corrosive and highly flexible space holder materials. Mater Design 2014;64: 324–9.
[58] Shapovalov V. Porous metals. MRS Bull 1994;19:24–8.
[59] Liu Y, Li Y, Zhang H. Fabrication of lotus-structured porous magnesium with GASAR process. Acta Metal Sin 2004;40:1121–6.
[60] Wan J, Li YX, Liu Y. Effect of gas pressure on pore distribution of lotus-type porous magnesium fabricated by unidirectional solidification. Chinese J Nonferrous Met 2007; 17:200–6.

[61] Hyun SK, Suzuki S, Nakajima H. Fabrication of lotus-type porous magnesium by continuous casting process. In: MetFoam 2007 – Proceedings of the 5th International Conference on porous metals and metallic foams; 2008. p. 233–5.
[62] Hoshiyama H, Ikeda T, Nakajima H. Fabrication of lotus-type porous magnesium and its alloys by unidirectional solidification under hydrogen atmosphere. High Temp Mater Process 2007;26:303–16.
[63] Liu XH, Liu XF, Xie JX. The investigation of fabrication processing for lotus-type porous magnesium by the in-situ reaction and unidirectional solidification method. Procedia Eng 2012:270–8.
[64] Tane M, Nakajima H. Fabrication of lotus-type porous magnesium using hydrogen decomposed from MgH_2. In: MetFoam 2007 – Proceedings of the 5th International Conference on porous metals and metallic foams; 2008. p. 241–4.
[65] Tane M, Nakajima H. Fabrication of porous magnesium with directional pores through use of hydrogen thermally decomposed from MgH_2 powders during unidirectional solidification. J Mater Res 2008;23:849–55.
[66] Zahrani MM, Meratian M, Kabiri Y. Innovative processing of lotus-type porous magnesium through thermal decomposition of wood. Mater Lett 2012;85:14–7.
[67] Renger K, Kaufmann H. Vacuum foaming of magnesium slurries. Adv Eng Mater 2005; 7:117–23.
[68] Kaya M. A study on microstructure and fabrication of porous Mg-10Al alloy. Mater Manuf Process 2012;27:605–8.
[69] Lefebvre LP, Banhart J, Dunand DC. Porous metals and metallic foams: current status and recent developments. Adv Eng Mater 2008;10:775–87.
[70] Koizumi T, Kido K, Kita K, Mikado K, Gnyloskurenko S, Nakamura T. The improvement of mechanical properties of metallic foams by carbonates as a foaming agent. J Jpn Inst Met 2011;75:355–60.
[71] Plorin T, Bormann D, Heidenblut T, Bach FW. Investigations into manufacturing composite profiles having local magnesium-foam reinforcements. Germany Adv Mater Res 2010:129–60.
[72] Neu T, Mukherjee M, Moreno FG, Banhart J. Magnesium and magnesium alloy foams. In: 7th International Conference on porous metals and metallic foams (MetFoam 2011); 2012. p. 133.
[73] Wen C, Yamada Y, Shimojima K, Chino Y, Hosokawa H, Mabuchi M. Porous bioresorbable magnesium as bone substitute. In: 2nd Osaka International Conference on platform science and technology for advanced magnesium alloys. Osaka, Japan: Materials Science Forum; 2003. p. 1001–6.
[74] Zhuang H, Han Y, Feng A. Preparation, mechanical properties and in vitro biodegradation of porous magnesium scaffolds. Mater Sci Eng C 2008;28:1462–6.
[75] Hao GL, Han F, Li W. Processing and mechanical properties of magnesium foams. J Porous Mater 2009;16:251–6.
[76] Hao GL, Xu QP, Han FS. Low-frequency damping behavior of porous magnesium. In: 2nd International Conference on advances in materials and manufacturing processes, ICAMMP 2011. Guilin, China: Advanced Materials Research; 2012. p. 2002–7.
[77] Hao GL, Han FS, Wu J, Wang SF. Mechanical and damping properties of porous AZ91 magnesium alloy. Powder Metall 2007;50:127–31.
[78] Han F, Hao G, Wang X, Wei X. Characterisation of mechanical and damping properties of porous AZ91 Mg alloy. In: MetFoam 2007 – Proceedings of the 5th International Conference on porous metals and metallic foams; 2008. p. 375–8.

[79] Aghion E, Yered T, Perez Y, Gueta Y. The prospects of carrying and releasing drugs via biodegradable magnesium foam. Adv Eng Mater 2010;12:B374–9.
[80] Čapek J, Vojtěch D. Effect of sintering conditions on the microstructural and mechanical characteristics of porous magnesium materials prepared by powder metallurgy. Mater Sci Eng C 2014;35:21–8.
[81] Čapek J, Vojtěch D. Properties of porous magnesium prepared by powder metallurgy. Mater Sci Eng C 2013;33:564–9.
[82] Čapek J, Vojtěch D. Porous magnesium for medical applications – influence of powder size on mechanical properties. Key Eng Mater 2014:342–5.
[83] Hao GL, Han FS, Wu J, Wang XF. Damping properties of porous AZ91 magnesium alloy reinforced with copper particles. Mater Sci Technol 2007;23:492–6.
[84] Cay H, Xu H, Li Q. Mechanical behavior of porous magnesium/alumina composites with high strength and low density. Mater Sci Eng A 2013;574:137–42.
[85] Seyedraoufi ZS, Mirdamadi S. Synthesis, microstructure and mechanical properties of porous Mg-Zn scaffolds. J Mech Behav Biomed Mater 2013;21:1–8.
[86] Zhang X, Li X, Li J, Sun X. Processing, microstructure and mechanical properties of biomedical magnesium with a specific two-layer structure. Prog Nat Sci Mater Int 2013.
[87] Kitazono K, Kikuchi Y, Sato E, Kuribayashi K. Processing of closed-cell magnesium foams. Mater Sci Forum 2007:1839–44.
[88] Kikuchi Y, Kakehi K, Kitazono K, Sato E, Kuribayashi K. Magnesium foam produced from bulk AZ31 magnesium alloy sheets. In: PRICM 5: the Fifth Pacific Rim International Conference on advanced materials and processing. Beijing, China: Materials Science Forum; 2005. p. 501–4.
[89] Mehara K, Kobashi M, Kanetake N. Fabrication of magnesium foam by precursor method using machined chips. In: PRICM 6: the 6th Pacific Rim International Conference on advanced materials and processing. Jeju Island, South Korea: Advanced Materials Research; 2007. p. 905–8.
[90] Okumura H, Watanabe K, Kamado S, Kojima Y. Manufacturing of porous magnesium alloy by pulse electric current sintering process and their compressive properties. Mater Sci Forum 2003:1019–24.
[91] Okumura H, Watanabe K, Kamado S, Kojima Y. Fabrication of porous magnesium alloys by pulse electric current sintering process using machined chips. Mater Trans 2003;44: 595–600.
[92] Morgenthal I, Andersen O, Kostmann C, Stephani G, Studnitzky T, Witte F, et al. Highly porous magnesium alloy structures and their properties regarding degradable implant application. Adv Eng Mater 2014;16:309–18.
[93] Zhang X, Li X-W, Li J-G, Sun X-D. Preparation and mechanical property of a novel 3D porous magnesium scaffold for bone tissue engineering. Mater Sci Eng C 2014;42:362–7.
[94] Tan L, Gong M, Zheng F, Zhang B, Yang K. Study on compression behavior of porous magnesium used as bone tissue engineering scaffolds. Biomed Mater 2009;4.
[95] Baumgärtner F, Duarte I, Banhart J. Industrialization of powder compact foaming process. Adv Eng Mater 2000;2:168–74.
[96] Avedesian MM, Baker H. ASM specialty handbook: magnesium and magnesium alloys. ASM International; 1999. p. 274.
[97] Gu X, Zheng Y, Cheng Y, Zhong S, Xi T. In vitro corrosion and biocompatibility of binary magnesium alloys. Biomaterials 2009;30:484–98.
[98] Witte F, Kaese V, Haferkamp H, Switzer E, Meyer-Lindenberg A, Wirth CJ, et al. In vivo corrosion of four magnesium alloys and the associated bone response. Biomaterials 2005; 26:3557–63.

[99] Wang YM, Wang FH, Xu MJ, Zhao B, Guo LX, Ouyang JH. Microstructure and corrosion behavior of coated AZ91 alloy by microarc oxidation for biomedical application. Appl Surf Sci 2009;255:9124–31.
[100] Zainal Abidin NI, Atrens AD, Martin D, Atrens A. Corrosion of high purity Mg, Mg2Zn0.2Mn, ZE41 and AZ91 in Hank's solution at 37°C. Corrosion Sci 2011;53: 3542–56.
[101] Malekani J, Schmutz B, Gu Y, Schuetz M, Yarlagadda PK. Biomaterials in orthopedic bone plates: a review. In: Proceedings of the 2nd Annual International Conference on materials science, metal & manufacturing (M3 2011). Global Science and Technology Forum; 2011. p. 71–7.
[102] Nair LS, Laurencin CT. Biodegradable polymers as biomaterials. Prog Polym Sci 2007; 32:762–98.
[103] Ding Y, Wen C, Hodgson P, Li Y. Effects of alloying elements on the corrosion behavior and biocompatibility of biodegradable magnesium alloys: a review. J Mater Chem B 2014;2:1912–33.
[104] Peng Q, Huang Y, Zhou L, Hort N, Kainer KU. Preparation and properties of high purity Mg-Y biomaterials. Biomaterials 2010;31:398–403.
[105] Verstraeten SV, Aimo L, Oteiza PI. Aluminium and lead: molecular mechanisms of brain toxicity. Arch Toxicol 2008;82:789–802.
[106] Stulikova I, Smola B. Mechanical properties and phase composition of potential biodegradable Mg-Zn-Mn-base alloys with addition of rare earth elements. Mater Charact 2010;61:952–8.
[107] Rosalbino F, De Negri S, Saccone A, Angelini E, Delfino S. Bio-corrosion characterization of Mg-Zn-X (X = Ca, Mn, Si) alloys for biomedical applications. J Mater Sci Mater Med 2010;21:1091–8.
[108] Huan ZG, Leeflang MA, Zhou J, Fratila-Apachitei LE, Duszczyk J. In vitro degradation behavior and cytocompatibility of Mg-Zn-Zr alloys. J Mater Sci Mater Med 2010;21: 2623–35.
[109] Mushahary D, Sravanthi R, Li Y, Kumar MJ, Harishankar N, Hodgson P, et al. Zirconium, calcium, and strontium contents in magnesium based biodegradable alloys modulate the efficiency of implant-induced osseointegration. Int J Nanomedicine 2013;8: 2887–902.
[110] Witte F, Feyerabend F, Maier P, Fischer J, Störmer M, Blawert C, et al. Biodegradable magnesium-hydroxyapatite metal matrix composites. Biomaterials 2007;28:2163–74.
[111] Alvarez-Lopez M, Pereda MD, Del Valle JA, Fernandez-Lorenzo M, Garcia-Alonso MC, Ruano OA, et al. Corrosion behaviour of AZ31 magnesium alloy with different grain sizes in simulated biological fluids. Acta Biomater 2010;6:1763–71.
[112] Shahzad M, Waqas H, Rafi-ud-din, Qureshi AH, Wagner L. The roles of Zn distribution and eutectic particles on microstructure development during extrusion and anisotropic mechanical properties in a Mg-Zn-Zr alloy. Mater Sci Eng A 2014;620:50–7.
[113] Ferreira PC, Piai KDA, Takayanagui AMM, Segura-Muñoz SI. Aluminum as a risk factor for Alzheimer's disease. Rev Lat Am Enfermagem 2008;16:151–7.
[114] Frumkin H, Louise J. Toxicolgical profile for aluminum. Atlanta: US HHS Research Report, ATSDR; 2008.
[115] Wen Z, Wu C, Dai C, Yang F. Corrosion behaviors of Mg and its alloys with different Al contents in a modified simulated body fluid. J Alloys Compounds 2009;488:392–9.
[116] Liang SM, Ma YQ, Chen RS, Han EH. Effect of composition on the microstructure and mechanical properties of Mg-Al-Zn alloys. Magnesium Technol 2008:331–6.

[117] Song G, Atrens A. Corrosion mechanisms of magnesium alloys. Adv Eng Mater 1999;1: 11–33.
[118] Zhou W, Shen T, Aung NN. Effect of heat treatment on corrosion behaviour of magnesium alloy AZ91D in simulated body fluid. Corrosion Sci 2010;52:1035–41.
[119] Kirkland NT, Lespagnol J, Birbilis N, Staiger MP. A survey of bio-corrosion rates of magnesium alloys. Corrosion Sci 2010;52:287–91.
[120] Gao J, Wu S, Qiao L, Wang Y. Corrosion behavior of Mg and Mg-Zn alloys in simulated body fluid. Trans Nonferrous Met Soc China (English Edition) 2008;18:588–92.
[121] Zhang S, Li J, Song Y, Zhao C, Zhang X, Xie C, et al. In vitro degradation, hemolysis and MC3T3-E1 cell adhesion of biodegradable Mg-Zn alloy. Mater Sci Eng C 2009;29: 1907–12.
[122] Brandão-Neto J, Stefan V, Mendonça BB, Bloise W, Castro AVB. The essential role of zinc in growth. Nutr Res 1995;15:335–58.
[123] Post JI, Eibl JK, Ross GM. Zinc induces motor neuron death via a selective inhibition of brain-derived neurotrophic factor activity. Amyotroph Lateral Scler 2008;9:149–55.
[124] Cao P, Qian M, St John DH. Effect of manganese on grain refinement of Mg–Al based alloys. Scr Mater 2006;54:1853–8.
[125] Sajuri ZB, Miyashita Y, Hosokai Y, Mutoh Y. Effects of Mn content and texture on fatigue properties of As-Cast and extruded AZ61 magnesium alloys. Int J Mech Sci 2006; 48:198–209.
[126] Huang X, Suzuki K, Watazu A, Shigematsu I, Saito N. Effects of manganese on microstructure and mechanical properties of AZ31 magnesium alloy processed by differential speed rolling. Mater Sci Forum 2007:283–6.
[127] Erikson KM, Syversen T, Aschner JL, Aschner M. Interactions between excessive manganese exposures and dietary iron-deficiency in neurodegeneration. Environ Toxicol Pharmacol 2005;19:415–21.
[128] Walker J, Shadanbaz S, Woodfield TBF, Staiger MP, Dias GJ. Magnesium biomaterials for orthopedic application: a review from a biological perspective. J Biomed Mater Res B Appl Biomater 2014;102:1316–31.
[129] Harandi SE, Mirshahi M, Koleini S, Idris MH, Jafari H, Kadir MRA. Effect of calcium content on the microstructure, hardness and in-vitro corrosion behavior of biodegradable Mg-Ca binary alloy. Mater Res 2013;16:11–8.
[130] Li Z, Gu X, Lou S, Zheng Y. The development of binary Mg-Ca alloys for use as biodegradable materials within bone. Biomaterials 2008;29:1329–44.
[131] Erdmann N, Angrisani N, Reifenrath J, Lucas A, Thorey F, Bormann D, et al. Biomechanical testing and degradation analysis of MgCa0.8 alloy screws: a comparative in vivo study in rabbits. Acta Biomater 2011;7:1421–8.
[132] Denkena B, Witte F, Podolsky C, Lucas A. Degradable implants made of magnesium alloys. In: Proc 5th Euspen Int Conf, Montpellier, France; 2005.
[133] Wan Y, Xiong G, Luo H, He F, Huang Y, Zhou X. Preparation and characterization of a new biomedical magnesium-calcium alloy. Mater Design 2008;29:2034–7.
[134] Park RS, Kim YK, Lee SJ, Jang YS, Park IS, Yun YH, et al. Corrosion behavior and cytotoxicity of Mg-35Zn-3Ca alloy for surface modified biodegradable implant material. J Biomed Mater Res B Appl Biomater 2012;100B:911–23.
[135] Park S-H, Um Y-S, Kum C-H, Hur B-Y. Thermophysical properties of Al and Mg alloys for metal foam fabrication. Colloids Surf A 2005;263:280–3.
[136] Gandel DS, Birbilis N, Easton MA, Gibson MA. Influence of manganese, zirconium and iron on the corrosion of magnesium. In: 50th Annual Conference of the Australasian corrosion Association 2010: corrosion and prevention; 2010. p. 875–85.

[137] El-Moneim AA, Akiyama E, Ismail KM, Hashimoto K. Corrosion behaviour of sputter-deposited Mg-Zr alloys in a borate buffer solution. Corrosion Sci 2011;53:2988−93.
[138] Mushahary D, Wen C, Kumar JM, Harishankar N, Pande G, Hodgson P, et al. Effect of Collagen type-I on the rate of osseointegration of Ca-containing biodegradable Mg-Zr based alloys. Eur Cells Mater 2013;26:22.
[139] Witte F. The history of biodegradable magnesium implants: a review. Acta Biomater 2010;6:1680−92.
[140] Li Y, Wong CS, Wen C, Hodgson P. Biodegradable Mg-Zr-Ca alloys for bone implant materials. Mater Technol 2012;27:49−51.
[141] Yamamoto A, Honma R, Sumita M. Cytotoxicity evaluation of 43 metal salts using murine fibroblasts and osteoblastic cells. J Biomed Mater Res 1998;39:331−40.
[142] Pang S, Liu Y, Li H, Sun L, Li Y, Zhang T. New Ti-based Ti-Cu-Zr-Fe-Sn-Si-Ag bulk metallic glass for biomedical applications. J Alloys Compounds 2015;625:323−7.
[143] Chen Q, Thouas GA. Metallic implant biomaterials. Mater Sci Eng R 2014;87:1−57.
[144] Nowag S, Frangville C, Multhaup G, Marty JD, Mingotaud C, Haag R. Biocompatible, hyperbranched nanocarriers for the transport and release of copper ions. J Mater Chem B 2014;2:3915−8.
[145] Sengupta J, Ghosh S, Datta P, Gomes A, Gomes A. Physiologically important metal nanoparticles and their toxicity. J Nanoscience Nanotechnol 2014;14:990−1006.
[146] Roy S, Pal S. Characterization of silane coated hollow sphere alumina-reinforced ultra high molecular weight polyethylene composite as a possible bone substitute material. Bull Mater Sci 2002;25:609−12.
[147] Thamaraiselvi T, Rajeswari S. Biological evaluation of bioceramic materials-a review. Carbon 2004;24:172.
[148] Warashina H, Sakano S, Kitamura S, Yamauchi K-I, Yamaguchi J, Ishiguro N, et al. Biological reaction to alumina, zirconia, titanium and polyethylene particles implanted onto murine calvaria. Biomaterials 2003;24:3655−61.
[149] Karageorgiou V, Kaplan D. Porosity of 3D biomaterial scaffolds and osteogenesis. Biomaterials 2005;26:5474−91.
[150] Seo OH, Jeong MJ, Jung IY, Hur BY. Comparative study on TiH_2 and $CaCO_3$ for fabrication of Mg alloy foams. Mater Sci Forum 2008:273−6.
[151] Léon Y, León CA. New perspectives in mercury porosimetry. Adv Colloid Interface Sci 1998;76−77:341−72.
[152] Hutmacher DW. Scaffolds in tissue engineering bone and cartilage. Biomaterials 2000; 21:2529−43.
[153] Wu Z, Tang T, Guo H, Tang S, Niu Y, Zhang J, et al. In vitro degradability, bioactivity and cell responses to mesoporous magnesium silicate for the induction of bone regeneration. Colloids Surf B Biointerfaces 2014;120:38−46.
[154] Svehla M, Morberg P, Zicat B, Bruce W, Sonnabend D, Walsh WR. Morphometric and mechanical evaluation of titanium implant integration: comparison of five surface structures. J Biomed Mater Res 2000;51:15−22.
[155] Harvey EJ, Bobyn JD, Tanzer M, Stackpool GJ, Krygier JJ, Hacking SA. Effect of flexibility of the femoral stem on bone-remodeling and fixation of the stem in a canine total hip arthroplasty model without cement. J Bone Joint Surg A 1999;81:93−107.
[156] Lewandrowski KU, Bondre SP, Gresser JD, Wise DL, Tomford WW, Trantolo DJ. Improved osteoconduction of cortical bone grafts by biodegradable foam coating. Bio-Med Mater Eng 1999;9:265−75.

[157] Zimmer G, Rohrhofer A, Lewis K, Goessl A, Hoffmann O. The surface microporosity of ceramic biomaterials influences the resorption capacity of osteoclasts. J Biomed Mater Res A 2013;101:3365–71.
[158] Paganias CG, Tsakotos GA, Koutsostathis SD, MacHeras GA. Osseous integration in porous tantalum implants. Indian J Orthop 2012;46:505–13.
[159] Bobe K, Willbold E, Morgenthal I, Andersen O, Studnitzky T, Nellesen J, et al. In vitro and in vivo evaluation of biodegradable, open-porous scaffolds made of sintered magnesium W4 short fibres. Acta Biomater 2013;9:8611–23.
[160] Ryan G, Pandit A, Apatsidis DP. Fabrication methods of porous metals for use in orthopaedic applications. Biomaterials 2006;27:2651–70.
[161] Gibson LJ. The mechanical behaviour of cancellous bone. J Biomech 1985;18:317–28.
[162] Yamada Y, Shimojima K, Sakaguchi Y, Mabuchi M, Nakamura M, Asahina T, et al. Effects of heat treatment on compressive properties of AZ91 Mg and SG91A Al foams with open-cell structure. Mater Sci Eng A 2000;280:225–8.
[163] Liao HT, Chen YY, Lai YT, Hsieh MF, Jiang CP. The osteogenesis of bone marrow stem cells on mPEG-PCL-mPEG/hydroxyapatite composite scaffold via solid freeform fabrication. BioMed Res Int 2014;2014.
[164] Lin CY, Kikuchi N, Hollister SJ. A novel method for biomaterial scaffold internal architecture design to match bone elastic properties with desired porosity. J Biomech 2004;37:623–36.
[165] Witwicka H, Hwang SY, Odgren PR. The structure of bone. Reference module in biomedical sciences. Elsevier; 2014.
[166] Hulbert SF, Young FA, Mathews RS, Klawitter JJ, Talbert CD, Stelling FH. Potential of ceramic materials as permanently implantable skeletal prostheses. J Biomed Mater Res 1970;4:433–56.
[167] Stangl R, Rinne B, Kastl S, Hendrich C, Wennerberg A, Richards RG, et al. The influence of pore geometry in CP Ti-implants – a cell culture investigation. Eur Cells Mater 2001;2:1–9.
[168] Kuboki Y, Jin Q, Kikuchi M, Mamood J, Takita H. Geometry of artificial ECM: sizes of pores controlling phenotype expression in BMP-induced osteogenesis and chondrogenesis. Connect Tissue Res 2002;43:529–34.
[169] Akay G, Birch MA, Bokhari MA. Microcellular polyHIPE polymer supports osteoblast growth and bone formation in vitro. Biomaterials 2004;25:3991–4000.
[170] Kobashi M, Maehara K, Kanetake N. Effect of thermal condition on blowing behavior and pore morphology of porous magnesium. J Jpn Inst Light Met 2009;59:261–4.
[171] Gibson LJ, Ashby MF. Cellular solids: structure and properties. Cambridge: University Press; 1999.
[172] Körner C, Singer RF. Processing of metal foams – challenges and opportunities. Adv Eng Mater 2000;2:159–65.
[173] Müller U, Imwinkelried T, Horst M, Sievers M, Graf-Hausner U. Do human osteoblasts grow into open-porous titanium? Eur Cells Mater 2006;11:8–15.
[174] Zardiackas LD, Parsell DE, Dillon LD, Mitchell DW, Nunnery LA, Poggie R. Structure, metallurgy, and mechanical properties of a porous tantalum foam. J Biomed Mater Res 2001;58:180–7.
[175] Hofmann S, Hagenmüller H, Koch AM, Müller R, Vunjak-Novakovic G, Kaplan DL, et al. Control of in vitro tissue-engineered bone-like structures using human mesenchymal stem cells and porous silk scaffolds. Biomaterials 2007;28:1152–62.

[176] Joly P, Duda GN, Schöne M, Welzel PB, Freudenberg U, Werner C, et al. Geometry-driven cell organization determines tissue growths in scaffold pores: consequences for fibronectin organization. PLoS One 2013;8.
[177] Sobral JM, Caridade SG, Sousa RA, Mano JF, Reis RL. Three-dimensional plotted scaffolds with controlled pore size gradients: effect of scaffold geometry on mechanical performance and cell seeding efficiency. Acta Biomater 2011;7:1009–18.
[178] Kuboki Y, Jin Q, Takita H. Geometry of carriers controlling phenotypic expression in BMP-induced osteogenesis and chondrogenesis. J Bone Joint Surg A 2001; 83A(Suppl. 1):S105–15.
[179] Sampath TK, Reddi AH. Importance of geometry of the extracellular matrix in endochondral bone differentiation. J Cell Biol 1984;98:2192–7.
[180] An Y, Wen C, Hodgson P, Yang C. Investigation of cell shape effect on the mechanical behaviour of open-cell metal foams. Comput Mater Sci 2012;55:1–9.
[181] Arifvianto B, Zhou J. Fabrication of metallic biomedical scaffolds with the space holder method: a review. Materials 2014;7:3588–622.
[182] Bekoz N, Oktay E. Effects of carbamide shape and content on processing and properties of steel foams. J Mater Process Technol 2012;212:2109–16.
[183] Zhang J, Wu L, Jing D, Ding J. A comparative study of porous scaffolds with cubic and spherical macropores. Polymer 2005;46:4979–85.
[184] Yang C, Zhang Y, Rolfe BF. Special finite element-based unit cell approach for the prediction of mechanical properties of foamed titanium. In: Advances in heterogeneous material mechanics 2008 – Proceedings of the 2nd International Conference on heterogeneous material mechanics (ICHMM 2008); 2008. p. 329–33.
[185] Pinto P, Peixinho N, Silva F, Soares D. Compressive properties and energy absorption of aluminum foams with modified cellular geometry. J Mater Process Technol 2014;214: 571–7.
[186] Van Bael S, Chai YC, Truscello S, Moesen M, Kerckhofs G, Van Oosterwyck H, et al. The effect of pore geometry on the in vitro biological behavior of human periosteum-derived cells seeded on selective laser-melted Ti6Al4V bone scaffolds. Acta Biomater 2012;8:2824–34.
[187] Chu TMG, Orton DG, Hollister SJ, Feinberg SE, Halloran JW. Mechanical and in vivo performance of hydroxyapatite implants with controlled architectures. Biomaterials 2002; 23:1283–93.
[188] Jin QM, Takita H, Kohgo T, Atsumi K, Itoh H, Kuboki Y. Effects of geometry of hydroxyapatite as a cell substratum in BMP-induced ectopic bone formation. J Biomed Mater Res 2000;51:491–9.
[189] Park C, Nutt SR. Metallographic study of GASAR porous magnesium. Mater Res Soc Symp Proc 1998:315–20.

Metal scaffolds processed by electron beam melting for biomedical applications

3

A. Ataee[2], *Y. Li*[2], *G. Song*[3], *C. Wen*[1,2]
[1]Swinburne University of Technology, Hawthorn, Victoria, Australia; [2]RMIT University, Melbourne, Victoria, Australia; [3]CSIRO Manufacturing Flagship, Clayton, Victoria, Australia

3.1 Introduction

The numbers of orthopedic operations, including osteoplastic and joint replacement surgeries, are increasing every year. Millions of people undergo surgeries to receive orthopedic implants worldwide. It is estimated that more than 4 million adults in the United States currently live with a total knee replacement [1], and around 100,000 people in Australia require joint replacement surgery every year [2]. However, there is a major issue that causes patients to go through revision surgeries that are due to bone resorption and loosening of the implant. The procedure includes removing the old implant and inserting a new one that leads to additional risks, suffers, and costs to the patient.

To have a successful implant, the following three major issues must be overcome [3–7]:

- poor osseointegration,
- lack of biological anchorage for bone tissue ingrowth, and
- loosening of the implant due to bone resorption caused by a stiffness mismatch between the implanted material and bone.

The reason for the first and second issues is a weak interfacial bonding between the implant and the bone, which is the consequence of the differences in morphologies of the implant and bone. As a solution, for nearly four decades, porous coatings have been used to provide surface anchorage between orthopedic implant devices and the adjoining bone to improve implant fixation by encouraging bone tissue ingrowth [8–10]. These methods mostly include the addition of metal beads to a solid implant surface by a diffusion bonding process, thermal spraying, sintering of cellular metals, mesh arrays, and metallic foams to implant surfaces [11].

To address the third issue, it has been reported that open cellular foams or scaffolds can have significantly reduced stiffness or elastic moduli with a reduction in density [12,13]. Over the last few decades, achievements have been made to design and manufacture porous scaffolds that mimic the architecture and mechanical behavior of natural bone. The porous scaffolds also provide the potential for complete bone ingrowth and ensure a long-term biological fixation [4,14]. A variety of production methods have

Metallic Foam Bone. http://dx.doi.org/10.1016/B978-0-08-101289-5.00003-2

been developed to fabricate open cellular foams or scaffolds. The most common methods include sintering loose metal powders or fibers, the space holder sintering method, vapor deposition, rapid prototyping, and electro discharge compaction [15]. The first two sintering methods produce nonhomogenous porous structures while the vapor deposition and rapid prototyping methods have the advantage of producing homogeneous porous structures. Moreover, the rapid prototyping and electro discharge compaction methods can be used to produce functionally graded structures.

To date, Ti alloys, in particular Ti-6Al-4V, have been the material of choice for load-bearing implant applications [5,6,14,16–18]. While great progress has been made in the production of biocompatible scaffolds, several challenges still exist for conventional manufacturing techniques [19]:

1. It is hard to achieve an open cellular porous structure with a high degree of interconnected porosity, defined pore shape, specified pore size, and graded porosity distribution.
2. Standard mass-produced implants do not work well for maxillofacial and skull surgeries or for patients having abnormal anatomy. In these situations, patient-customized implants are preferred.
3. The traditional machining has a limitation when implants with complex shapes are required, particularly when a production of thin wall implants or significant material removal are necessary.
4. Fabrication of titanium alloy scaffolds with conventional techniques (such as casting) is difficult due to its high melting point (above 1650°C), high chemical affinity to atmospheric gases, and reactions with most mold materials [20].

Advances in metal powder bed fusion-based additive manufacturing (AM) have enabled the successful production of metallic parts from prealloyed powders, including stainless steels, maraging steels, cobalt–chromium alloys, titanium alloys, etc. [21]. In particular, for biomedical applications, electron beam melting (EBM), or selective electron beam melting, and selective laser melting (SLM) have eliminated the number of manufacturing constraints in shape, size, and internal structure and made it possible to fabricate implants that adapt to the physical and mechanical requirements of the region of implantation. This chapter focuses on the application of EBM in the manufacturing of biomedical implants.

3.2 Electron beam melting used in biomedical manufacturing

3.2.1 Device description

High-power electron beam has been used for many years to heat treat and for welding, soldering, and machining materials [22]. The first patent describing electron beam as an energy source for the direct manufacturing of 3D bodies was published in 1993 [23]. In 1997, the EBM process was commercialized by the Swedish company Arcam AB, which manufactured and distributed a series of EBM machines called S12, A2, A1, A2XX, Q10, and Q20 during 2002–2013 [24].

EBM is a kind of AM method that is classified as a powder bed fusion technique and is operationally similar to the rastering of an electron beam in a scanning electron microscope.

An EBM machine consists of a control panel and a processing chamber, which is equipped with a turbo pump for evacuation. Fig. 3.1 shows the schematic of an EBM machine.

The electron beam gun is located in an electron beam column above the build chamber that generates the electron beam by heating a tungsten filament to a temperature ranging from 1900K to 2200K and accelerating it to a velocity of 0.1−0.5 times the speed of light using an accelerating voltage of 60 kV. The generated electron beam then runs down in a so-called drift tube while the first lens corrects for astigmatism and produces a circular electron beam with a Gaussian energy distribution. Then the electromagnetic coil/lens focuses the beam to a small spot from around 0.1−1 mm on the powder bed, and finally the deflection lens orients the beam from one position to another on the powder bed.

When the electron beam hits the powder particles in the building chamber, it releases kinetic energy as thermal energy and increases the temperature. Depending on the power of the electron beam, the powder particles are completely molten in a certain range of area and layer thickness. This method can make fully dense metal parts and maintain the characteristics of the material [25−28].

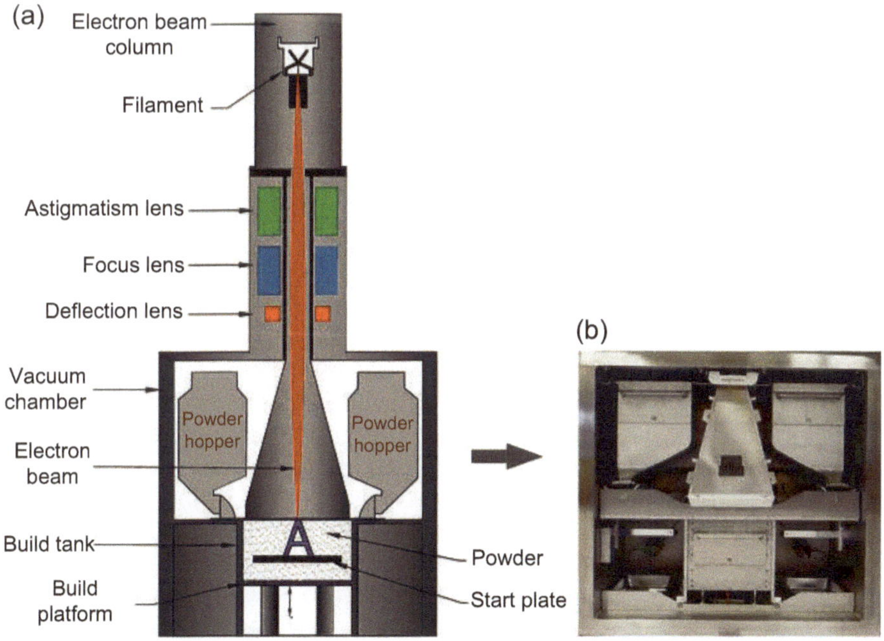

Figure 3.1 (a) Schematic of an electron beam melting machine and (b) an image from inside of an Arcam A1 processing chamber [24].

In order to prevent the scattering of electron beam in collisions with gas atoms, the build chamber is kept under a vacuum of approximately 1×10^{-4} to 1×10^{-5} mbar during the process, and the electron gun is kept under a vacuum of approximately 1×10^{-6} mbar. It has the additional benefit of preventing high-temperature oxidation (specifically for reactive metals such as titanium) and eliminating vaporized impurities incorporated in the metal powder, making it a suitable method for the molding of high-quality metal products. Moreover, the vacuum acts as an insulator and helps to keep the process at an elevated temperature [29]. Generally, all conductive materials can be processed by EBM, but the popular materials are titanium and some of its alloys, cobalt–chromium alloys, and steels.

The production chamber consists of a building tank with an adjustable build platform (base plate), two powder hoppers, and a rake system for spreading the powders. The build table is the area where the powder is spread over by the rake, and it moves down along the Z-axis as the build progresses step by step. The hoppers hold the powder stock material.

To manufacture a component using an EBM device, similar to the SLM method, a 3D design of the component is created by conventional CAD software and an STL (stereolithography) model is generated to use in the EBM device as an input file. Then slice data is created by dividing the model into equal intervals in the direction of the height or build axes. Subsequently, suitable processing parameters for the model, such as the scanning speed and scanning strategy (a combination of the scanning pattern, which defines the cross-section of the layer and the related process parameters), electron beam current, and preheating temperature, should be selected.

At the beginning of the process, the base plate is heated by the electron beam from room temperature to a temperature around 475°C for processing Ti-6Al-4V, as shown in Fig. 3.2.

Then for 10 min the degassing process happens to remove species (for example, water vapor from the surface of the base plate); afterward, the temperature of the build plate increases until it reaches the initial preheating temperature (734°C for Ti-6Al-4V). Then the build table moves by 1 layer thickness, a layer of metal powder spreads homogeneously on the build platform, and the main process starts, as shown in Fig. 3.3.

Each layer is processed in four distinct steps. The powder bed is preheated up close to the melting point (conventionally 600 to 900°C or roughly up to 0.8 T_m [31]), using a defocused electron beam or a relatively low beam current and a high scan speed. The preheating step slightly sinters the metal powder to improve the conductivity and cohesion of particles and to prevent powder spreading in the chamber (powder cloud) due to negative charge buildup [32]. It also helps to decrease the thermal gradient during the process and residual stress in the finished part [33]. After the preheating step, the electron beam scans the powder surface to melt the metal powder according to the slice data and solidifies it into the desired shape. Once the first layer has been melted, the build plate descends by 1 layer

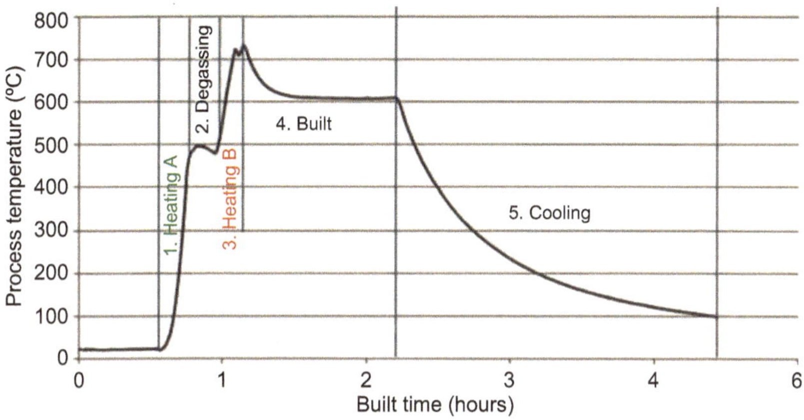

Figure 3.2 Sample diagram of build temperature versus time obtained from the thermocouple located at the bottom of the build plate of the A2 Arcam system [30].

thickness (generally 100 and 50 μm), and additional metal powder is supplied from hoppers and spread/raked over the previously solidified layer. The process is repeated to directly achieve the 3D shape close to that of the imported CAD one [32,34,35].

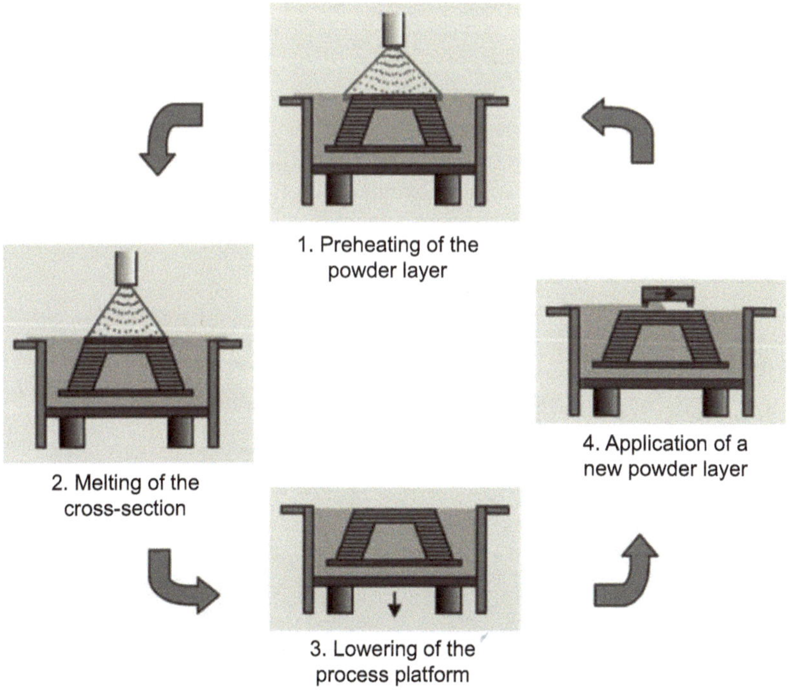

Figure 3.3 Layer-by-layer generation of a component [20].

After the building step, the part is cooled down either under vacuum or helium. The parts will be cleaned from partly molten and remaining powders by powder blasting with the same powder and blowing, and the powders will be recovered to be reused.

In contrast to the SLM method, in which the detection and focus of the photons are conducted by mirrors, in the EBM system, the electron beam is focused and oriented by electromagnetic lenses, which can provide high scanning speeds and a high positioning accuracy with a scan speed of up to 8000 m/s and a high build rate of up to 120 cm^3/h [24,36,37].

It should be mentioned that although there are some differences between the Arcam EBM machine models (for example, recent versions have been equipped with multibeam technology as well as improvements in precision, scanning strategy, and build rate), the steps described above are basically the same.

3.2.2 Electron beam and powder interaction

While both SLM and EBM are complex 3D printing technologies and involve many different physical phenomena, the interactions between the beam and powder layer in EBM are substantially different from SLM, as shown in Figs. 3.4 and 3.5, respectively [38]. Moreover, the penetration depth of an electron beam is several times greater than a laser beam with little change in beam width. This makes it possible to perform a high-density molding, even when using materials with a high melting point of around 2000°C [35,39].

3.2.3 Process parameters

In EBM, a number of process parameters, such as beam speed/speed function, focus offset, beam current (beam power, W), line offset (hatch distance), scanning speed (mm/s), and layer thickness (mm) can be adjusted or optimized to achieve different

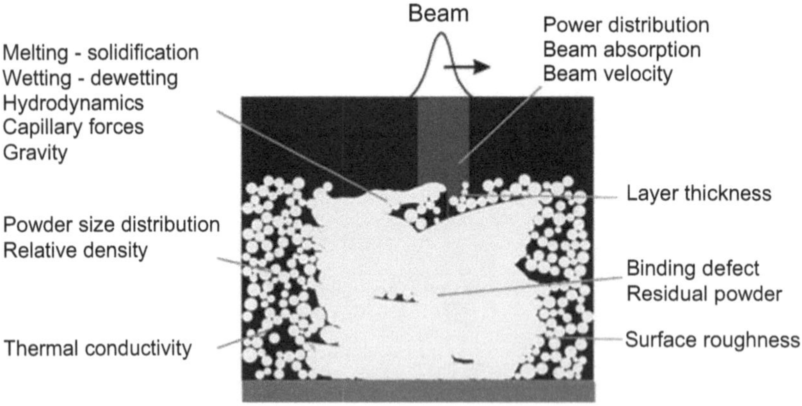

Figure 3.4 Physical aspects of electron beam–powder interaction [40].

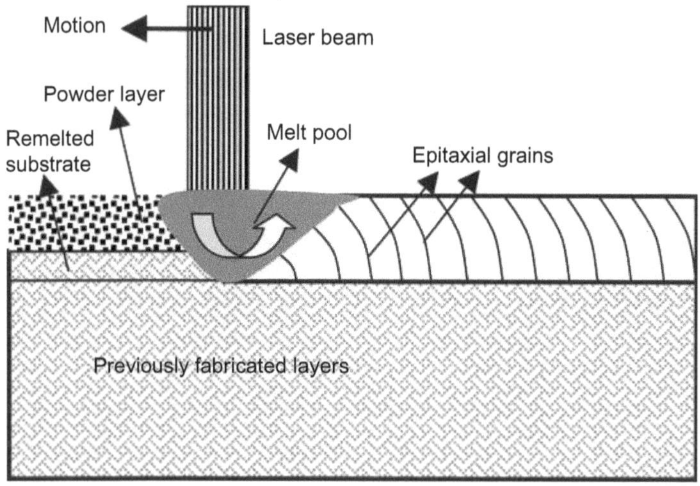

Figure 3.5 Laser powder interaction [38].

microstructures and mechanical properties [33,41]. These parameters affect the energy density, which describes the average applied energy per volume of material during an EBM process.

The experimental quantity of electron beam density (EBD) is described by [42]

$$\mathrm{EBD}\left(\mathrm{J/mm^3}\right) = \frac{\text{Beam power}(W)}{\text{Scan speed}(r) \times \text{hatch distance } (l) \times \text{Layer thickness}(t)} \tag{3.1}$$

where beam power (W) = current (I) × voltage (V). An Arcam machine works at 60 KV so beam power relates directly to current (I).

The influence of energy density on the properties of manufactured parts has been discussed by a number of studies [39,43,44]. One can adjust the process parameters (beam speed, beam current, and focus offset) manually or just use a predefined algorithm recommended by the manufacturer, called the Arcam build theme. The manual method is not used to fabricate bulk parts; however, it is used quite often to produce parts with small features such as fine lattice structures. For example, one of the predefined algorithms is to adjust the beam speed near the edge of a part to prevent overheating, and a sample manual setting for the fabrication of bulk Ti-6Al-4V can use the parameters as beam speed 900 mm/s, beam current 7.5 mA, and focus offset 19 mA [45].

3.2.3.1 Speed function index

Speed function index, or speed factor (SF), is a process variable that relates to the actual beam scanning speed (beam speed) and beam current. Gong et al. [46] studied the effects of different SFs and beam speed on the microstructure of the build parts and showed that to fabricate a part with higher densities, the energy density needs to be increased either by a higher beam power or a lower layer thicknesses. This goal is not reachable just by lowering the spot velocity, as the heat transfer losses are also increased [47]. On the other hand, a greater heat load (J/mm^3) causes more thermal strains and a significant deformation of the layer.

Practically, it is difficult to measure the beam size in the EBM process, and therefore to optimize the beam size or the beam focal conditions, a different focus offset condition should be investigated systematically [31]. However, the scanning speed cannot be directly adjusted, and the SF has little practical use when the process operates using an Arcam build theme [48]. It is dynamically controlled by a "speed function" during the building process to achieve the correct melt pool size.

3.2.3.2 *Focus offset*

Focus offset is a major processing parameter during the EBM process that affects the energy density and can be explained as an offset of the focal plane from its zero position [21]. Increasing the focus offset value increases the beam diameter and leads to a decrease in energy density while a reduction in the focus offset value results in a concentrated electron beam spot and a deeper melting depth [21,49].

3.2.3.3 *Line offset or overlap*

As discussed by Faidel et al. [47], a particular overlap size is available for better surface roughness and a lower porosity with different layer thicknesses. When the overlap is too small (see Fig. 3.6), the metal particles cannot fully fuse together. The stability of the part decreases, and the number and size of the defects increase at once. On the other hand, high overlap leads to the accumulation of heat in the part and thermal deformation of the layer of the part, and this results in more defects.

For example, a typical scan setting would be two contours having a line offset of 0.3 mm. If we consider the melt pool size to be around 1 mm in diameter, it means that the melted profiles will overlap one another by 0.7 mm (see Fig. 3.6).

3.2.3.4 *Beam current*

The selection of the beam current and scan speed depends on the part geometry. Thin-walled delicate features are melted by lower beam currents in the range of 5−10 mA while large and bulky areas might be melted by a higher scanning speed using higher beam currents in the range of 20−30 mA [19].

As discussed by Attar [50], for low scan line energy, the walls are formed with defects. By increasing the input energy, the width of the walls increases, the wall surface quality improves, and the appearance of nonconnected layers is suppressed (see Fig. 3.7).

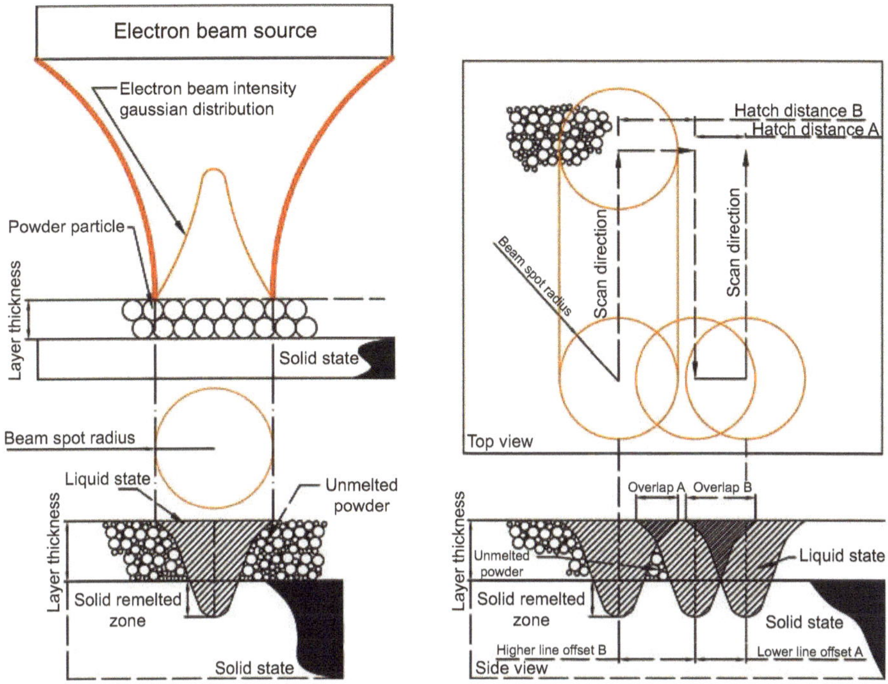

Figure 3.6 Schematic of the electron beam melting process: the effects of line offset and overlap. (It is clear that increasing the line offset from A to B leads to a decrease in the size of overlap B to overlap A, which causes trap of unmelted powder inside the part.)

3.2.3.5 *Preheating temperature*

While there is a general rule to preheat the powder close to the melting point (conventionally 600–900°C, or roughly up to 0.8 T_m during EBM [31]), this step has a significant effect on the final microstructural and mechanical properties of the build part. For Ti-6Al-4V, applying a preheating temperature above 677°C results in a coarse microstructure associated with a decrease in mechanical properties [51].

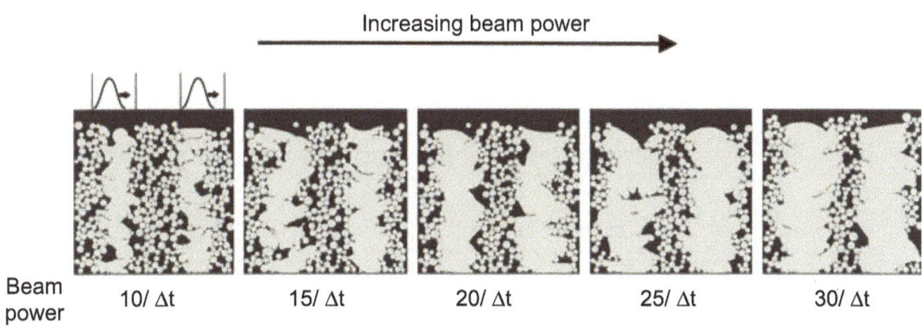

Figure 3.7 Effect of line energy on wall quality (2.0 × 2.0 mm cells), beam width: 350 μm, scan speed: $0.1\Delta x/\Delta t$, layer thickness: 100 μm [50].

3.2.3.6 Layer thickness

One of the key process parameters for all layer-based AM processes is the layer thickness. The layer thickness can be varied between 50 and 150 μm and depends on the type of the machine, powder particle size, and other process parameters. The layer thickness strongly affects the geometric accuracy of the fabricated part [50]. It is also observed that a lower layer thickness exhibits less sensitivity to energy input defects [31] while the quality of the walls decreases intensely with an increasing layer thickness. Furthermore, for layer thicknesses less than 70 μm, the surface quality is not improved further.

To increase the production accuracy and velocity, it is recommended to adapt the powder size in such a way that monolayers of particles are applied during the build process [40]. The typical layer thickness for Arcam machines is accepted to be 100 μm.

3.2.3.7 Scanning strategy

Scanning strategy can be described as a combination of the scanning pattern, which defines the cross-section of the layer, and the related process parameters. The scanning pattern describes the geometric track of the electron beam to melt the cross-section. Layers to be melted are divided into two regions: a polygon line, which describes the boundary of the profile or outlining, and parallel vector lines to fill in the profile that is called the hatch [44]. Fig. 3.8 shows a typical Arcam scanning strategy for fabrication of Ti-6Al-4V bulk samples [52].

The scanning strategy and the scan speed affect the microstructure and porosity of fabricated parts. Puebla et al. [53] showed that the Young's modulus (or stiffness) of the EBM-processed Ti-6Al-4V sample is reduced along with the tensile properties and hardness due to an increase in the residual porosity and the existence of unsintered powder volumes within the layers.

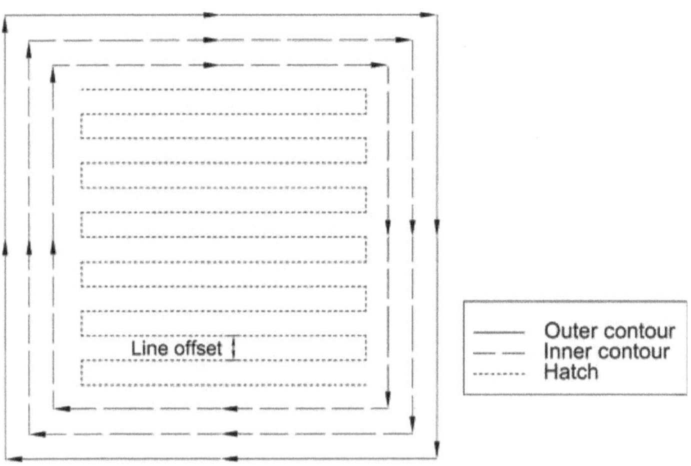

Figure 3.8 Arcam default scanning strategy [52].

3.2.3.8 Powder specification

Similar to any other powder-based production processes, the flowability and packing of the corresponding layer affect the efficiency and the quality of the fabricated part. Powder flowability is a complex issue that is influenced by a number of parameters, including cohesive strength (powder flowability through hoppers), compressibility (bulk density), wall friction, internal friction, electrostatic and van der Waals forces, surface tension, and interlocking characteristics. The flowability improves significantly with sphericity, and crushed and irregular powders result in poor flow behavior. Although bimodal size distribution is ideal for the EBM process because it can promote layer filling and densification and improves beam energy coupling [31], the electrostatic charge would easily influence fine powder and small particles, resulting in the spreading of powder above the building platform [54]. Unfortunately, there is not much research available into the effect of particle morphology on the process efficiency and properties of fabricated parts.

For certain ranges of materials, the Arcam Company provides both the base material powder and the recommended process parameters. Sample powders of Ti-6Al-4V ELI from Arcam have a spherical morphology with a bulk density of no more than 2.7 g/cm^3. Gong et al. [21,55] reported that Arcam powder had a particle size distribution between 46.94 μm (D10) and 99.17 μm (D90) with a mean volume diameter of 72.69 μm (Fig. 3.9). The particle size was almost normally distributed, but a minor percentage of particles with a diameter larger than 100 μm existed.

It should be noted that the EBM process does not change the composition of the powder [56], but during the powder recovery process, the oxygen content of the recycled powder may increase and affect the mechanical properties. For example, for Ti-6Al-4V, as reported by Koike et al. [57], the nominal oxygen contents of recycled powder increased roughly three times of the nominal content, from ~0.12% to 0.34%. Consequently, this might result in higher microhardness and a lower elongation, tensile strength, and yield strength of the build parts.

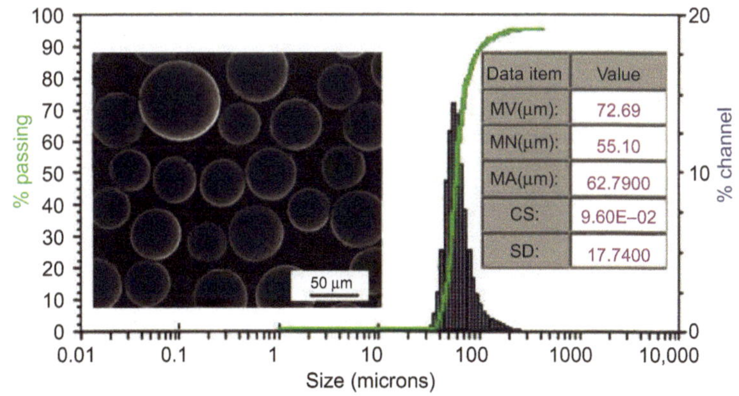

Figure 3.9 Arcam Ti-6Al-4V ELI powder specifications [55]. MV, MN, MA, CS and SD stand for mean diameter of the volume distribution, mean diameter of the number distribution, mean diameter of the area distribution, calculated surface (M^2/cc), and standard deviation in microns, respectively.

3.2.4 Advantages of electron beam melting technology

AM technologies utilizing laser or EBM avoid the need for toolings such as jigs, molds, and fixtures. Also, fabrication of optimized and complex patterns that are especially applicable in automotive, aerospace, and biomedical products becomes much easier. Specifically, EBM can manufacture open-cellular scaffolds with specified stiffness, a free-form exterior, and complex graded interior structures joined to fully dense components, which are hard or impossible to fabricate by conventional cutting tools and technologies [11]. Moreover, it is economical to use EBM for ranges of low to large batches in a short period with low material waste and low residual stress [58]. The EBM process is 95% energy efficient, which is 5−10 times greater than laser technology [34]. Furthermore, EBM technology can be a cost-effective and time-saving method for fabricating a prototype, custom implant, and instrument of orthopedic medical devices [19,59].

3.2.5 Disadvantages of electron beam melting technology

Basically, working with EBM processes is expensive [60], and despite the potential advantages over conventional manufacturing methods, there are a number of critical process deficiencies such as process stability, part defects, and quality variations in the EBM build parts [61].

3.2.5.1 Residual stress

Residual stress is the first potential defect when we use a high-powered energy source. It is observed that application of a high intensity or focused beam and the fast cooling rate in the layered-based AM processes leads to the formation of a large thermal gradient over the part [62] and can lead to bending/deforming during the building process, which influences the dimensional accuracy. While thermal gradients and subsequently residual stresses can be reduced by preheating during EBM, this phase slightly sinters the powder bed and increases its strength, making it difficult to remove the loose powder from the parts. In particular, this becomes an issue in the fabrication of cellular parts [63].

3.2.5.2 Balling

Attar [50] explained the balling issue as the formation of small spheres of solidified materials, having the approximate size of the beam diameter. Melt ball formation (Fig. 3.10(a)), or balling, happens when a low-energy density is transmitted from the electron beam into the powder. For example, a low beam power, high scanning speed, high layer thickness, or high level of oxygen might cause melt pool instability, and then the surface tension of the molten liquid can exceed the wetting ability of the previously solidified layer, forming a melted ball [64,65]. The appearance of melt balls prevents the process from continuation due to a rough and bumpy surface of the top layer [39] and results in the formation of volumetric defects, primarily a lack of fusion and a poor surface finish [50].

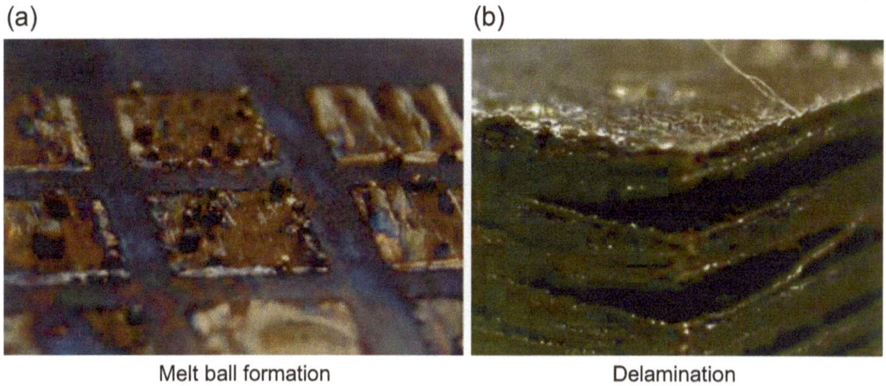

Figure 3.10 (a) Melt ball formation and (b) delamination defects in the electron beam melting process [39].

3.2.5.3 Delamination and cracking

Delamination defects occur when the induced residual stress is greater than the binding abilities between the top layer and the previous one due to a temperature gradient for various reasons (Fig. 3.10(b)), for example, when energy is being inserted into the material in a particularly nonuniform way, such as the selective melting process, or when the design is complicated [50]. While delamination highly depends on the scanning strategy (Fig. 3.11), building over loose powder, creating overhanging surfaces, may also cause delamination, buckling, and warping of cellular structures. This happens due to a significant decrease in the amount of conductive heat transfer in comparison to building over previously melted powder and bulk conductivity [66].

3.2.5.4 Porosity

Gas porosity mainly originates from trapped gas, but larger defects can also arise when there is a lack of powder fusion. The porosity due to trapped gas can be identified by its

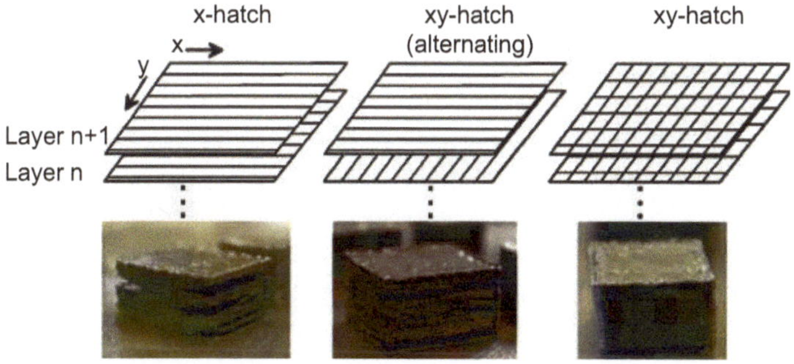

Figure 3.11 Effects of the scanning strategy on layer connection [44].

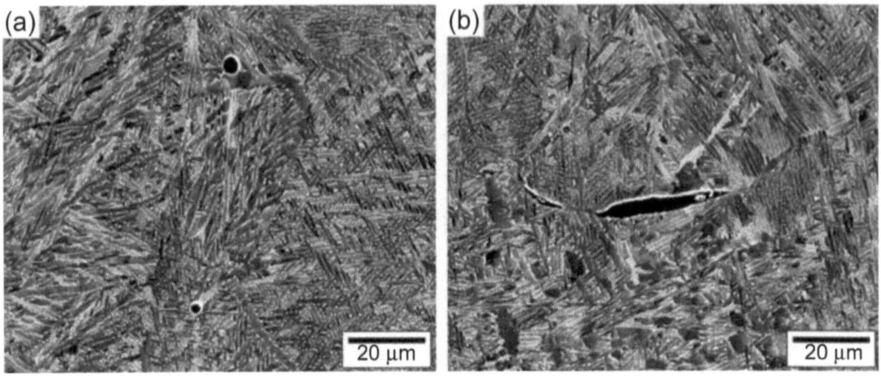

Figure 3.12 Different types of pores: (a) spherical pores due to trap of gas and (b) irregular large pores due to a lack of powder diffusion [52].

rounded (spherical) shape within the compact part, but the porosity due to a lack of powder fusion is larger and irregular, as shown in Fig. 3.12 [21,52,67].

Typically, a higher heat input and a larger overlap of the contour scan lines can reduce the gas porosity defects by allowing for more opportunity for gas bubbles to escape from the bigger melt pool [52].

3.2.5.5 Stair-stepping effect

The stair-stepping effect occurs in all layer-based AM processes and affects the part surfaces that are sloped on the building platform. This effect strongly depends on the orientation of a part surface during the process and has an enormous impact on the resulting surface quality and part accuracy, especially for sloped and round surfaces, in comparison to the CAD model [68].

Attar [50] schematically showed the stair-stepping issue and its effects on surface roughness in layer-based AM (Fig. 3.13). The stair-stepping effect decreases by reducing the layer thickness.

3.2.5.6 Rough surface and accuracy

In EBM, process parameters can noticeably influence the surface roughness of a fabricated part [69]. It is worth noting that the EBM technique produces rougher surfaces with a rippled exterior appearance in comparison to the SLM method (Fig. 3.14) [57].

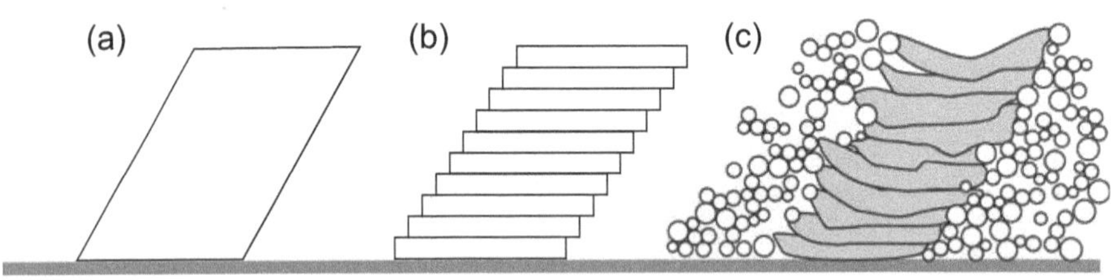

Figure 3.13 Stair-stepping effect: (a) designed or CAD model, (b) sliced model created for additive manufacturing based on layer thickness, and (c) actual results of a fabricated part [50].

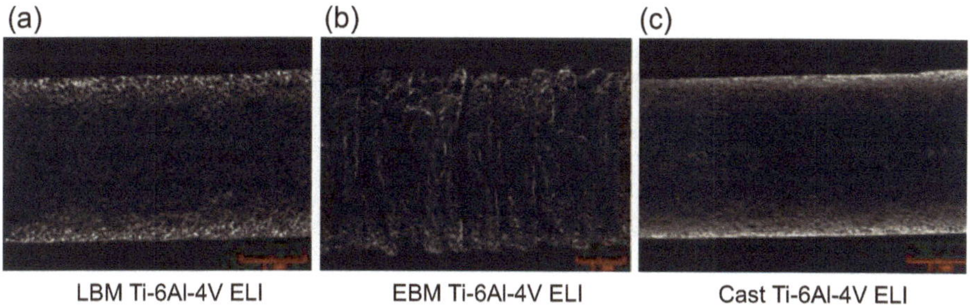

Figure 3.14 Comparison of surface roughness on cylinders made by different methods: (a) laser beam melting, (b) electron beam melting, and (c) casting [57]. *EBM*, electron beam melting; *LBM*, laser beam melting.

The influence of the energy density value on the surface quality of steel (H13) is also illustrated in Fig. 3.15. It can be seen that to achieve a certain surface quality only a range of EBDs should be considered [44].

The EBM method operates by melting and assembling sliced layers of a CAD model on each other; therefore any nonhorizontal, nonupward-facing surface tends to be rough. While the decrease in the layer thickness can increase the surface quality, it requires a longer construction time [50]. Powder size variation can also lead to better compactness and better surface roughness. It is reported that a smaller powder size distribution and a narrower diameter range result in a better surface quality [50], and bimodal powder size distribution can improve the powder packing that enhances beam energy coupling [31] and decreases the surface roughness [50].

Safdar et al. [69] reported that the roughness (Ra) of fabricated Ti-6Al-4V parts increases with an increasing beam current and sample thickness and decreases with an increase in offset focus and scan speed. Also, it is observed that the arrangement of the components or even part orientation inside the chamber can affect the surface roughness by changing the amount of heat accumulation between them [70,71].

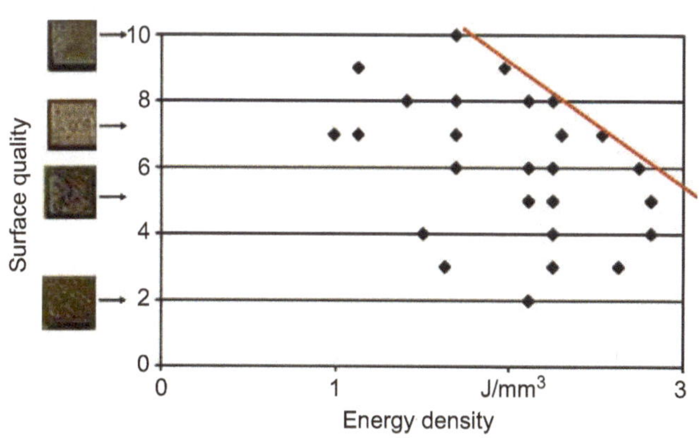

Figure 3.15 Effects of energy density on the surface quality of steel (H13) [44].

However, a poor overall surface finish and defects on bottom-facing surfaces typically occur with the EBM process due to the surface tension of the molten metal [63].

3.3 Achievements in the design and fabrication of biocompatible scaffolds

The success of the biological fixation of implants depends on the topology, architecture, and surface characteristics of the implanted material. The surface characteristics of materials affect the osteoblast adhesion on biomaterials; therefore the porosity and pore size of the biomaterial play a critical role in the bone ingrowth in vivo.

The most important structural characteristic of scaffolds affecting the mechanical properties is the volume fraction of the solid material or the relative density (ρ^*/ρ), which is defined as the ratio of the density of the foam to that of the solid [13]. The fraction of pore space in the scaffold, the porosity, equals $(1-(\rho^*/\rho))$. The porosity can also be expressed as pore volume, pore volume fraction, cumulative pore volume, or pore frequency [7]. The pore diameter is defined as the diameter of a sphere whose volume equals the pore volume.

It is reported that the minimum pore size required for improving osseointegration is 300 μm [72]. It is accepted that the porosity should be above 60%, and pore size ranges of 300–800 μm may have better bone tissue ingrowth [3,14,73,74]. Although a higher porosity allows for increased bone ingrowth [75], the upper limit in porosity and pore size must be defined by constraints that refer to the mechanical properties of the implant related to bone tissue.

Surface roughness is another factor that can affect attachment, proliferation, and differentiation of human fatal osteoblasts [76]. For different Ti-6Al-4V porous surfaces produced by the EBM process, Ponader et al. [69] found that cell proliferation decreased significantly on porous surfaces with higher Ra values, and the best surface roughness for cell proliferation was Ra $\leq$ 24.9 μm.

It is ideal to design a scaffold having a biomimetic structure, but there are still a number of restrictions from manufacturing such as the manufacturability of desired lattice shapes and sizes (e.g., strut size, strut angle [77,78]), desired material with a certain mechanical property, inevitable anisotropy [79], and high cost. So any developments in this area have to be considered as a multiobjective optimization process.

Since many options (different types, shapes, and sizes of unit cells) for a porous structure are possible in the design of biomaterial scaffolds using AM techniques, or specifically EBM, a number of analytical and numerical approaches were developed in the field of biomaterials to investigate and optimize the mechanical properties of cellular structures [80–85].

A simulation of a complex EBM method in which the effects of EBM process parameters on the heat distribution of the build part are considered has also been performed by a number of studies [30,39,40,50,86,87], and extensive studies have been carried out on manufacturing issues in the production of nonstochastic scaffolds using EBM. For example Cansizoglu et al. [78] designed and fabricated regular meshes of

Ti-6Al-4V and showed that the building orientation and angle affect the properties of the lattice structures. They revealed that the smallest strut dimension that can be fabricated without further process optimization is approximately 0.7 mm in diameter and recommended that the strut angle cannot be less than approximately 20 degree when using 0.7 mm-diameter struts. Li et al. [56] fabricated an open and fully interconnected Ti-6Al-4V scaffold with a porosity of 60%, which exhibits a yield strength, Young's modulus, and ultimate compressive strength of 194.6 MPa, 4.25 GPa, and 222.6 MPa, respectively. Murr et al. [88] demonstrated that fully dense monolithic orthopedic device prototypes having complex but regular mesh arrays can be fabricated by EBM from Ti-6Al-4V. Koike et al. [57] compared Ti-6Al-4V ELI specimens fabricated by SLM and EBM methods and indicated that EBM-fabricated parts showed slightly lower strength than SLM and wrought specimens. They made a dumbbell-shaped specimen directly by EBM for tensile tests. Hrabe et al. [89] fabricated porous Ti-6Al-4V scaffolds over a range of relative densities (0.17−0.40) and pore sizes (500−1500 μm). Li et al. [90] have studied the effects of cell shape on the mechanical properties of additively manufactured Ti-6Al-4V meshes with different unit cells (cubic, G7, and rhombic dodecahedron), and porosities ranged from 58% to 88%. Yamanaka et al. [91] developed a weak-textured microstructure of commercially pure titanium (CP-Ti) by EBM and showed that it is possible to use EBM to produce components having isotropic tensile properties, which cannot be obtained by conventional processes.

While the above mentioned studies were performed on the production of general nonstochastic scaffolds, other studies have been carried out in the manufacturing of custom or patient-specific implants and scaffolds. For example, Harrysson et al. [19] and Murr et al. [92] discussed the fabrication of patient-specific knee implants using EBM. Heinl et al. [20,93] fabricated nonstochastic Ti-6Al-4V structures with interconnected macroporosity for biomedical and bone substitute applications. Harrysson et al. [94] also used EBM for fabricating custom hip implants with titanium and predefined mechanical properties. Acetabular cups and heads made from Ti-6Al-4V scaffolds for orthopedic implants have also been described by Marin et al. [60,95].

Chahine et al. [96] fabricated the root-form implant and the abutment as one piece for dental implants using porous Ti-6Al-4V and showed that the mechanical properties of the polished parts were comparable to its wrought counterpart. A cost analysis and fabrication of metal coping of Ti-6Al-4V for the metal ceramic crown restoration in dental applications were performed by Syam et al. [25,26]. They showed that the EBM process could achieve a 100% dense coping, and the production of an enormous number of coping in one EBM cycle makes this process competitive to the conventional methods.

Investigation into the applications of EBM in the manufacture of skull bones and craniofacial scaffolds has also been performed [71,97−99]. For example, Parthasarathy et al. [71] fabricated a range of porous titanium scaffolds and discussed the microstructural and surface characterizations. The components with porosities around 50−70% satisfied the mechanical strength requirements needed for craniofacial applications and showed that the mechanical properties, especially the strength, depend on the strut size apart from the porosity.

Most of the current studies on open cellular nonstochastic porous structures are focused on regular lattice-based geometries, such as cubic [85,100], diamond [83,85], honeycomb [101], pyramidal [102], octahedral [103], rhombic dodecahedron [104], and kelvin polyhedral/tetrakaidecahedron [105]. It has been reported that lattices with straight-edged struts and pores and sharp turns cannot provide a biomorphic environment suitable for cell attachment, migration, and proliferation [106,107]. These scaffolds would not exhibit good manufacturability in SLM and EBM in large unit cell structures (cell sizes of more than 5 mm) consisting of vertical and diagonal straight struts. Moreover, low-volume fractions as resultant long overhangs will lead to thermal deformation [108].

Triply periodic minimal surfaces (TPMSs) have been shown to be a promising approach in the design of scaffolds due to their outstanding mechanical and biological features [84,106,109]. For example, Yan et al. [109] investigated the fabrication of interconnected and high-porosity gyroid and diamond TPMS lattices having pore sizes in the range of 560−1600 μm and 480−1450 μm by the SLM method from Ti-6Al-4V. They found that the TPMS lattices with 80−95% porosity showed a similar porosity with trabecular bone, and the related elastic modulus was in the range of 0.12−1.25 GPa. Also, they indicated that the elastic moduli of the Ti-6Al-4V TPMS lattices having a porosity ranging from 5 to 10% were the same as the modulus of cortical bone.

3.4 Metallurgy and mechanical properties of electron beam melting-manufactured parts

The incremental layer-by-layer melt and solidification process accompanying the laser or electron beam AM of precursor powders differs fundamentally from conventional manufacturing methods. Mechanical properties of parts produced by EBM are intensely dependent on their microstructure, and by adjusting and optimizing beam-scan parameters and scan strategies it is possible to achieve superior microstructural and mechanical properties incrementally rather than by bulk cast or wrought product posttreatment [41,59]. The mechanical properties of Ti-6Al-4V parts manufactured by the EBM method and the minimum requirements of the ASTM standard for surgical implants are listed in Table 3.1. It can be seen that more than the specified requirements are reachable.

Generally in the EBM process, the phase transformation from the liquefied temperature to room temperature happens in three steps:

1. solidification from melt pool temperature (~1800°C) to isothermal hold at a preheating temperature (~700°C),
2. holding of the build at the preheating temperature (~700°C), and
3. slow cooling from the preheating temperature (~700°C) to room temperature.

The solidification rate is determined by process parameters such as beam speed, focus parameters, part geometries, and dimensions as well as the associated heat

Table 3.1 Comparison of some mechanical properties of electron beam melting-manufactured Ti-6Al-4V bulk samples with requirements of ASTM standards for surgical implants

Bulk samples							
Material	**Method**	**YS (MPa)**	**TS (Mpa)**	**EL (%)**	**E (GPa)**	**Hardness (GPa)**	**Remarks and references**
Ti-6Al-4V	EBM	1130	1180	16–25	–	3.6–3.9	Machined [112]
Ti-6Al-4V	EBM	884–939	994–1032	12–14	–	–	Machined [51]
Ti-6Al-4V	EBM	834	950	14	–	3.1	Machined [111]
Ti-6Al-4V ELI	EBM	–	928–1028	14	121	–	As built and polished [96]
Ti-6Al-4V ELI	EBM	930	970	16	120		Arcam [112]
Ti-6Al-4V ELI	Cast	>758	>860	>8	–	–	ASTM F1108 min. requirements [113]
Ti-6Al-4V ELI	Wrought	>795	>860	>10	–	–	ASTM F136 min. requirements [114]
Ti-6Al-4V	Wrought	>869–825	>930–895	>10			ASTM F1472 min. requirements [115]

YS, TS, EL, and E stand for yield strength, tensile strength, elongation, and modulus of elasticity, respectively.

conduction and cooling rates. For example, for Ti-6Al-4V, a variation in the cooling rate promotes α-phase growth and affects the dislocation density and α-to-α' (martensite) phase changes, which cause changes in the mechanical property. Strength and ductility can be improved by fine or equiaxed microstructure while a coarse or lamellar microstructure exhibits decreased strength and ductility.

Moreover, the EBM process shows a directional solidification. For Ti-6Al-4V, it can produce a broad range of characteristic crystallographic phases: α (hcp), β (bcc), γ' (hcp-martensite), and γ'' (fcc-orthorhombic) and phase microstructures, which for conventional wrought and cast billets require complex thermomechanical processing [41,92,116,117]. Safdar et al. [118] observed columnar grains of prior β phase growing along the build direction on EBM-fabricated components from Ti-6Al-4V, and Murr et al. [119] described the columnar architectures in a range of precursor metal powders such as Co-base and Ni-base superalloys as well as Cu.

Murr [41] discussed the metallurgical aspects of AM using EBM on a number of metals and alloys and compared their mechanical properties with samples manufactured by wrought or casting methods. For example, to compare wrought and EBM build Ti-6Al-4V parts, both microstructures are dominated by acicular α-phase (hcp) grains surrounded by β-phase (bcc), which is dark in contrast, although the wrought alloy contains some equiaxed α-grains (see Fig. 3.16). For thin (1 mm)

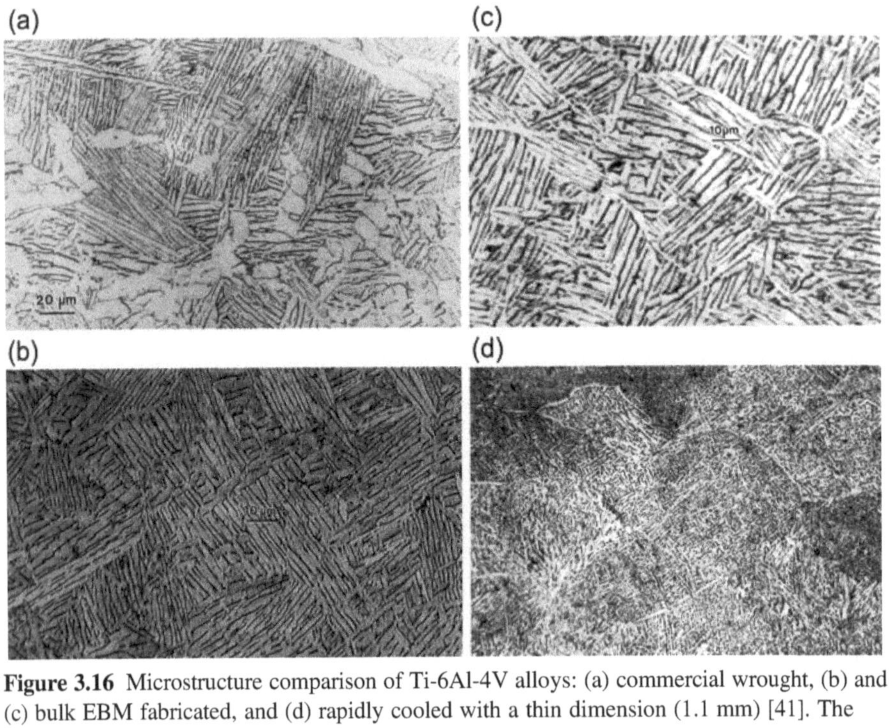

Figure 3.16 Microstructure comparison of Ti-6Al-4V alloys: (a) commercial wrought, (b) and (c) bulk EBM fabricated, and (d) rapidly cooled with a thin dimension (1.1 mm) [41]. The magnification of (c) and (d) is the same.

sample dimensions, a rapid cooling creates α' martensite (hcp) having tiny interphase dimensions [41].

It is also observed that by performing hot isostatic pressing, the microstructure slightly coarsens and results in a minor decrease in strength and a little increase in elongation at the fracture point but significantly improved fatigue life [27,51].

3.5 Overview of challenges and future research directions

EBM processing: while significant advancements have been made in the area of EBM, a number of issues, such as the effect of process parameters and scanning strategies on the mechanical property, lattice design parameters (morphology, lattice structure, size), effects of powder alloying elements, particle size distribution, and spacing issues, are still not fully known. Moreover, the interaction between mechanical properties, bone ingrowth, and manufacturing parameters is not well understood.

Mechanical properties of scaffolds processed by EBM: there is extensive research on the characterization of the mechanical properties of the samples made by EBM; however, most of the research focused only on compressive studies under different loading conditions. Further research is needed in comprehensive numerical and experimental investigations on the mechanical properties such as compression, bending, tension, torsion, wear, and fatigue strength and their anisotropy.

Materials processed by EBM: most of the EBM research in the biomedical field has been carried out on CP-Ti and Ti-6Al-4V using Arcam-provided prealloyed powders and its recommended process parameters. CP-Ti scaffolds may exhibit inadequate mechanical properties while Ti-6Al-4V contains aluminum and vanadium, which are not entirely biocompatible. Therefore EBM of new biocompatible titanium alloys that are free of toxic elements, while also displaying a combination of excellent mechanical properties and corrosion resistance, are highly desirable. This includes research into novel composition design, powder processing, new EBM-processing parameters, and characterization as well as evaluation of microstructure, mechanical properties, corrosion resistance, and in vitro and in vivo biocompatibilities.

Acknowledgments

This research is financially supported by the National Health and Medical Research Council through grant GNT1087290.

References

[1] Weinstein AM, Rome BN, Reichmann WM, Collins JE, Burbine SA, Thornhill TS, et al. Estimating the burden of total knee replacement in the United States. J Bone Joint Surg 2013;95:385–92.

[2] Annual report Australian orthopedic association national joint replacement registry-hip and knee arthroplasty. Adelaide: AOA; 2015.
[3] Nouri A, Hodgson PD, Wen CE. Biomimetic porous titanium scaffolds for orthopaedic and dental applications. Biomimetics Learn Nat 2010;36.
[4] Wen CE, Xiong JY, Li YC, Hodgson PD. Porous shape memory alloy scaffolds for biomedical applications: a review. In: 3rd International symposium on functional materials 2009. ISFM; 2009. Jinju2010.
[5] Wen CE, Yamada Y, Shimojima K, Chino Y, Asahina T, Mabuchi M. Processing and mechanical properties of autogenous titanium implant materials. J Mater Sci Mater Med 2002;13:397−401.
[6] Wen CE, Mabuchi M, Yamada Y, Shimojima K, Chino Y, Asahina T. Processing of biocompatible porous Ti and Mg. Scr Mater 2001;45:1147−53.
[7] Lewis G. Properties of open-cell porous metals and alloys for orthopaedic applications. J Mater Sci Mater Med 2013;24:2293−325.
[8] Bobyn JD, Pilliar RM, Binnington AG, Szivek JA. The effect of proximally and fully porous-coated canine hip stem design on bone modeling. J Orthop Res 1987;5:393−408.
[9] Bobyn JD, Stackpool GJ, Hacking SA, Tanzer M, Krygier JJ. Characteristics of bone ingrowth and interface mechanics of a new porous tantalum biomaterial. J Bone Joint Surg Ser B 1999;81:907−14.
[10] Hacking SA, Bobyn JD, Toh KK, Tanzer M, Krygier JJ. Fibrous tissue ingrowth and attachment to porous tantalum. J Biomed Mater Res 2000;52:631−8.
[11] Murr LE, Gaytan SM, Medina F, Lopez H, Martinez E, MacHado BI, et al. Next-generation biomedical implants using additive manufacturing of complex cellular and functional mesh arrays. Philos Trans R Soc A Math Phys Eng Sci 2010;368:1999−2032.
[12] Gibson LJ. Modelling the mechanical behavior of cellular materials. Mater Sci Eng A 1989;110:1−36.
[13] Gibson LJ, Ashby MF. Cellular solids: structure and properties. 2nd ed., 1st pbk. ed. with corr. ed. Cambridge (New York): Cambridge University Press; 1999.
[14] Wen CE, Yamada Y, Shimojima K, Chino Y, Hosokawa H, Mabuchi M. Novel titanium foam for bone tissue engineering. J Mater Res 2002;17:2633−9.
[15] Ryan G, Pandit A, Apatsidis DP. Fabrication methods of porous metals for use in orthopedic applications. Biomaterials 2006;27:2651−70.
[16] Long M, Rack HJ. Titanium alloys in total joint replacement—a materials science perspective. Biomaterials 1998;19:1621−39.
[17] Niinomi M. Recent metallic materials for biomedical applications. Metall Mater Trans A 2002;33:477−86.
[18] Wang K. The use of titanium for medical applications in the USA. Mater Sci Eng A 1996; 213:134−7.
[19] Harrysson OLA, Cormier DR. Direct fabrication of custom orthopedic implants using electron beam melting technology. Advanced manufacturing technology for medical applications. John Wiley & Sons, Ltd.; 2006. p. 191−206.
[20] Heinl P, Rottmair A, Körner C, Singer RF. Cellular titanium by selective electron beam melting. Adv Eng Mater 2007;9:360−4.
[21] Gong H, Rafi K, Starr T, Stucker B. The effects of processing parameters on defect regularity in Ti-6Al-4V parts fabricated by selective laser melting and electron beam melting. In: 24th International SFF symposium − an additive manufacturing conference, SFF 2013; 2013. p. 424−39.
[22] Cline HE, Anthony TR. Heat treating and melting material with a scanning laser or electron beam. J Appl Phys 1977;48:3895−900.

[23] Larson R. Method and device for producing three-dimensional bodies. Google Patents 1994.
[24] Arcam. Arcam webpage. 2015.
[25] Syam WP, Al-Shehri HA, Al-Ahmari AM, Al-Wazzan KA, Mannan MA. Preliminary fabrication of thin-wall structure of Ti6Al4V for dental restoration by electron beam melting. Rapid Prototyp J 2012;18:230−40.
[26] Syam WP, Al-Ahmari AM, Mannan MA, Al-Shehri HA, Al-Wazzan KA. Metallurgical, accuracy and cost analysis of Ti6Al4V dental coping fabricated by electron beam melting process. Innovative developments in virtual and physical prototyping. CRC Press; 2011. p. 375−83.
[27] Luca F, Emanuele M, Pierfrancesco R, Alberto M. Microstructure and mechanical properties of Ti-6Al-4V produced by electron beam melting of pre-alloyed powders. Rapid Prototyp J 2009;15:171−8.
[28] Murr LE, Gaytan SM, Medina F, Martinez E, Martinez JL, Hernandez DH, et al. Characterization of Ti−6Al−4V open cellular foams fabricated by additive manufacturing using electron beam melting. Mater Sci Eng A 2010;527:1861−8.
[29] Biamino S, Penna A, Ackelid U, Sabbadini S, Tassa O, Fino P, et al. Electron beam melting of Ti−48Al−2Cr−2Nb alloy: microstructure and mechanical properties investigation. Intermetallics 2011;19:776−81.
[30] Neira Arce A. Thermal modeling and Simulation of electron beam melting for rapid prototyping on Ti6Al4V alloys [Ph.D.]. Ann Arbor: North Carolina State University; 2012.
[31] Murr LE, Martinez E, Amato KN, Gaytan SM, Hernandez J, Ramirez DA, et al. Fabrication of metal and alloy components by additive manufacturing: examples of 3D materials science. J Mater Res Technol 2012;1:42−54.
[32] Karlsson J. Optimization of electron beam melting for production of small components in biocompatible titanium grades. 2015.
[33] Denis C, Ola H, Harvey W. Characterization of H13 steel produced via electron beam melting. Rapid Prototyp J 2004;10:35−41.
[34] Hiemenz J. Electron beam melting. Adv Mater Process 2007;165:45−6.
[35] Niinomi M, Narushima T, Nakai M. Advances in metallic biomaterials processing and applications. Berlin, Heidelberg: Springer Berlin Heidelberg; 2015.
[36] Arcam. Arcam A2 catalog. Arcam AB; 2015.
[37] Arcam. Arcam Q10 catalog. Arcam AB; 2015.
[38] Das S. Physical aspects of process control in selective laser sintering of metals. Adv Eng Mater 2003;5:701−11.
[39] Zäh MF, Lutzmann S. Modelling and simulation of electron beam melting. Prod Eng Res Devel 2010;4:15−23.
[40] Carolin K, Andreas B, Elham A. Fundamental consolidation mechanisms during selective beam melting of powders. Model Simul Mater Sci Eng 2013;21:085011.
[41] Murr LE. Metallurgy of additive manufacturing: examples from electron beam melting. Addit Manuf 2015;5:40−53.
[42] Kruth JP, Kumar S, Vaerenbergh JV. Study of laser-sinterability of ferro-based powders. Rapid Prototyp J 2005;11:287−92.
[43] Hrabe N, Quinn T. Effects of processing on microstructure and mechanical properties of a titanium alloy (Ti−6Al−4V) fabricated using electron beam melting (EBM), part 2: energy input, orientation, and location. Mater Sci Eng A 2013;573:271−7.
[44] Zah M, Kahnert M. The effect of scanning strategies on electron beam sintering. Prod Eng Res Devel 2009;3:217−24.

[45] Hrabe NW, Heinl P, Bordia RK, Körner C, Fernandes RJ. Maintenance of a bone collagen phenotype by osteoblast-like cells in 3D periodic porous titanium (Ti-6Al-4V) structures fabricated by selective electron beam melting. Connect Tissue Res 2013;54:351–60.
[46] Gong X, Lydon J, Cooper K, Chou K. Beam speed effects on Ti-6Al-4V microstructures in electron beam additive manufacturing. J Mater Res 2014;29:1951–9.
[47] Faidel D, Jonas D, Natour G, Behr W. Investigation of the selective laser melting process with molybdenum powder. Addit Manuf 2015;8:88–94.
[48] Hrabe N, Quinn T. Effects of processing on microstructure and mechanical properties of a titanium alloy (Ti–6Al–4V) fabricated using electron beam melting (EBM), part 1: distance from build plate and part size. Mater Sci Eng A 2013;573:264–70.
[49] Schwerdtfeger J, Singer RF, Körner C. In situ flaw detection by IR-imaging during electron beam melting. Rapid Prototyp J 2012;18:259–63.
[50] Attar E. Simulation of selective electron beam melting processes. 2011.
[51] Al-Bermani SS, Blackmore ML, Zhang W, Todd I. The origin of microstructural diversity, texture, and mechanical properties in electron beam melted Ti-6Al-4V. Metall Mater Trans A 2010;41:3422–34.
[52] Tammas-Williams S, Zhao H, Léonard F, Derguti F, Todd I, Prangnell PB. XCT analysis of the influence of melt strategies on defect population in Ti–6Al–4V components manufactured by selective electron beam melting. Mater Charact 2015;102:47–61.
[53] Puebla K, Murr LE, Gaytan SM, Martinez E, Medina F, Wicker RB. Effect of melt scan rate on microstructure and macrostructure for electron beam melting of Ti-6Al-4V. Mater Sci Appl 2012;3:259–64.
[54] Kahnert M, Lutzmann S, Zah MF. Layer formations in electron beam sintering. In: 18th Solid freeform fabrication symposium, SFF 2007; 2007. p. 88–99.
[55] Gong H. Generation and detection of defects in metallic parts fabricated by selective laser melting and electron beam melting and their effects on mechanical properties [Electronic Theses and Dissertations. Paper 515]. 2013.
[56] Li X, Wang CT, Zhang WG, Li YC. Properties of a porous Ti-6Al-4V implant with a low stiffness for biomedical application. Proc Inst Mech Eng Part H J Eng Med 2009;223:173–8.
[57] Koike M, Greer P, Owen K, Lilly G, Murr L, Gaytan SM, et al. Evaluation of titanium alloys fabricated using rapid prototyping technologies-electron beam melting and laser beam melting. Materials 2011;4:1776–92.
[58] Murr LE, Gaytan SM, Ramirez DA, Martinez E, Hernandez J, Amato KN, et al. Metal fabrication by additive manufacturing using laser and electron beam melting technologies. J Mater Sci Technol 2012;28:1–14.
[59] Christensen A, Kircher R, Lippincott A. Qualification of electron beam melted (EBM) Ti6AI4V-ELI for orthopedic applications. In: Medical device materials IV: materials and processes for medical devices conference 2007. Palm Desert, CA; 2008. p. 48–53.
[60] Marin E, Lanzutti A, Turchet S, Fusi S, Pressacco M, Fedrizzi L. Structural and mechanical characterization of highly porous biomaterials in commercially pure titanium for orthopedic arthroplasty: trabecular titaniumtm. Metall Ital 2011;103:27–36.
[61] Gong X, Anderson T, Chou K. Review on powder-based electron beam additive manufacturing technology. Manuf Rev 2014;1:2.
[62] Vrancken B, Wauthle R, Kruth JP, Van Humbeeck J. Study of the influence of material properties on residual stress in selective laser melting. In: 24th International SFF symposium – an additive manufacturing conference, SFF 2013; 2013. p. 393–407.

[63] Williams C, Cochran J, Rosen D. Additive manufacturing of metallic cellular materials via three-dimensional printing. Int J Adv Manuf Technol 2011;53:231–9.
[64] Gusarov AV, Yadroitsev I, Bertrand P, Smurov I. Heat transfer modelling and stability analysis of selective laser melting. Appl Surf Sci 2007;254:975–9.
[65] Li R, Liu J, Shi Y, Wang L, Jiang W. Balling behavior of stainless steel and nickel powder during selective laser melting process. Int J Adv Manuf Technol 2012;59:1025–35.
[66] Kruth JP, Mercelis P, Van Vaerenbergh J, Craeghs T. Feedback control of selective laser melting. In: Proceedings of the 3rd international conference on advanced research in virtual and rapid prototyping: virtual and rapid manufacturing advanced research virtual and rapid prototyping; 2007. p. 521–7.
[67] Gaytan SM, Murr LE, Medina F, Martinez E, Lopez MI, Wicker RB. Advanced metal powder based manufacturing of complex components by electron beam melting. Mater Technol 2009;24:180–90.
[68] Arabnejad S, Burnett Johnston R, Pura JA, Singh B, Tanzer M, Pasini D. High-strength porous biomaterials for bone replacement: a strategy to assess the interplay between cell morphology, mechanical properties, bone ingrowth and manufacturing constraints. Acta Biomater 2016, 345–356.
[69] Safdar A, He HZ, Wei LY, Snis A, Chavez De Paz LE. Effect of process parameters settings and thickness on surface roughness of EBM produced Ti-6Al-4V. Rapid Prototyp J 2012;18:401–8.
[70] Jamshidinia M, Kovacevic R. The influence of heat accumulation on the surface roughness in additive manufacturing by electron beam melting® (EBM). In: Proceedings – ASPE 2014 spring topical meeting: dimensional accuracy and surface finish in additive manufacturing; 2014. p. 45–50.
[71] Parthasarathy J, Starly B, Raman S, Christensen A. Mechanical evaluation of porous titanium (Ti6Al4V) structures with electron beam melting (EBM). J Mech Behav Biomed Mater 2010;3:249–59.
[72] Frosch K-H, Barvencik F, Viereck V, Lohmann CH, Dresing K, Breme J, et al. Growth behavior, matrix production, and gene expression of human osteoblasts in defined cylindrical titanium channels. J Biomed Mater Res Part A 2004;68A:325–34.
[73] Karageorgiou V, Kaplan D. Porosity of 3D biomaterial scaffolds and osteogenesis. Biomaterials 2005;26:5474–91.
[74] Berner A, Woodruff MA, Lam CXF, Arafat MT, Saifzadeh S, Steck R, et al. Effects of scaffold architecture on cranial bone healing. Int J Oral Maxillofac Surg 2014;43:506–13.
[75] Li JP, Habibovic P, van den Doel M, Wilson CE, de Wijn JR, van Blitterswijk CA, et al. Bone ingrowth in porous titanium implants produced by 3D fiber deposition. Biomaterials 2007;28:2810–20.
[76] Ponader S, Vairaktaris E, Heinl P, Cv W, Rottmair A, Körner C, et al. Effects of topographical surface modifications of electron beam melted Ti-6Al-4V titanium on human fetal osteoblasts. J Biomed Mater Res Part A 2008;84A:1111–9.
[77] Williams C. Design and development of a layer-based additive manufacturing process for the realization of metal parts of designed mesostructure. Georgia Institute Technology; 2008.
[78] Cansizoglu O, Harrysson O, Cormier D, West H, Mahale T. Properties of Ti–6Al–4V non-stochastic lattice structures fabricated via electron beam melting. Mater Sci Eng A 2008;492:468–74.
[79] Yamaguchi M, Johnson DR, Lee HN, Inui H. Directional solidification of TiAl-base alloys. Intermetallics 2000;8:511–7.

[80] Li K, Gao XL, Subhash G. Effects of cell shape and cell wall thickness variations on the elastic properties of two-dimensional cellular solids. Int J Solids Struct 2005;42:1777–95.
[81] Li K, Gao XL, Subhash G. Effects of cell shape and strut cross-sectional area variations on the elastic properties of three-dimensional open-cell foams. J Mech Phys Solids 2006; 54:783–806.
[82] Luxner MH, Stampfl J, Pettermann HE. Numerical simulations of 3D open cell structures – influence of structural irregularities on elasto-plasticity and deformation localization. Int J Solids Struct 2007;44:2990–3003.
[83] Ahmadi SM, Campoli G, Amin Yavari S, Sajadi B, Wauthle R, Schrooten J, et al. Mechanical behavior of regular open-cell porous biomaterials made of diamond lattice unit cells. J Mech Behav Biomed Mater 2014;34:106–15.
[84] Kadkhodapour J, Montazerian H, Raeisi S. Investigating internal architecture effect in plastic deformation and failure for TPMS-based scaffolds using simulation methods and experimental procedure. Mater Sci Eng C 2014;43:587–97.
[85] Kadkhodapour J, Montazerian H, Darabi AC, Anaraki AP, Ahmadi SM, Zadpoor AA, et al. Failure mechanisms of additively manufactured porous biomaterials: effects of porosity and type of unit cell. J Mech Behav Biomed Mater 2015;50:180–91.
[86] Mohammadhosseini A, Masood SH, Fraser D, Jahedi M. Residual stresses and deformations in electron beam melting process using finite element analysis. Adv Mater Res 2012:789–92.
[87] Jamshidinia M, Kong F, Kovacevic R. Numerical modeling of heat distribution in the electron beam melting® of Ti-6Al-4V. J Manuf Sci Eng 2013;135:061010.
[88] Murr LE, Gaytan SM, Medina F, Lopez MI, Martinez E, Wicker RB. Additive layered manufacturing of reticulated Ti-6Al-4V biomedical mesh structures by electron beam melting. In: 25th Southern Biomedical Engineering Conference 2009. Miami, FL; 2009. p. 23–8.
[89] Hrabe NW, Heinl P, Flinn B, Körner C, Bordia RK. Compression-compression fatigue of selective electron beam melted cellular titanium (Ti-6Al-4V). J Biomed Mater Res Part B Appl Biomater 2011;99 B:313–20.
[90] Li SJ, Xu QS, Wang Z, Hou WT, Hao YL, Yang R, et al. Influence of cell shape on mechanical properties of Ti-6Al-4V meshes fabricated by electron beam melting method. Acta Biomater 2014;10:4537–47.
[91] Yamanaka K, Saito W, Mori M, Matsumoto H, Chiba A. Preparation of weak-textured commercially pure titanium by electron beam melting. Addit Manuf 2015, 105–109.
[92] Murr LE, Amato KN, Li SJ, Tian YX, Cheng XY, Gaytan SM, et al. Microstructure and mechanical properties of open-cellular biomaterials prototypes for total knee replacement implants fabricated by electron beam melting. J Mech Behav Biomed Mater 2011;4: 1396–411.
[93] Heinl P, Müller L, Körner C, Singer R, Müller F. Cellular Ti–6Al–4V structures with interconnected macro porosity for bone implants fabricated by selective electron beam melting. Acta Biomater 2008;4:1536–44.
[94] Harrysson O, Hosni Y, Nayfeh J. Custom-designed orthopedic implants evaluated using finite element analysis of patient-specific computed tomography data: femoral-component case study. BMC Musculoskelet Disord 2007;8.
[95] Marin E, Fusi S, Pressacco M, Paussa L, Fedrizzi L. Characterization of cellular solids in Ti6Al4V for orthopedic implant applications: trabecular titanium. J Mech Behav Biomed Mater 2010;3:373–81.
[96] Chahine G, Koike M, Okabe T, Smith P, Kovacevic R. The design and production of Ti-6Al-4V ELI customized dental implants. JOM 2008;60:50–5.

[97] Parthasarathy J. In: Raman S, Starly B, Shehab R, Landers T, Siddique Z, editors. Design, analysis and fabrication of porous titanium implants using electron beam melting for craniofacial applications; 2009 [ProQuest Dissertations Publishing].
[98] Parthasarathy J, Starly B, Raman S. A design for the additive manufacture of functionally graded porous structures with tailored mechanical properties for biomedical applications. J Manuf Process 2011;13:160–70.
[99] Parthasarathy J. 3D modeling, custom implants and its future perspectives in craniofacial surgery. Ann Maxillofac Surg 2014;4:9–18.
[100] Campoli G, Borleffs MS, Amin Yavari S, Wauthle R, Weinans H, Zadpoor AA. Mechanical properties of open-cell metallic biomaterials manufactured using additive manufacturing. Mater Des 2013;49:957–65.
[101] Babaee S, Jahromi BH, Ajdari A, Nayeb-Hashemi H, Vaziri A. Mechanical properties of open-cell rhombic dodecahedron cellular structures. Acta Mater 2012;60: 2873–85.
[102] Ptochos E, Labeas G. Shear modulus determination of cuboid metallic open-lattice cellular structures by analytical, numerical and homogenisation methods. Strain 2012; 48:415–29.
[103] Sun J, Yang Y, Wang D. Mechanical properties of Ti-6Al-4V octahedral porous material unit formed by selective laser melting. Adv Mech Eng 2012;4.
[104] Horn TJ, Harrysson OLA, Marcellin-Little DJ, West HA, Lascelles BDX, Aman R. Flexural properties of Ti6Al4V rhombic dodecahedron open cellular structures fabricated with electron beam melting. Addit Manuf 2014;1–4:2–11.
[105] Zargarian A, Esfahanian M, Kadkhodapour J, Ziaei-Rad S. Effect of solid distribution on elastic properties of open-cell cellular solids using numerical and experimental methods. J Mech Behav Biomed Mater 2014;37:264–73.
[106] Rajagopalan S, Robb RA. Schwarz meets Schwann: design and fabrication of biomorphic and durataxic tissue engineering scaffolds. Med Image Anal 2006;10:693–712.
[107] Spalazzi JP, Dionisio KL, Jie J, Lu HH. Osteoblast and chondrocyte interactions during coculture on scaffolds. Eng Med Biol Mag IEEE 2003;22:27–34.
[108] Yan C, Hao L, Hussein A, Raymont D. Evaluations of cellular lattice structures manufactured using selective laser melting. Int J Mach Tools Manuf 2012;62:32–8.
[109] Yan C, Hao L, Hussein A, Young P. Ti–6Al–4V triply periodic minimal surface structures for bone implants fabricated via selective laser melting. J Mech Behav Biomed Mater 2015;51:61–73.
[110] Murr LE, Esquivel EV, Quinones SA, Gaytan SM, Lopez MI, Martinez EY, et al. Microstructures and mechanical properties of electron beam-rapid manufactured Ti–6 Al–4V biomedical prototypes compared to wrought Ti–6Al–4V. Mater Charact 2009; 60:96–105.
[111] Tan X, Kok Y, Tan YJ, Descoins M, Mangelinck D, Tor SB, et al. Graded microstructure and mechanical properties of additive manufactured Ti-6Al-4V via electron beam melting. Acta Mater 2015;97:1–16.
[112] Arcam. Ti6Al4V ELI titanium alloy catalog. 2016.
[113] ASTM F110. Standard specification for Titanium-6Aluminum-4Vanadium alloy castings for surgical implants. West Conshohocken (PA): ASTM International; 2014.
[114] ASTM F136. Standard specification for wrought Titanium-6Aluminum-4Vanadium ELI (extra low interstitial) alloy for surgical implant applications. West Conshohocken (PA): ASTM International; 2013.

[115] ASTM F1472-14. Standard specification for wrought Titanium-6Aluminum-4Vanadium alloy for surgical implant applications (UNS R56400). West Conshohocken (PA): ASTM International; 2014.

[116] Murr LE, Quinones S, Gaytan SM, Lopez MI, Rodela A, Martinez EY, et al. Microstructure and mechanical behavior of Ti−6Al−4V produced by rapid-layer manufacturing, for biomedical applications. J Mech Behav Biomed Mater 2009;2:20−32.

[117] Murr LE, Gaytan S, Medina F, Martinez E, Hernandez DH, Martinez L, et al. Effect of build parameters and build geometries on residual microstructures and mechanical properties of Ti-6Al-4V components built by electron beam melting (EBM). In: 20th Annual International Solid Freeform Fabrication Symposium, SFF 2009; 2009. p. 374−97.

[118] Safdar A, Wei LY, Snis A, Lai Z. Evaluation of microstructural development in electron beam melted Ti-6Al-4V. Mater Charact 2011;65:8−15.

[119] Murr LE, Martinez E, Gaytan S, Ramirez D. Contributions of light microscopy to contemporary materials characterization: the new directional solidification. Metallogr Microstruct Anal 2012;1:45−58.

Titanium foam for bone tissue engineering

4

T. Matsushita [1], S. Fujibayashi [2], T. Kokubo [1]
[1]Chubu University, Kasugai, Aichi, Japan; [2]Kyoto University, Kyoto, Japan

4.1 Introduction

Attempts have been made to use a variety of materials for tissue engineering scaffolds, including organic polymers, ceramics, and metals. Organic polymers and ceramics have been mainly used for biodegradable scaffolds, while metals have been used for load-bearable scaffolds. In terms of the metals used for implants, stainless steel, Co–Cr–Mo alloys, and titanium (Ti) metal and its alloys have been mainly used because of their high chemical durability and mechanical strength. Among them, Ti metal and its alloys exhibit better biological compatibility with living tissue as well as having an elastic modulus close to that of bone tissue [1,2]. In particular, when a large amount of pores is introduced into them, their elastic modulus approaches that of bone tissue, resulting in better mechanical compatibility. In addition, it was found that Ti metal and its alloys can exhibit osteoconductivity, bone formation in contact with bone, and osteoinductiviy, ectopic bone formation, when subjected to certain chemical and heat treatments, as described in Chapter 6. Therefore Ti foam is expected to play an important role in bone tissue engineering.

A porous layer can be induced to form on Ti or its alloys by fiber sintering [3], plasma spraying of Ti particles, or certain other methods. This porous layer forms on medical devices such as hip joints and is useful for fixing medical devices to the surrounding bone by a mechanical interlocking mechanism. When the porous layer is subjected to chemical and heat treatments for inducing bioactivity, the hip joint becomes tightly bonded to the surrounding bone. Such bioactive hip joints have been clinically used in Japan since 2007, as described in Chapter 6.

In addition, a large volume, 3D porous Ti body may also be used as a prosthesis for large bone defects in orthopedic and craniomaxillofacial surgery. Such devices require an external structure that exactly fits defects of complex shape and must also have an internal pore structure that is regulated in terms of size, arrangement, and connectivity so as to have mechanical and biological properties compatible with the surrounding tissue.

3D Ti foams have been fabricated mainly by a sintering of metallic powders containing volatile materials [4,5]. This technique is simple, but it is not easily applied to the fabrication of a device having a complex outer form. Additive manufacturing methods such as selective laser melting (SLM) and selective electron beam melting have been developed [6–8]. By these techniques, even devices with a complex outer form and a tightly regulated internal structure are easily fabricated.

Metallic Foam Bone. http://dx.doi.org/10.1016/B978-0-08-101289-5.00004-4

The present authors also fabricated Ti foams for spinal interbody fusion by using these two types of techniques and subjected them to chemical and heat treatments for inducing their bioactivity. The resultant products were implanted into rabbit tibia in order to evaluate bioactivities such as bone bonding and osteoconductivity and were implanted into the muscle of a dog to evaluate their oeteoinductivities. On the basis of these results, spinal fusion devices made of Ti foam were first applied to the canine spine and then five patients.

The results of these trials are provided in the following.

4.2 Materials

4.2.1 Titanium foam prepared by the powder sintering method

4.2.1.1 Method

In this technique, Ti metal powders are mixed with granules of volatile material as a space holder at an appropriate ratio, pressed into a mold, and finally heat-treated, as shown in Fig. 4.1. Commercially pure Ti metal powders less than 45 μm in size and 30 μm in average size, which were prepared by gas atomization, were used in our experiments. Although various kinds of volatile materials, such as ammonium hydrogen carbonate [4] and wax [9], can be used as the space holder, crushed granules of ammonium hydrogen carbonate 250–500 or 500–1400 μm in size were used in our experiments. The mixture of the Ti metal powder and granules of ammonium hydrogen carbonate was pressed in a mold and heat-treated for 2 h at various temperatures ranging from 1200–1400°C under a 10^{-5} Torr vacuum [10]. The ammonium hydrogen carbonate was evaporated during the heat treatment, leaving connected pores in which the size was determined by the size of the granules.

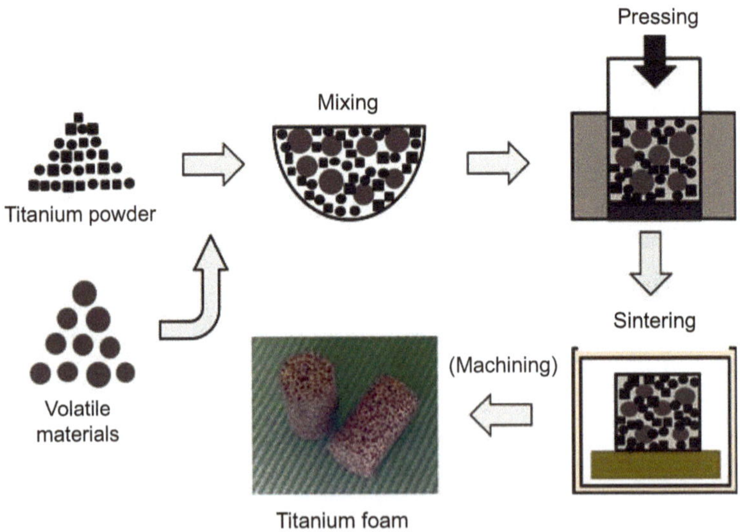

Figure 4.1 Fabrication of titanium (Ti) foam by the powder sintering method.

4.2.1.2 Structure

Fig. 4.2 shows scanning electron micrographs under different magnitudes of a fractured surface of Ti foam prepared by a powder sintering method using a space holder 250−500 μm in size. Macropores 250−500 μm in size as well as middle-sized pores approximately 50 μm in size are evident in the lower magnification on the left. In addition, a middle-sized pore is observed at the bottom of the macropore, and micropores are observable in the cell wall in the higher magnification photograph on the right. The macropores are connected through the middle-sized pores. The amount of interconnected pores decreased with an increasing Ti content.

Computerized tomography (CT) images of cross-sections of the Ti foam prepared by the powder sintering method using different space holders 500−1400 μm in size are shown in Fig. 4.3. The gray tone image shows the Ti metal, and the black tone image shows the macropores connected by channels more than 50 μm in size [11]. The white

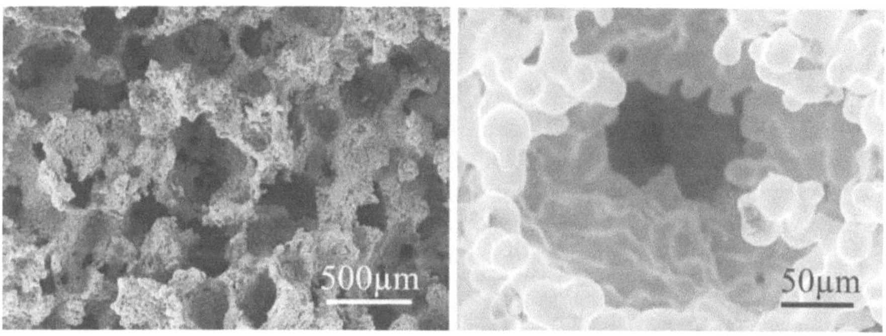

Figure 4.2 Scanning electron micrograph images of sintered foam made of commercially pure titanium (Ti) under different magnifications.

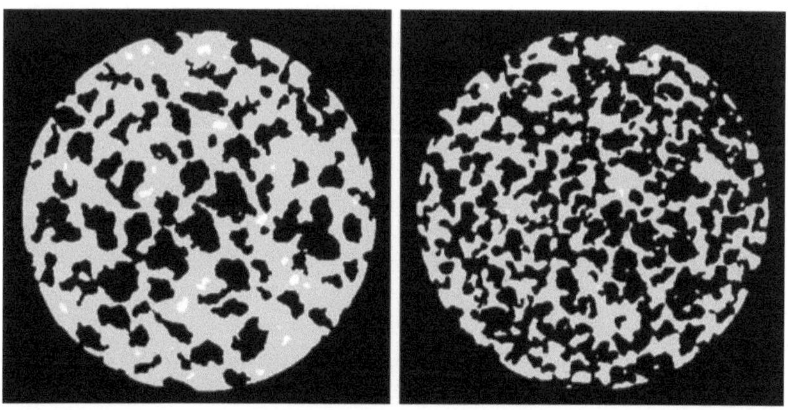

Figure 4.3 Computerized tomography images of sintered titanium (Ti) foam with a porosity of 46.3% (left) and 56.3% (right). The black color in the circle shows pores connected by channels that are more than 50 μm in size.

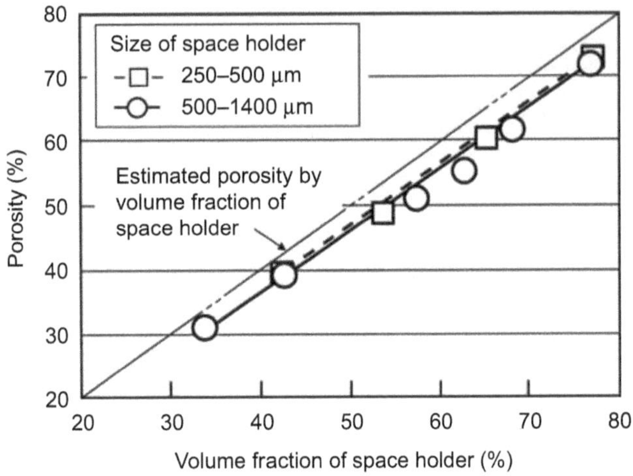

Figure 4.4 The effect of the volume fraction of the space holder on porosity.

tone image with isolated small spots shows closed pores. The amount of interconnected pores increased with an increasing amount of the space holder.

The porosity of the obtained Ti foam was determined by the size and weight of the sintered body. The relative Ti foam porosity prepared by the powder sintering method using space holders of different size is plotted in Fig. 4.4 against the volume fractions of the space holder in the starting mixtures. It can be seen from Fig. 4.4 that the porosity of the Ti foam increases in proportion to the volume of the space holder fraction, irrespective of its size. However, the measured porosities were lower than the values estimated from the volume fraction of the space holder by 4–5%.

The average macropore size determined by CT imaging of the Ti foam sintered at 1400°C for 2 h was 268 μm when 69% of the space holder granules were 250–500 μm in size, while it was 333 μm on average when 70% of the space holder granules were 500–1400 μm in size. The pore size increased with the increasing size of the space holder granules but only slightly. The porosity and the pore size of the Ti foam decreased with increasing temperature and the time allowed for the heat treatment. Fig. 4.5 shows some examples of Ti foam containing pores of different volumes and sizes prepared by the powder sintering method.

4.2.2 Titanium foam prepared by the selective laser melting method

4.2.2.1 Method

As described in Section 4.2.1, Ti foam with pores of different volumes and sizes can be easily fabricated by the powder sintering method. However, this method is not readily applicable to devices with complex outer forms. In contrast with this, the SLM method not only can be easily applied to even complex outer forms, but it is also able to control the complex internal porous structure.

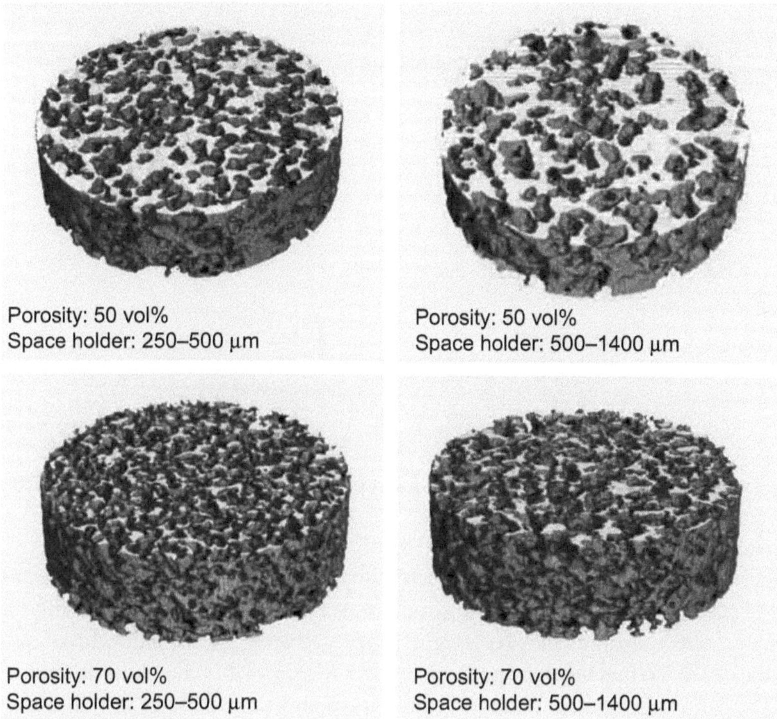

Figure 4.5 Titanium (Ti) foams containing different amounts of connected pores in different sizes that were fabricated by the powder sintering method using different volumes and sizes of space holders.

Fig. 4.6 shows Ti foam fabrication carried out by the SLM method. In this method, a 3D image of the target foam is horizontally sliced into thin layers of 2D images. According to this sliced data, laser beam scans were performed on the Ti metal powder layer sprinkled on a table. As a result, the metal powders are selectively melted and solidified, forming a 2D profile of one cross-section. In the next step, the platform moves vertically downward, allowing the deposition of an unmelted Ti powder layer. Again the laser beam selectively melts the second layer, and this process is continued repeatedly to construct the final 3D structure. In this process, the ratio of the laser beam power to its scan speed is required to be sufficiently high for complete melting of the Ti powders. For example, it should be larger than 0.5 W/mm/s for making a dense Ti cube $9 \times 9 \times 9$ mm^3 in size [12]. Various types of Ti foams fabricated by SLM methods in our laboratory are shown in Fig. 4.7. They were fabricated using an SLM apparatus (EOSINT M 270) and commercially pure Ti powders $\leq$45 μm in grain size of Grade 2. The power of the laser beam was 120 W and its scanning speed was 200 mm/s. The scanning interval was 180 mm and the beam offset was 180 μm [12].

4.2.2.2 Structure

In the powder sintering method, the volume and size of the pores can be controlled by the volume and size of the space holder material, but the shape and spatial arrangement of the pores cannot be controlled. In contrast, in the case of SLM, not only the volume

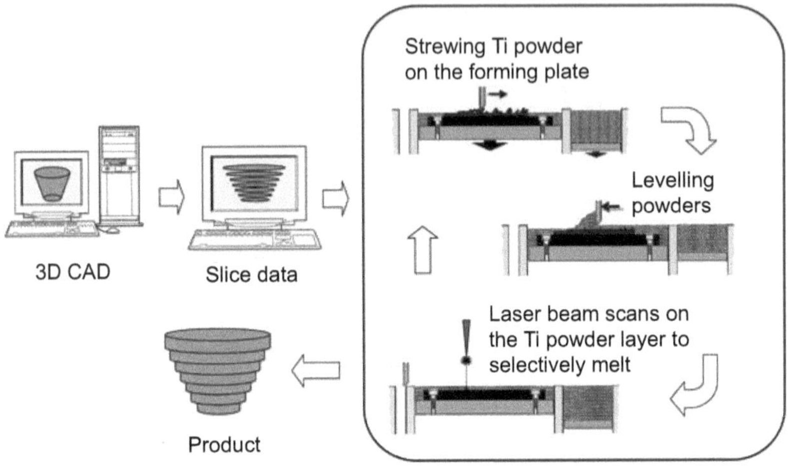

Figure 4.6 The fabrication of titanium (Ti) foam by the selective laser melting method.

and size but also the shape and spatial are controllable based on the requirements of the designed structure. For example, the structure of a foam containing uniformly distributed interconnected pores can be roughly approximated by a diamond-like structure consisting of a connected tetrapod, as shown in Fig. 4.8. The volume and size of the pores can be varied by changing the length and the diameter of the arm of the tetrapod. With increasing arm diameter, both the volume and size of the pores decrease. An increase in the arm length increases the pore size, while a decrease in the arm length decreases it, without changing the pore volume. Table 4.1 shows the relative pore size and porosity of Ti foams fabricated by the SLM method in our laboratory, which were originally designed to be 900, 600, or 300 μm in pore size and 65% in porosity. The obtained pore sizes were larger than the designed values by 2–14%. The obtained porosities were larger or smaller than the designed values by

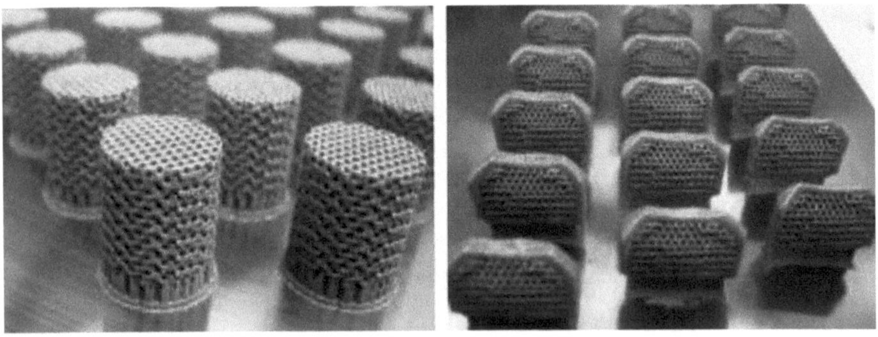

Figure 4.7 Cylindrical foams (left) and interbody spinal fusion devices (right) fabricated using the selective laser melting method.

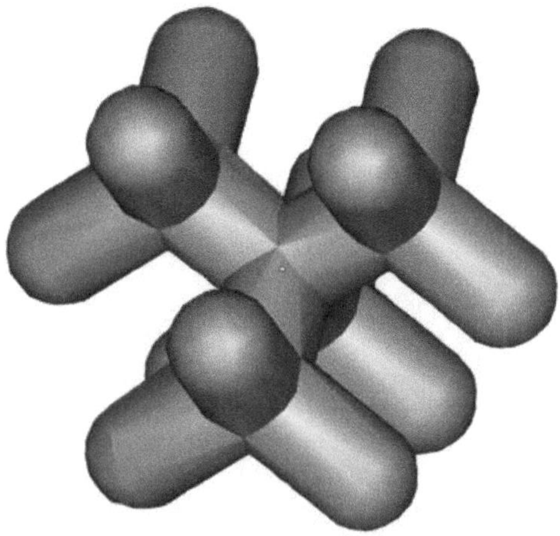

Figure 4.8 A porous structure unit having four cylindrical struts, named the diamond structure.

1.5–5%. The deviation of the obtained values from the designed values may be minimized by modifying the fabrication conditions.

One problem with the SLM method is the formation of an incomplete melting zone around the melted portion. The central part of the strut is completely melted by laser beam irradiation. However, an incompletely melted zone inevitably forms at the periphery of the melted part, as shown in Fig. 4.9. The partially melted Ti particles are loosely bonded to the melted central portion of the strut in the incompletely melted zone. If the fabricated foam is heat-treated at approximately 1300°C in an argon gas atmosphere, the partially molten Ti particles are fairly coagulated, resulting in a smoother surface [12].

4.3 Mechanical properties of titanium foams

4.3.1 Titanium foam prepared by the powder sintering method

Fig. 4.10 presents the relative compressive strength and porosity of Ti foams fabricated by the powder sintering method as a function of the sintering temperature.

Table 4.1 Comparison of pore size and porosity of foams fabricated by the selective laser melting method with those of designed

	Pore size (μm)		Porosity (%)	
Specimen	**Designed**	**Fabricated**	**Designed**	**Fabricated**
(A)	900	919	65.5	63.5
(B)	600	627	65.5	66.6
(C)	300	343	65.5	59.8

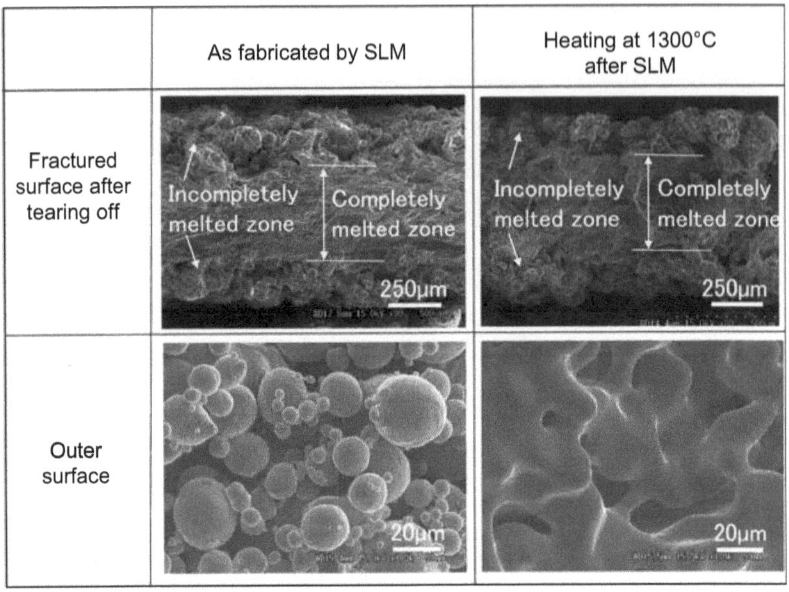

Figure 4.9 Scanning electron micrograph images of outer and fractured surfaces of a sheet fabricated using the selective laser melting method (SLM).

The compressive strengths were measured for cylindrical specimens 6 mm in diameter and 6 mm in length at a crosshead speed of 1 mm/min, according to ISO 13314. The 0.2% yield strength was taken as the compressive strength. It is evident from Fig. 4.10 that the compressive strength of the Ti foam increases with increases in the sintering temperature, while the porosity decreases.

Fig. 4.11 shows the 0.2% yield strength of Ti foams fabricated by the powder sintering method, where Ti powders of Grade 2 (A) or 3 (B), containing different amounts

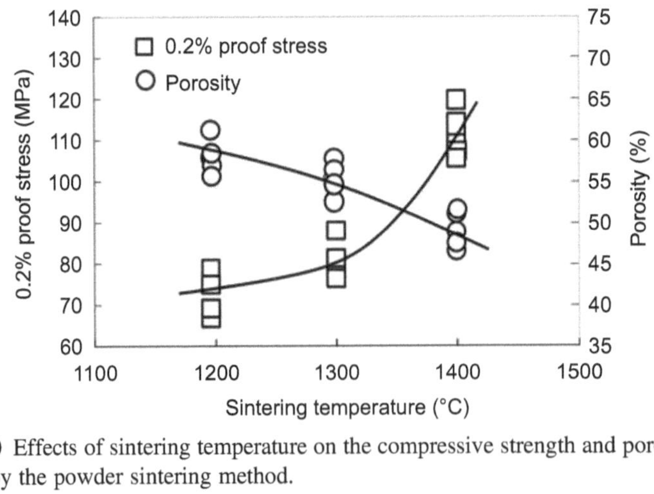

Figure 4.10 Effects of sintering temperature on the compressive strength and porosity of foam fabricated by the powder sintering method.

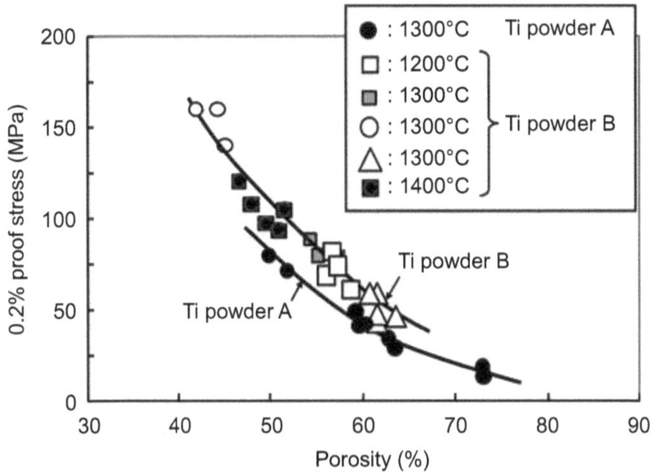

Figure 4.11 Strength of commercially pure titanium (Ti) foams manufactured by powder sintering at elevated temperatures.

of space holders, were sintered at different temperatures as a function of their porosity. It can be seen from Fig. 4.11 that the relative compressive strength of the Ti foams is determined by the amount of the space holder, but not by the sintering temperature, and that for both the A and B powders the compressive strength decreased with increasing porosity, although the decrease in A was a little lower than for the latter. This might be attributed to a higher amount of impurities, such as oxygen and iron, in powder B.

The elastic modulus of dense Ti metal is approximately 100 GPa, which is much higher than that of human cortical bone at 15–20 GPa. This difference in the elastic modulus causes abnormal stress on the surrounding bone so as to make the implant fixation unstable. The elastic modulus of Ti foams can be decreased by increasing the porosity, reaching 10 to 5 GPa at the porosity of 45–55%, as shown in Fig. 4.12. Therefore Ti foams exhibit a better compatibility to the bone mechanically than the dense titanium metal foam.

4.3.2 Titanium foam prepared by the selective laser melting method

The mechanical strength of the foams that were fabricated by the SLM method having different structures is shown in Fig. 4.13 as a function of the porosity. The relative mechanical strength of the foams fabricated by powder sintering is also shown in Fig. 4.13 for comparison [13]. Number 1 represents the data for the foams consisting of lattice structures with different wall thicknesses larger than 1 mm. Number 2 represents the data on a porous specimen designed by modifying a CT image of a cancellous bone of a 48-year-old female. Number 3 is that of another cancellous bone of a 48-year-old female. Number 4 is the data on the stacking of a hollow cubic unit cell.

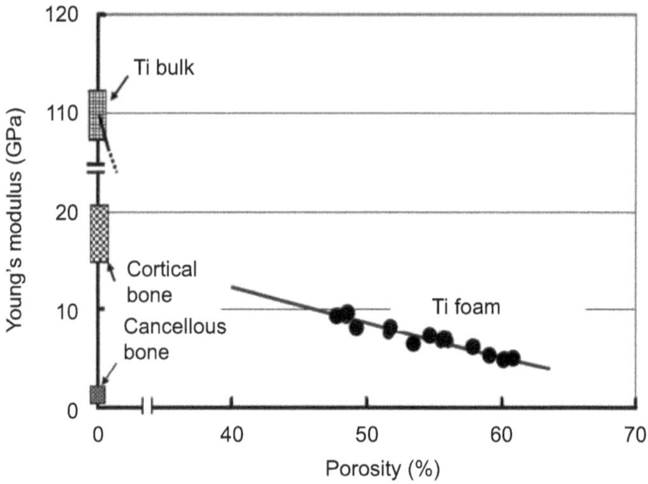

Figure 4.12 Young's modulus of commercially pure titanium (Ti) foam in comparison with bones.

Number 5 (A), (B), and (C) are the data on porous samples consisting of (A), (B), and (C) in Table 4.1. All of them decreased in strength with increasing porosity. However, the strengths of Numbers 2, 3, and 4 were lower than Number 1 at the corresponding porosity. This might be attributed to the lower thickness of the cell wall, which was less than 1 mm in Numbers 2, 3, 4, and 5 [14]. On the other hand, the strength is higher than that of the powder sintering product at the corresponding porosity.

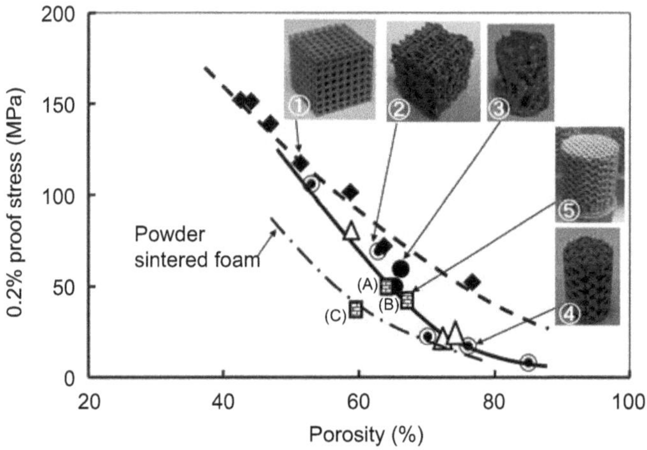

Figure 4.13 Compressive strength of various types of porous structures fabricated by the selective laser melting method in comparison with powder sintered foam.
Reproduced from Matsushita T, Fujibayashi S, Sasaki K. Additive manufacturing in titanium: porous devices for medical application. J Jpn Soc Technol Plast 2015;56:112–17. [Japanese] with permission from JSTP.

4.4 Biological properties of titanium foam

4.4.1 Osteoconductivity

Bone growth into connected pores in contact with bone without any intervention of fibrous tissue is termed osteoconduction. Ti foams in general are hardly penetrated with newly grown bone. However, they are deeply penetrated with newly grown bone (osteoconduction) when they are subjected to specific surface treatments such as NaOH and heat, NaOH, $CaCl_2$, heat, and water, and H_2SO_4/HCl and heat, respectively, as described in Chapter 6. Therefore, for example, a porous Ti layer that formed on the surface of an artificial hip joint subjected to NaOH and heat treatment to induce bioactivity becomes penetrated with new bone. It was confirmed that this kind of porous Ti layer was penetrated with newly grown bone so as to become tightly fixed to the surrounding bone [15–17].

Although the thickness of these porous layers is generally less than 1 mm, bone ingrowth into deeper regions occurs in the entire porous body, if its pore sizes are appropriate [18]. Takemoto et al. fabricated a Ti foam 50% in porosity and 300 μm in average pore size by a powder sintering method [19]. It was subjected to a 5 M NaOH treatment at 60°C for 24 h, 0.5 mM HCl at 40°C for 24 h, and a final heat treatment at 600°C for 1 h. As shown in Fig. 4.14, it was confirmed 3 months after implantation into the lumbar of a beagle dog that bony tissue had grown into the pores in the central portion of the foam. In contrast, the bone hardly grew into the pores of the foam

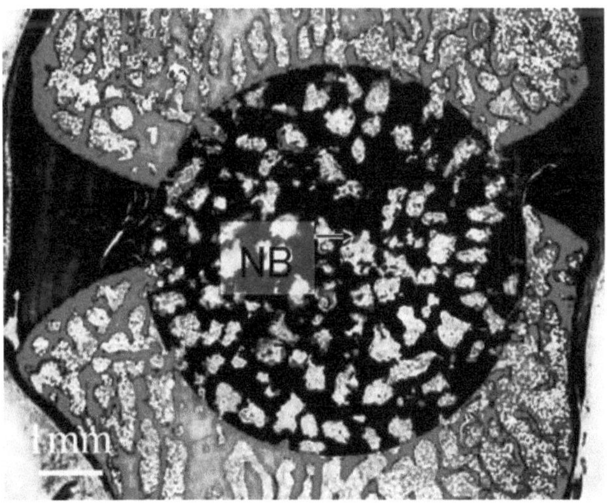

Figure 4.14 Bone formation in titanium (Ti) foam subjected to an NaOH–HCl–heat treatment, 3 months after implantation into a beagle dog. *NB*, new bone.
Reproduced from Takemoto M, Fujibayashi S, Neo M, So K, Akiyama N, Matsushita T, et al. A porous bioactive titanium implant for spinal interbody fusion: an experimental study using a canine model. J Neurosur Spine 2007;7:435–43 with permission from the American Association of Neurological Surgeons.

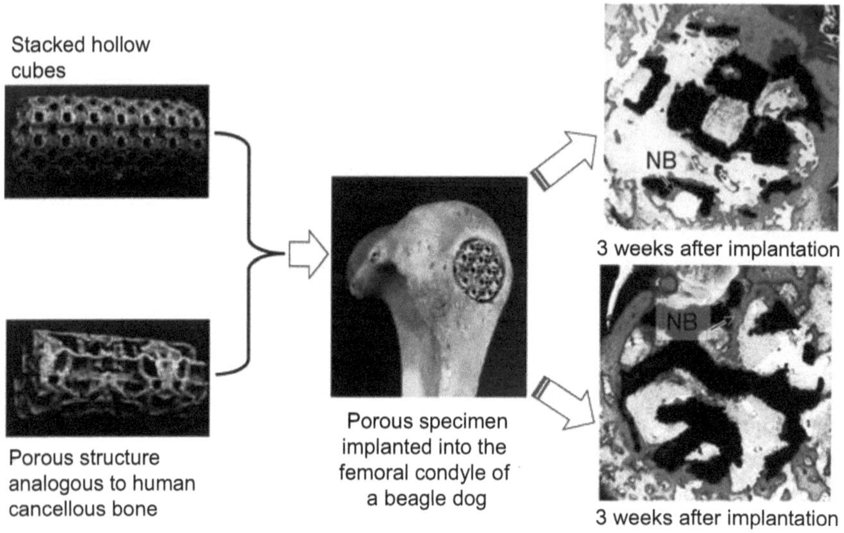

Figure 4.15 Bone growth into a porous cylindrical specimen prepared by the selective laser melting method and bioactive treatments. *NB*, new bone.

not subjected to the chemical and heat treatments. The bone−implant contact area was 35% for the treated foam, whereas it was only 11% for the untreated foam.

The cylindrical specimens 6 mm in diameter and 15 mm in length of the Ti foams with different porous structures that are shown in Fig. 4.15 were fabricated by the SLM method under the conditions described in Section 4.2. They were implanted into the metaphysis of the femoral condyle of mature male rabbits before and after the chemical and heat treatments described above. It was found 3 weeks later that bone had grown into the deeper regions of the treated foams, whereas it penetrated into only a shallow region in the untreated foams.

4.4.2 Osteoinductivity

It is known that some porous bioactive ceramics such as hydroxyapatite exhibit not only osteoconductivity but also osteoinductivity, that is, ectopic bone formation.

Fujibayashi et al. prepared two kinds of porous Ti with different pore structures; one was fabricated by a plasma-spraying method of Ti powders and another was prepared by pressing Ti wire into a mold [20]. One half of each of these specimens was subjected to a 5 M NaOH treatment at 60°C for 24 h and a subsequent heat treatment at 600°C for 1 h, while the other half was left untreated. Specimens of $5 \times 5 \times 7$ mm^3 in size were implanted into the dorsal muscles of mature beagle dogs. It was found 12 months later that new bone had formed only in the porous material that was fabricated by the plasma-spraying method and subjected to the chemical and heat treatments.

Takemoto et al. fabricated porous Ti metals by a plasma-spraying method that were 41% in porosity and 300–500 μm in pore size and subjected them to three different kinds of chemical and heat treatments [21]. The alkali- and heat- treatment was the same NaOH and heat treatment described above as a work by Fujibayashi et al. The water–AH treatment consists of an initial NaOH treatment, a water treatment at 40°C for 48 h, and a final heat treatment. The HCl–AH treatment consists of an initial NaOH treatment, a 0.5 mM HCl treatment at 40°C for 24 h, and a final heat treatment. These specimens were implanted in the dorsal muscles of mature beagle dogs. At 3 months after implantation, there was obvious bone formation with osteocytes and marrow-like tissue observed in the central part of the implant in the HCl–AH group, although only a small amount of bone-like tissue was seen in the central part of the water–AH group implant, and there was no bone formation but some vascular invasion found in the central part of the implant in the AH group. At 12 months after implantation, the new bone area on a cross-section of the specimen had become enlarged. Especially in the HCl–AH group, the new bone was observed in an area extending from the central part to the periphery. This superior osteoinductive ability displayed by the HCl–AH group was considered to be due to both the chemical and topographic effects exerted on the Ti surface. The HCl treatment removes sodium ions from the sodium titanate phase to form Ti oxide after a subsequent heat treatment. A bimodal distribution of micropores 0.1 μm and 0.1–1 μm in size appears on the Ti surface after an HCl treatment.

Kawai et al. fabricated Ti foams 60% in porosity and 250–300 μm in average pore size by a powder sintering method and subjected them to an H_2SO_4/HCl mixed acid solution treatment at 70°C for 1 h, followed by a heat treatment at 600°C for 1 h [22]. The acid and heat-treated specimens as well as the specimens that were only heat-treated, which were 6 mm in diameter and 15 mm in length, were implanted into the dorsal muscles of mature beagle dogs. It was found 12 months later that the acid and heat-treated specimen displayed bone formation in its porous structure, while

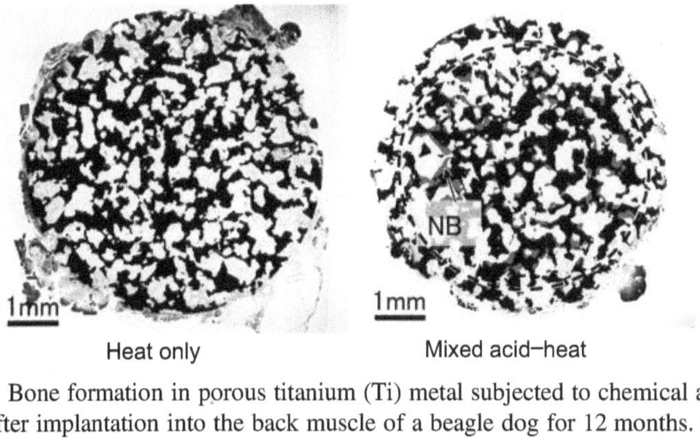

Figure 4.16 Bone formation in porous titanium (Ti) metal subjected to chemical and heat treatments after implantation into the back muscle of a beagle dog for 12 months. Chemical and heat-treated porous Ti cylinders show new bone in central pores. *NB*, new bone. Reproduced from Kawai T, Takemoto M, Fujibayashi S, Tanaka M, Yamaguchi S, Pattanayak DK, et al. Osteoinduction on acid and heat treated porous Ti metal samples in canine muscle. PLoS One 2014;9:e88366.

the specimen that was heat-treated alone did not display it, as shown in Fig. 4.16. Both of the specimens precipitate rutile on their surfaces. However, the former forms apatite on its surface in a simulated body fluid, whereas the latter does not. This indicates that apatite formation plays an important role in exhibiting osteoinductivity.

On the other hand, Fukuda et al. fabricated Ti foams containing square longitudinal channels that were 500, 600, 900, or 1200 μm on the diagonal using the SLM method. Cylindrical specimens, 3.3 mm in diameter and 15 mm in length, were implanted into the dorsal muscle of mature beagle dogs before and after the NaOH, HCl, and heat treatments described above [23]. It was found that bony tissue formed in the foams subjected to the chemical and heat treatments, showing that bone was able to form even in this kind of channel structure in periods greater than 16 weeks after the implantation, as shown in Fig. 4.17, and that channels 500−600 μm on the diagonal are most favorable for osteoinduction among the channels examined. The untreated foam did not show any bone formation.

4.5 Applications of titanium foam in orthopedics

4.5.1 Device design and clinical trials for lumbar interbody fusion

A simple cage of Ti metal has been used for lumbar interbody fusion. However, it does not bond to the surrounding bone. In order to fix it to the surrounding bone, an autogenic bone graft is needed, which often leads to complications. If a Ti foam subjected to chemical and heat treatment effective for inducing bioactivity were to be used instead of the simple cage, it would be expected to bond to the surrounding bone without the need for an autogenic bone graft.

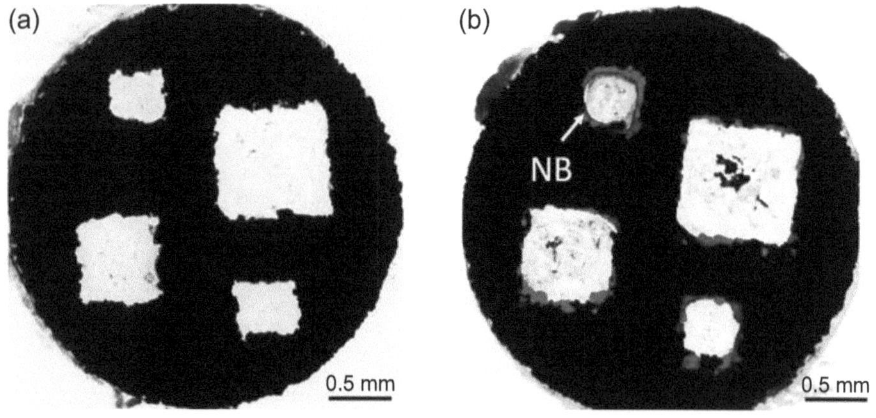

Figure 4.17 Bone induced in the channels of untreated and bioactive-treated specimens implanted in the dorsal muscle of a beagle dog: (a) no bone formation in the untreated specimen and (b) bone formation in the bioactive-treated specimen. *NB*, new bone.
Reproduced from Fukuda A, Takemoto M, Saito T, Fujibayashi S, Neo M, Pattanayak DK, et al. Osteoinduction of porous Ti implants with a channel structure fabricated by selective laser melting. Acta Biomater 2011;7:2327−36 with permission from Elsevier.

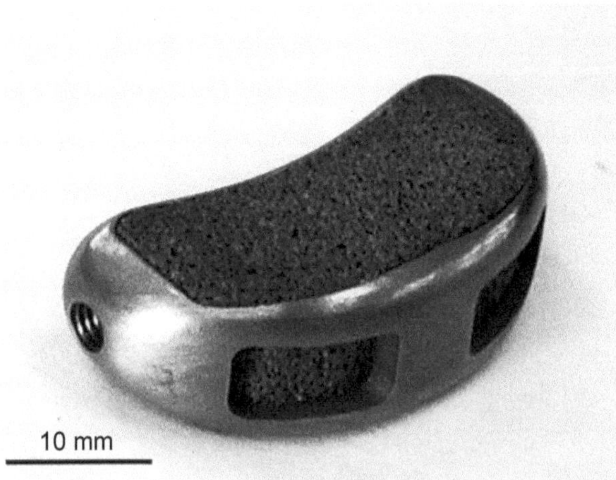

Figure 4.18 Device of bioactive titanium (Ti) foam for lumbar interbody fusion.

In our clinical trials for lumbar interbody fusion using Ti foam fabricated by the powder sintering method, a thin dense outer frame was used around the foam to improve handling during surgery, as shown in Fig. 4.18. The outer frame had windows to decrease the effective elastic modulus and screw holes for fixing surgical instruments. This device was subjected to the NaOH, HCl, and heat treatments described above for inducing bioactivity. It did not exhibit any cracks or residual deformation, even after it was subjected to repetitive loads of compressive force of 10 kN at 4-Hz for 10^6 cycles.

The clinical trial was performed at Kyoto University Hospital for five patients with degenerative unstable lumbar lesions [24]. Clinical assessments were performed using the Japanese Orthopedic Association (JOA) back pain evaluation questionnaire score. Bone union was judged using CT and simple functional X-ray image assessment. The average JOA score of 15.8 points (12−21) before the operation was improved to 26.6 points (18−29) within 1 year after the operation. The improvement rate of the JOA score was 85.8%. Patient satisfaction was 87.4%, and back problems and leg pains were clearly improved at an early date after the operation in every patient. In all cases, bony union was achieved, and the period required for bony union was 3.6 months on average. No adverse events were observed. Autogenic bone graft was not required. The safety and efficacy of bioactive Ti foam devices in lumbar interbody fusion were confirmed. It should be noted that in certain cases a gap that appeared between the device and the vertebral body just after the operation was filled with new bone 12 months after the original operation, as shown in Fig. 4.19.

4.5.2 Device design and clinical trials for anterior cervical discectomy and fusion

Fig. 4.20 shows the design procedure of a device used for anterior cervical discectomy and fusion [13]. A cervical spine structure was built from CT images, after which a

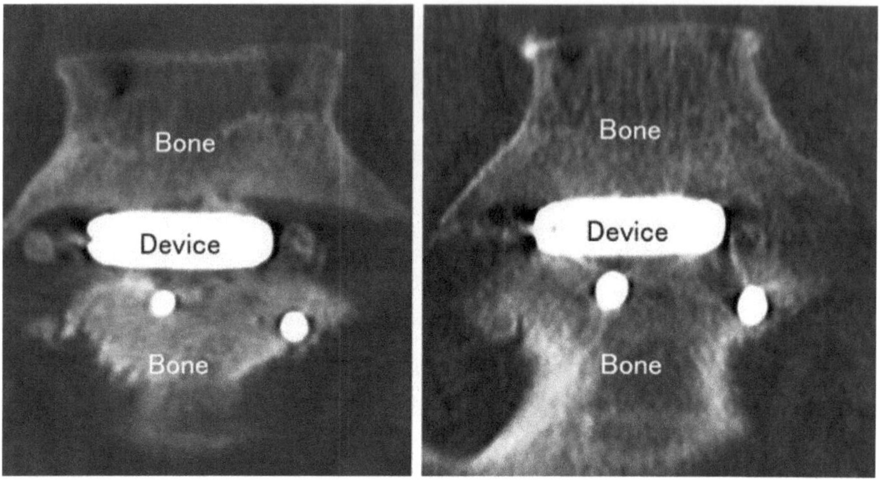

Figure 4.19 Coronal computerized tomography images taken immediate postoperatively and at 12 months. The immediate postoperative image (left) shows an apparent gap between the titanium (Ti) foam and the vertebral bone. The 12-month image (right) demonstrates complete gap filling and direct bone bonding to the Ti foam.

frame fit to the intervertebral disc was designed. The frame is made of dense Ti metal, as in the case of lumbar interbody fusion. A porous structure 600 μm in pore diameter and 65% in porosity was placed into the inside of this frame. Using this design, the device was analyzed by the finite element method to confirm the strength under a

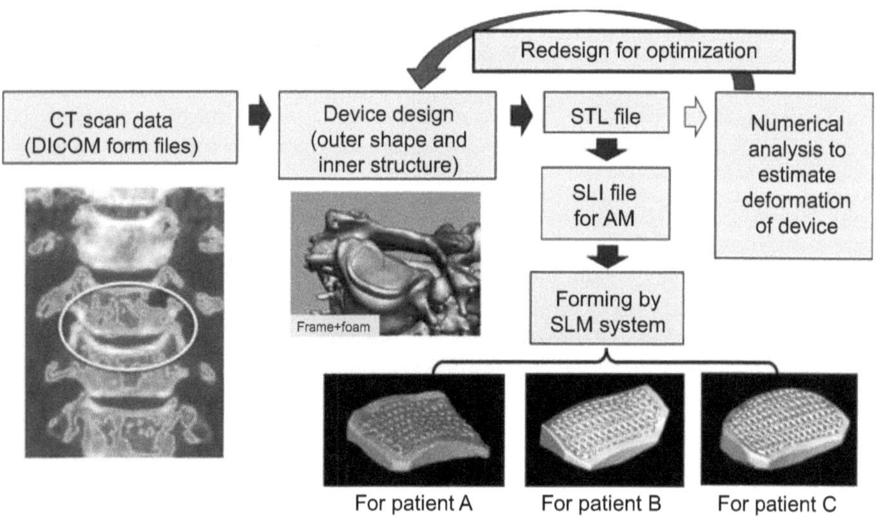

Figure 4.20 Flow chart of the selective laser melting process to fabricate devices for anterior cervical discectomy and fusion. *SLM*, Selective laser melting method; *STL*, Standard Triangulated Language; *SLI*, Slice layer Interface.
Reproduced from Matsushita T, Fujibayashi S, Sasaki K. Additive manufacturing in titanium: porous devices for medical application. J Jpn Soc Technol Plast 2015;56:112–17. [Japanese] with permission from JSTP.

load of 5 kN. The stress and deformation were within the range of tolerance of the material. The design data were converted to an Standard Triangulated Language file. The devices were fabricated by SLM under the conditions described in Section 4.2.2. The obtained device was subjected to the NaOH, HCl, and heat treatments for inducing bioactivity.

The clinical trial was performed at Kyoto University Hospital for five patients with degenerative unstable cervical lesions with symptoms of tingling and numbness of the hands as well as difficulty in walking.

Clinical assessments were made by the cervical myelopathy evaluation questionnaire score and improvement rate of the JOA. Image assessments of bone union were made using CT and simple functional X-ray. The preoperative average JOA score of 12.1 points (10.5–15) improved to 16.1 points (14.5–16.5) by 1 year after the operation, and the improvement rate of the JOA score was 79.8%. In all cases, autogenic bone graft proved unnecessary. The bone union rate was 80%, and no adverse events were observed. Fig. 4.21 shows an X-ray of the device installed in the cervical spine [13]. The portion of the device fits into the indented shape formed by the top and bottom surfaces of the vertebral end plates and is stably held between them. The results show that when a device made with SLM and induced bioactivity is employed, autogenic bone graft is not required.

4.6 Future trends

The demand for custom-made medical care has dramatically increased, including that for individually tailored medical devices. In order to meet this demand, such devices need to be prepared so as to match each patient and each disease, with the additional

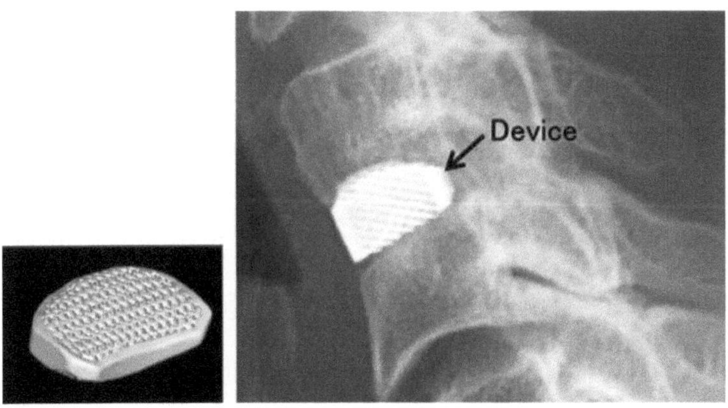

Figure 4.21 Bioactive porous device fabricated by selective laser melting (left) and postoperative lateral radiograph (right).
Reproduced from Matsushita T, Fujibayashi S, Sasaki K. Additive manufacturing in titanium: porous devices for medical application. J Jpn Soc Technol Plast 2015;56:112–17. [Japanese] with permission from JSTP.

constraint that they must be supplied quickly and inexpensively. In addition, if devices with complicated shapes and structures that previously could not be fabricated by conventional manufacturing processes were to be made readily available, a new type of innovative medical care would come into existence.

In this section, the future of various types of Ti foam is discussed. Foam is superior to bulk material in terms of elastic modulus, because the modulus of a porous material is easily altered by modulating the pore structure. However, the strength of a porous material is lower than that of a bulk metal. Therefore it is a matter of vital importance to continue the effort to balance the strength and effective elastic modulus of these devices. A porous material can be used as a prosthesis material in which the deformation is almost the same as that of surrounding bone.

Ti foams of the same porosity and pore size can be fabricated by either the powder sintering or SLM method. The characteristics of each are summarized in Table 4.2. One of the differences between them is the required thickness of the struts. When a fine and thin porous material is desired, it is preferable to use a powder sintering method, even though multiple steps are required.

In order to use a porous material clinically, safety must be secured from the viewpoints of both strength and reliability. From the economic point of view, a reduction of the manufacturing cost and shortening of the delivery time are essential for meeting the clinical need. A manufacturing process such as SLM is extremely useful in achieving these goals.

At present, since an additive manufacturing technique is more flexible in responding to a wide variety of structural needs and is able to meet the requirements for single-piece

Table 4.2 Characteristics of commercially pure titanium foams fabricated by powder sintering and selective laser melting

Item	Powder sintered foam	Selective laser melted foam
Porosity	10–90%	10–90%
Pore size	Up to 800 μm	100 μm–2 mm
Strut thickness	10 μm–3 mm	More than 300 μm
Microstructural character	Macropore and micropore on the struts	Macropore and powder deposited on the struts or micropore on the struts created during heating at 1300°C
Interconnected pores	More than 50% of porosity necessary	Easy to be fully interconnected pores
Bone ingrowth	Better in the foam with interconnected pores and bioactivity	Better in the foam with bioactivity
Preparation route	Multiple steps	One step

production more easily than the powder sintering method, it is advantageous for medical applications. However, it is essential for practical applications that the equipment cost be reduced, the reliability increased, and the quality of the product be assured from the powder metallurgical point of view.

Porous materials subjected to treatments for inducing bioactivity are useful for the stable fixation of the device and shortening the healing period. As described in this chapter, both osteoconduction and osteoinduction are observed in bioactive Ti foams.

Chemical and heat treatments are able to induce bioactivity over the entire surface of a device, even if it is one of complicated structure and shape, in contrast with conventional methods such as the plasma-spraying of hydroxyapatite, which can activate only a very limited surface area.

In addition, in medical applications of porous materials, it is also critical to develop software to accurately design a device to fit to the afflicted part of the body using CT images of the affected area. Once a convenient design process is made available, medical devices with a porous and dense structure for large bone defects will become a reality. It is expected that devices composed of bioactive porous and solid materials will come to be widely used in orthopedics as well as oral maxillofacial surgeries.

References

[1] Niinomi M, Hattori T, Morikawa K, Kasuga T, Suzuki A, Fukui H, et al. Development of low rigidity β-type titanium alloy for biomedical applications. Mater Trans 2002;43: 2970–7.

[2] Ozaki T, Matsumoto H, Watanabe S, Hanada S. Beta Ti alloys with low Young's modulus. Mater Trans 2004;45(8):2776–9.

[3] Weiss MB. Titanium fiber-mesh metal implant. J Oral Implantol 1986;12:498–507.

[4] Wen CE, Yamada Y, Shimojima K, Chino Y, Hosokawa H, Mabuchi M. Novel titanium foam for bone tissue engineering. J Mater Res 2002;17:2633–9.

[5] Oh IH, Nomura N, Masahashi N, Hanada S. Mechanical properties of porous titanium compacts prepared by powder sintering. Scripa Mater 2003;49:1197–202.

[6] Hollander DA, Walter MV, Wirtz T, Sellei R, Rohlfing BS, Paar O, et al. Structural, mechanical and in vitro characterization of individually structured Ti-6Al-4V produced by direct laser forming. Biomaterials 2006;27:955–63.

[7] Ryan GE, Pandit AS, Apatsidis DP. Fabrication methods of porous metals for use in orthopaedic applications. Biomaterials 2006;27:2651–70.

[8] Heinl P, Muller L, Korner C, Singer RF, Mulaer FA. Cellular Ti-6Al-4V structures with interconected macro prosity for bone implants fabricated by selective electron beam melting. Acta Biomater 2008;4:1536–44.

[9] Ryan GE, Pandit AS, Apatsidis DP. Porous titanium scaffolds fabricated using a rapid prototyping and powder metallurgy technique. Biomaterials 2008;29:3625–35.

[10] Pattanayak DK, Matsushita T, Doi K, Takadama H, Nakamura T, Kokubo T. Effect of oxygen content of porous titanium metal on its apatite-forming ability and compressive strength. J Mater Sci Eng C 2009;29:1974–8.

[11] Otsuki B, Takemoto M, Fujibayashi S, Neo M, Kokubo T, Nakamura T. Pore throat size and connectivity determine bone and tissue ingrowth into porous implants: three-dimensional micro-CT based structural analyses of porous bioactive titanium implants. Biomaterials 2006;27:5982–6000.

[12] Pattanayak DK, Fukuda A, Matsushita T, Takemoto M, Fujibayashi S, et al. Bioactive Ti metal analogous to human cancellous bone: fabrication by selective laser melting and chemical treatments. Acta Biomater 2011;7:1398–406.

[13] Matsushita T, Fujibayashi S, Sasaki K. Additive manufacturing in titanium: porous devices for medical application. J Jpn Soc Technol Plast 2015;56:112–7 [Japanese].

[14] Matsushita T, Pattanayak DK, Takemoto M, Fujibayashi S, Nakamura T, Sasaki K, et al. Compressive strength of porous titanium metal thin wall prepared by selected laser melting. J Jpn Soc Technol Plast 2013;54:601–5 [Japanese].

[15] Nishiguchi S, Kato H, Neo M, Oka M, Kim H-M, Kokubo T, et al. Alkali- and heat-treated porous titanium for orthopedic implants. J Biomed Mater Res 2001;54:198–208.

[16] Kawanabe K, Ise K, Goto K, Akiyama H, Nakamura T, et al. A new cementless total hip arthroplasty with bioactive titanium porous-coating by alkaline and heat treatments: average 4.8-year results. J Biomed Mater Res B Appl Biomater 2009;90B:476–81.

[17] So K, Kaneuji A, Matsumoto T, Matsuda S, Akiyama H. Is the bone-bonding ability of a cementless total hip prosthesis enhanced by alkaline and heat treatments? Clin Orthop Relat Res 2013;471:3847–55.

[18] Karageorgiou V, Kaplan D. Porosity of 3D biomaterial scaffolds and osteogenesis. Biomaterials 2005;26:5474–91.

[19] Takemoto M, Fujibayashi S, Neo M, So K, Akiyama N, Matsushita T, et al. A porous bioactive titanium implant for spinal interbody fusion: an experimental study using a canine model. J Neurosur Spine 2007;7:435–43.

[20] Fujibayashi S, Neo M, Kim HM, Kokubo T, Nakamura T. Osteoinduction of porous bioactive titanium metal. Biomaterials 2004;25:443–50.

[21] Takemoto M, Fujibayashi S, Neo M, Suzuki J, Matsushita T, Kokubo T, et al. Osteoinductive porous titanium implants: effect of sodium removal by dilute HCl treatment. Biomaterials 2006;27:2682–91.

[22] Kawai T, Takemoto M, Fujibayashi S, Tanaka M, Yamaguchi S, Pattanayak DK, et al. Osteoinduction on acid and heat treated porous Ti metal samples in canine muscle. PLoS One 2014;9:e88366.

[23] Fukuda A, Takemoto M, Saito T, Fujibayashi S, Neo M, Pattanayak DK, et al. Osteoinduction of porous Ti implants with a channel structure fabricated by selective laser melting. Acta Biomater 2011;7:2327–36.

[24] Fujibayashi S, Takemoto M, Neo M, Matsushita T, Kokubo T, et al. A novel synthetic material for spinal fusion: a prospective clinical trial of porous bioactive titanium metal for lumbar interbody fusion. Eur Spine J 2011;20:1486–95.

Titanium foam scaffolds for dental applications

5

A. Nouri
University of Toronto, Toronto, ON, Canada

5.1 Introduction

Nowadays, the development of novel materials and structures for improving functions and esthetics for patients is of paramount importance in dentistry. Reconstruction of oral function can significantly improve the quality of life for patients and decrease costs in the healthcare system, therefore new strategies and studies are certainly necessary to all areas of clinical dental practice. For this reason, materials science and biomedical engineering have further integrated into new interdisciplinary areas to address challenges in dentistry.

The demand for dental and maxillofacial implants has increased steadily with the aging of the global population. Dental implants placed in the oral cavity are used as a method of replacing missing teeth. Maxillofacial implants are associated with restoring form and/or function to the maxilla (upper jaw) and the face [1]. For edentulous patients (those who have partially or completely lost their teeth) the condition is not fatal or physically debilitating, but the replacement of missing teeth with dental implants appears to be necessary for several reasons. For edentulous patients, the reduction in chewing forces limits the type and quantity of food consumed and may cause secondary health consequences. Furthermore, gaps in the dentition for edentulous patients may result in speech defects. Most importantly, tooth loss is known to have deleterious consequences on the underlying periodontal tissues, particularly the alveolar bone, which eventually results in bone atrophy [1]. It is estimated that over 26% of people ages 65–74 in the United States are edentulous [2]. The number of implants placed each year reflects the ever-increasing popularity of implants as a treatment modality. There was a seven-fold increase in the number of implants placed between the years 2000 and 2006 [3]. In the United States alone, more than 5 million dental implants are inserted each year, and the number continues to rise with improvements in surgical technique, treatment planning, and implant longevity [4].

Among three major types of dental prostheses, namely removable dentures, fixed bridges, and dental implants, the latter is a winning choice for permanent replacement. The inability of removable dentures and fixed bridges to appropriately restore function has resulted in a rise in the popularity of dental implants as an effective way to replace missing teeth. Endosseous implants, which are also known as *intraosseous* and *endosteal implants*, are the most commonly used dental implants. Endosseous dental implants have been developed and improved continuously since the very early designs of Cherchève in the 1960s [5,6]. These implants are usually screw-shaped cylinders

Metallic Foam Bone. http://dx.doi.org/10.1016/B978-0-08-101289-5.00005-6

and are made of either metal, metal covered with ceramic, or ceramic materials. They are placed into the sockets of missing teeth, and, like the natural tooth root, must tolerate and transfer loads effectively from the tooth to the alveolar bone surrounding the socket. There are also blade-shaped endosseous implants consisting of a thin, blade-like metal framework. The blade is embedded into the bone while the other end protrudes through the mucosa into the oral cavity [7]. The modern endosseous screw-shaped implants emerged from the leading work of Per-Ingvar Brånemark in Sweden [8]. Since then, a wide variety of screw- or tooth-root-shaped endosseous implants have come into clinical use, and they have achieved remarkable clinical success. Brånemark developed and introduced the concept of a direct bone-to-metal interface, termed as "osseointegration" [9]. Osseointegration was defined as "a direct structural and functional connection between ordered, living bone and the surface of a load-carrying implant" [10].

Titanium (Ti) and its alloys are among the most common bone replacement materials and have been extensively used for dental implants owing to their high biocompatibility, excellent corrosion resistance, and suitable mechanical properties. Typically, dental implants are machined from Ti rods, and their surface is subsequently modified using different techniques, such as sandblasting [11], acid-etching [12], anodization [13], discrete calcium–phosphate crystal deposition [14], and chemical modification [15,16]. However, the existing Ti implants still pose several drawbacks. First, the bonding strength at the implant–bone interface is not high enough to secure stable and long-term fixation. Second, the mismatch of the elastic modulus between implants and bone tissue can lead to stress shielding, bone resorption, and poor osseointegration. Thus the success or failure of an implant is determined by how the mechanical stress at the bone–implant interface is transferred to the surrounding bones [17,18]. Not only can stress shielding result in the resorption of bone, but also a concentration of excessive stress will lead to the failure of a dental implant. Therefore to increase the success rate of dental implants, it is important to consider the stress generated on the surrounding supporting tissues in order to reduce bone resorption around osseointegrated implants and enhance the bone apposition to implanted Ti surfaces.

Today, most endosseous dental implants are screw-shaped. Screw-shaped implants will have increased stability in comparison to those with little variation on their surface. However, in patients with continuing bone resorption, long-term stable fixation of these implants is difficult to achieve [19]. A promising solution to this problem is to use implants with a porous structure. The use of porous metal implants for medical applications has two main advantages. First, the elastic modulus of porous metals is lower than that of dense metals, which helps to prevent the effect of stress shielding at the bone interface. Depending on the porosity, moduli can even be tailored to match the modulus of cortical or cancellous bones. Second, a porous implant can provide a structural support for the bone ingrowth to achieve durable biological fixation [17,20]. To ensure bone ingrowth and extensive transportation of body fluid through the porous scaffold, a substantial pore interconnectivity is necessary [21]. A schematic illustration of a porous dental implant in the mandible is shown in Fig. 5.1. Bone ingrowth in the porous surface means that a stable fixation of such dental implants is expected, even at a reduced implant length.

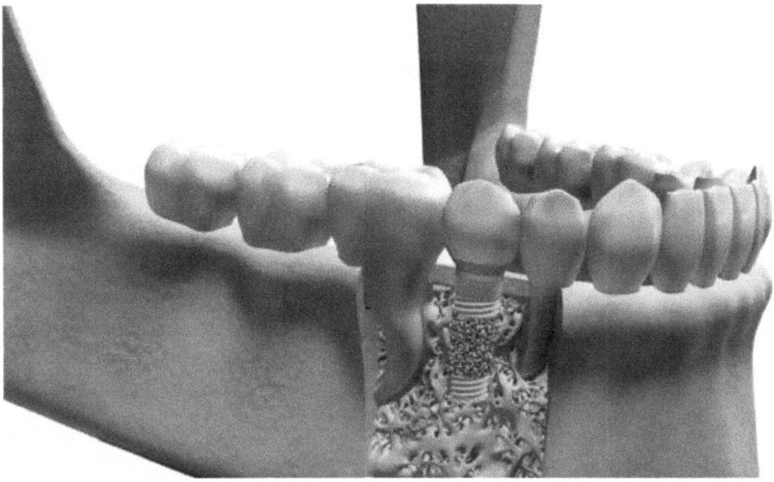

Figure 5.1 The porous dental implant is designed to be used in the mandible or maxilla to restore the function and aesthetics of missing teeth. After osteotomy preparation, the porous dental implant is inserted and immediately loaded. Following implant placement, primitive bone begins to form connections with the dental implant.
Courtesy of Zimmer Dental Inc.

Typically, porous Ti implants are categorized into three different types: (1) partly or fully porous-coated solid substrates, (2) fully porous materials, and (3) porous metal segments joined to solid metallic parts [20]. The ability of porous Ti scaffolds to have a wide range of stiffness and strength allows them to perform in a variety of applications. For example, thicker strut scaffolds (lower porosity) can be used in load-bearing regions (i.e., mandible cortical bone and dental abutment reconstruction regions), whereas thinner struts can be used for replacing cancellous bone and in nonload-bearing regions (i.e., cranial replacement) [22]. Accordingly, the architecture of a porous Ti scaffold is among the most important parameters that may affect cell response and ultimately determine cell fate [23].

This chapter provides an overview of the potentials, limitations, and challenges involved in using Ti foam scaffolds for dental applications. The chapter further aims to highlight some of the fundamental properties of porous dental implants, which allow for their enhanced osseointegration, stability, and effective dental rehabilitation.

5.2 Dental implants and materials

Due to the accessibility of the oral cavity, dental implants have one of the longest recorded histories among medical devices, and attempts to replace missing teeth with implanted materials dates back to ancient times [1,24]. It has been documented that over 4000 years ago, the ancient Chinese hammered bamboo pegs into the sockets of missing teeth [1]. There is clear archeological evidence that the Mayans were the first to use endosseous implants over 1400 years ago to support dental prostheses [25]. However, it was not until the 19th century that the implanted materials were reported experimentally and clinically in the dental literature [26]. In 1809, Maggiolo's implanted gold tooth roots into fresh extraction sockets failed after a period of time [27]. The failure of Maggiolo's gold implant propelled researchers in the late 1800, toward the use of alternative metals, including platinum posts coated with lead, gold, or iridium tubes, silver capsules, etc. [28].

The emergence of new materials and advancements in metallurgy in the 20th century led to an era of expanded surgical use of metallic implants. In the late 1930s, Venable and Stuck demonstrated the passivity of vitallium (Co—Cr—Mo alloy) for implant materials and subsequently made vitallium screws in root forms for dental implants [29,30]. The era of modern implant dentistry, however, was primarily built on orthopedic Ti research and later on adapted for dental implant applications largely due to the work of Brånemark and his colleagues in Göteburg, Sweden [8,9,31]. Beyond any doubt, Ti has unique properties among all metals in the periodic table, which truly makes it the material of choice for dental and maxillofacial implants.

5.2.1 Titanium and its alloys

Ti implants have revolutionized oral health care. They have been extensively used for both endosseous and subperiosteal (attaches on top of the jaw bone but underneath the gum tissue) implants. Endosseous implants have taken the form of rods, posts, and blades made of either commercially pure Ti (CP-Ti) or Ti alloys. The reason for the growing interest in Ti and its alloys in dentistry lies in their high degree of biocompatibility, suitable strength, and high corrosion resistance. Compared to other dental implants, the implants made of Ti are more durable, markedly lighter, and capable of withstanding high loads without undue deformation [32]. Ti dental implants are generally machined from billet stock of CP-Ti or Ti-based alloys. Dental crowns and bridge frameworks also can be machined from solid metal stock via computer-aided machining [33]. The Ti oxide layer (TiO_2) allows for bonding of fused porcelains, adhesive polymers, or, in the case of endosseous implants, plasma-sprayed or surface-nucleated apatite coatings for esthetic and surface modification purposes [33].

The American Society for Testing and Materials Committee F-4 on Materials for Surgical Implants has listed four grades of CP-Ti and two Ti alloys. CP-Ti, also referred to as unalloyed Ti, is classified into Grade-1, Grade-2, Grade-3, and Grade-4. The oxygen and iron (Fe) contents are increased from Grade-1 to Grade-4 [34]. The two alloys are Ti-6A1-4V and Ti-6A1-4V extra low interstitial. The four grades of unalloyed Ti as well as the aforementioned two alloys are the most commonly used implant materials in dentistry. A growing body of clinical evidence has revealed the excellent biocompatibility, tissue response, and predictability of all six of these commercially available endosseous implant biomaterials [34—36]. Before the 1996 update, the American Dental Association (ADA) Council on Scientific Affairs had not recommended endosseous implants for clinical practice [37]. In 1996, the ADA's Council on Scientific Affairs accepted the clinical trial of Ti-based endosseous implants to be carefully used for the treatment of selected patients [38]. In the case of patients with parafunctional habits (e.g., bruxism), the clinician should choose an implant made of a Ti alloy rather than CP-Ti Grade-1 [34]. As a result, some clinicians may feel more comfortable using a higher strength material, such as CP-Ti Grade-4 or a Ti alloy, if other factors of implant selection are equal.

In order to overcome the drawbacks of CP-Ti while retaining its advantages for bone replacement applications, many metallic elements have been considered to lower the elastic modulus and to show an appropriate immune response from the host tissue on implantation. Later generations of Ti implant materials have been developed with the following benefits: (1) higher β phase content and (2) more biocompatible alloying elements (less Al, Fe, V). Although the elastic modulus of α+ β type Ti alloy (e.g., Ti-6Al-4V) is much lower than those of stainless-steel and Co-based alloys, it is still considerably higher than that of cortical bone. The elastic moduli of β type Ti alloys are known to be smaller than those of α or α+ β type Ti alloys. In addition, β type Ti alloys show excellent cold workability and high strength. Thus the research and development of low-rigidity β type Ti alloys are gaining more attention for implant materials [39]. Many of these alloys contain a fairly large amount of Nb, tantalum (Ta), Zr, Mo, and/or Sn [40–43]. It has been reported that the Ti–Zr alloy exhibits enhanced mechanical stability compared to CP-Ti (Grade-4), with respect to fatigue strength and elongation. The ultimate tensile strength of Ti–Zr was found to be comparable to Ti-6Al-4V [44]. Ti-6Al-7Nb, which has been developed for surgical implants, is also attractive for dental applications [45].

Despite the outlined advantages of Ti and its alloys, some drawbacks still limit the potential use of Ti in biomedical applications. Ti is susceptible to crack propagation, which limits the service lifetime of Ti implants to only 10–15 years [46]. Another drawback of Ti is its poor machinability, which lies in its relatively low elastic modulus. This renders the manufacture of more complex pieces of dental implants difficult. Furthermore, it is usually challenging and dangerous to cast Ti, which is deterrent to the use of casting Ti in dental applications. At elevated temperatures, the metal fumes and oxidizes so rapidly that an almost explosive reaction may occur. For this reason, Ti is typically used in wrought form and machined to the desired implant shape [47].

5.2.2 Nickel–titanium shape memory alloys

Near equiatomic Ni–Ti alloys (also known as Nitinol), with a nickel content of 48–51%, have superior strength and high corrosion resistance. These alloys exhibit three properties that are not commonly observed in other metallic materials, including shape memory effect (SME), superelasticity, and high damping properties [48]. For SME, a large deformation can be fully recovered by a slight heating to return to its original shape. This phenomenon has been successfully exploited for many biomedical devices at the surgical site that are activated by body heat or external heat sources. Examples include minimally invasive instruments and cardiovascular self-expansion stents, which make use of pseudoelasticity to restore their designed shape after implementation [22]. In dentistry, a highly successful application example is dental orthodontic wire, which uses superelasticity characterized by a constant stress upon loading and unloading [49,50]. Other interesting application examples are dental implants and attachments for partial dentures, which use the SME [51]. Blade-type implants made of Ni–Ti have been used for patients who possess a comparatively narrow jaw bone structure in order to ensure tight initial fixation and to avoid accidental sinking on mastication with an open blade shape [51]. It was demonstrated that dental implants fabricated with gap-free abutments using a shape memory alloy showed significantly reduced bacterial leakage at the implant-abutment gap as compared to conventional implants. This improvement could alleviate clinical problems such as peri-implantitis and, thus, increase the long-term success of dental implants [52].

Although the presence of a protective Ti-based oxide layer acts as an effective barrier to Ni ion release, the high concentration of Ni in these alloys increases the risk of allergic reactions. Therefore the research and development of Ni-free Ti-based shape memory alloys composed of nontoxic elements have gained interest [53,54]. Takahashi et al. developed Ni-free Ti–Nb–Sn alloys to overcome the above drawback of Ni–Ti alloys [55]. The newly developed alloys exhibited SME at ambient temperature, whereas no appreciable superelasticity was observed.

Due to their unique properties, Ni–Ti alloys have also received increasing attention as potential materials for porous orthopedic implants [56–59]. Porous Ni–Ti alloys usually have a low elastic modulus (61–69 GPa), which can be further reduced by superelastic effect while maintaining a high strength [56,60]. Porous Ni–Ti with a 30–80% porosity exhibits elastic modulus values as low as that of cortical bone (12–17 GPa) or even cancellous bone (<3 GPa) [61]. A Nitinol with the superelastic property can be fabricated to have 70% porosity [62]. It was reported that the porous Ni–Ti materials bond very well to newly formed bone tissues and are suitable for clinical applications under load-bearing conditions [63].

5.3 Properties and characteristics of titanium foam scaffolds

Ti foam scaffolds for dental implant applications are designed based on many interrelated factors, including the geometry, alloys, surface properties, and various pore characteristics. The stability of the implant–bone interface, strength and rate of osseointegration, and the long-term success of dental implants are achieved by appropriate design and proper material selection. Although there is no specific implant design that meets all of the requirements in dental applications, implants can be engineered to maximize strength, interfacial stability, and load transfer. The following provides an overview of some of the key parameters for the long-term success of dental implants and, in particular, porous scaffolds.

5.3.1 Implant design

One of the most important factors to determine the success or failure of a dental implant is its overall dimensions, including length and diameter. The selection of implant dimensions depends on the width and depth of the bone into which the implant is to be placed [64]. In other words, there must be sufficient bone at the implant site to accommodate the selected implant. Dental implants are available in lengths ranging from 7.0–20 mm, although common usage ranges from 10–16 mm [65]. The success with 7-mm long implants led to the introduction of even shorter 5-mm long implants for use in the highly resorbed posterior mandible [66].

Many studies suggest that longer implants result in a higher success rate, possibly because the increased length of the bone–implant interfacial contact increases the potential for greater mechanical resistance to masticatory forces [67,68]. By contrast, shorter implants with a lower bone-to-implant contact may exhibit less resistance to occlusal (biting) forces and therefore are more susceptible to early failure [67]. It should be noted that implants longer than 18 mm also may be susceptible to failure, possibly due to the tendency for the bone to be overheated when a deep hole is drilled in it [68]. It has been suggested that stress levels for a given applied load are reduced on longer implants because of the greater surface area [65]. Consequently, the bone may experience less resorption and may be less prone to pathological complications following implant placement.

The implant diameter also contributes to the extent of bone-to-implant contact and to the level of resistance to occlusal forces, since the circumference of the implant increases with the diameter. Increasing the diameter for a given length of implant with the same design and structural characteristics would markedly increase the nominal surface area. Thus the degree of bone-to-implant contact surface increases with a concomitant increase in the resistance to occlusal forces [64]. The implant diameter also has a direct influence on the fatigue strength. Dental implants with small diameters have a higher tendency for fatigue fracture than dental implants with large diameters, particularly in the mandibular and maxillary posterior regions, where most fractures take place [69]. Most implants are approximately 4 mm in diameter. A diameter of at least 3.3 mm is usually recommended to ensure adequate implant strength. However, for low-load situations, such as mandibular incisor teeth, implants of 3-mm diameter are normally recommended [70].

Similarly, threaded implants or implants with porous surfaces have a greater surface area than a smooth cylinder. In the dental industry, most implants are parallel cylindrical or tapered cylindrical threaded designs [70]. In addition, most modern implants have a slightly rough surface that favors more rapid osseointegration. Although the surface porosity of the implant or the addition of a screw thread will weaken the implant itself and make it more prone to ion release and corrosion, the shortcomings are more than compensated for by their improved clinical performance [7,70]. The screw thread or surface porosity provides greater initial stability in the bone and allows the implant to be locked in place while the healing process occurs. It is notable that the thread geometry affects the distribution of stress forces around the implant. It was reported that implant stability is positively influenced by a decreased thread pitch, whereas excess helix angles, in spite of a faster insertion, may jeopardize the ability of implants to sustain the axial load [71,72]. A common thread pitch is 0.6 mm [70]. In poor bone-quality conditions, deeper threads seem to have a positive effect on primary stability [71]. An increase in the thread face angle will result in an increase in the shearing forces [73]. Designs of dental implants have begun to incorporate a tapered wall form. The tapered form implants require less space in the apical region, which allows them to be placed in narrow spaces or in narrow regions with labial or lingual concavities. They also possess a better stability for immediate placement and provide even distribution of compressive forces [73].

5.3.2 Biocompatibility

Biocompatibility is defined as the ability of a material to perform with an appropriate host response in a specific situation [74]. Practically, there is no material that is biocompatible for all applications. Therefore biocompatibility not only depends on the properties of the material but also should be defined by the location in which the material is used [75]. Dental materials may pose potential risks to various tissues such as cytotoxicity, generation of an adverse immune response, or activation of the blood clotting or complement pathways [76–78]. The biocompatibility of materials used in dental implants is evaluated by studying the reaction between the implant and the bone as well as between the implant and the soft tissue. Nevertheless, these evaluations are complex and comprehensive since adverse tissue reactions may occur in a variety of types. For example, the pulp/dentin test can be applied to determine the pulpal compatibility of a new material (local reaction), but it cannot be used to determine its allergenic potency [76].

In dentistry, alloys usually contain at least four metals, and often six or more. Thus dental alloys are metallurgically complex [79]. Metals that exhibit a high resistance to corrosion, such as Ti, Ta, Zr, Nb, and Pt, do not trigger a negative response of tissues. Even for these groups of metals, the type and amount of alloying elements have to be carefully optimized to elicit an appropriate immune response from the cells and the host tissue upon implantation. As one of the most commonly used Ti alloys for dental implants, Ti-6Al-4V has been a matter of dispute for the last few decades. The Ti-6Al-4V alloy has been used clinically since the 1950s. The release of both Al and V ions from this alloy has been found to be associated with long-term health problems, such as Alzheimer's disease, neuropathy, and osteomalacia [80,81]. Although soluble V as an alloying element has been reported to show toxic effects, no toxic reaction has been found for the use of the Ti-6Al-4V alloy in clinical practice [82]. Typically, ion releases from dental alloys are evaluated by in vitro studies, in which the alloy is subjected to different conditions such as galvanism, electrolyte bath, oral proteins, different pH levels, and brushing with toothpaste [79]. It is worth mentioning that a biocompatible alloy that does not cause any adverse reaction in cell cultures may cause problems in low pH conditions below plaque or crevices in the oral cavity. The low pH value in vivo may result in a more pronounced corrosion of the alloy than the neutral conditions in cell cultures [76]. In fact, cell culture studies indicate only whether potentially incompatible substances are released from a material at all.

The biocompatibility of dental materials is often evaluated based on cell culture and implantation studies. For cell culture studies, isolated cells derived from animal or human tissues are grown in culture plates and used for these tests. In addition to the frequent use of permanent cell lines such as mouse fibroblasts (L-929, 3T3) or human epithelial cells, other cells like gingival or pulp fibroblasts that are directly grown from explants of target tissues are also applied for toxicological studies of dental materials [83]. These cell cultures are incubated with the materials, and subsequently various parameters will be measured, including cell viability, protein synthesis, enzyme activity, or synthesis of inflammatory mediators. For implantation tests, materials are implanted subcutaneously, intramuscularly, or in the bone of an experimental animal. The tissue adjacent to the implant is investigated macroscopically and microscopically between 1 week and several months of implantation. The degree of inflammation surrounding the implant is assessed after a short implantation time, whereas in the case of an extended implantation period, the nature and quantity of the connective encapsulation will also be evaluated [76]. Another important biocompatibility test for the dentist is the pulp/dentin test. This test permits a better understanding of the processes of pulp reaction during the evaluation of a material [84]. The pulp compatibility of a material is investigated on the teeth of experimental animals or on human teeth that have to be extracted for orthodontic reasons [85]. In both cases, class V cavities are prepared without causing injury or trauma and are then filled with the test material. Varying from some days to several months, the teeth are removed and histologically prepared, and the pulps are microscopically evaluated for signs of acute or chronic inflammation and odontoblast reaction. Furthermore, the space between the test material and the cavity wall is investigated for bacterial penetration [86]. Given that each biocompatibility method reveals a number of disadvantages, data always need to be assessed together with findings from other tests, such as cell culture experiments and clinical studies.

5.3.3 Mechanical properties

The architectural structure of Ti foam scaffolds should not only ensure biological integration in the host tissue but also exhibit the desired biomechanical properties encountered in the dental environment. There are at least two different aspects associated with the significance of the mechanical properties of the scaffolds. First, the scaffold must be integrated mechanically to the host tissue upon implantation, i.e., it must be held in place, withstand the recurring loads, and adapt to the deformations and fluid shear stresses. Second, the scaffold should operate at the implantation site to provide the appropriate mechanical signals to the attached complexes of protein–cells in order for the cells to produce the expected extracellular material [18]. In general, the dental implant must be strong enough to withstand occlusal forces without deformation. A number of studies on occlusal force have been made. The maximum occlusal force that can be applied to teeth varies significantly between individuals, but generally it is larger for men than for women. Maximum occlusal forces of 350–440 N for women and 525–640 N for men have been reported [87]. It has also been noted that the maximum amount of force applied to molar teeth is usually several times larger than that being applied to the incisor region. On average, in the molar region it is from 230–450 N, on cuspids it is from 140–330 N, and it is from 88–250 N on incisors [88]. Typically, the desired mechanical strength should be based on the expected occlusal force ranges reported in the molar region.

Implant materials with a lower elastic modulus are more desirable, because the materials with low stiffness transmit forces to the bone better [34]. One of the interesting features of porous scaffolds is that their elastic modulus can be adjusted to be comparable with that of the bone tissue. This can be achieved by controlling the porosity, pore size, pore shape, and pore distribution. The introduction of a 3D porous surface implant has been successful in improving stress transfer from the implant to the bone interface, an improved stress distribution from the implant to the bone, and resultant lower stresses to the implant [89]. However, it should be noted that any alteration in the porous structure can also adversely affect other mechanical properties. For instance, the elastic modulus, yield strength, and ultimate compressive strength decrease with an increase of porosity.

Apart from the porosity and pore characteristics, the mechanical properties of Ti are also affected by a small amount of impurity. In particular, the amount of oxygen and nitrogen present with Ti is crucial for its mechanical properties such as hardness, strength, and ductility. Heated to a high temperature, Ti derives its strength from solution hardening by such elements as oxygen and nitrogen. The presence of these interstitial elements also leads to brittleness of Ti and its alloys [90–92].

The mechanical properties of an ideal porous Ti implant should match the properties of the maxilla, mandible, and, in particular, alveolar bones. Mechanical properties of bone vary widely from cancellous to cortical bone. The elastic modulus of cortical bone is between 5 and 23 GPa and that of cancellous bone is between 0.1 and 2 GPa. The compressive strength varies between 100 and 200 MPa for cortical bone and between 2 and 38 MPa for cancellous bone [93,94].

Zimmer Dental Inc. conducted an experiment to determine whether the friction caused by implant placement into a fresh extraction socket was capable of damaging porous implant surfaces. Implants with two different porous surfaces were evaluated: *Trabecular Metal* dental implants (fabricated by coating a vitreous carbon skeleton with Ta through a proprietary chemical vapor deposition coating process) and *Cancellous-Structured Titanium* (*CSTi*) dental implants (fabricated through a proprietary process that sinters CP-Ti powder onto a Ti or CoCr alloy substrate). In this study, the *Trabecular Metal* material and *CSTi* dental implants showed no evidence of abrasion or the release of metal debris into the osteotomy. In addition, both implants showed no deformation after implant placement [31]. The placement of *Trabecular Metal* dental implants in facial alveolar bone regeneration associated with immediate implant therapy has been reported [95]. It is notable that *Trabecular Metal* material is a 3D structure (with up to 80% porosity) similar to cancellous bone (Fig. 5.2). In the midsection of the implant, the *Trabecular Metal* material is made of Ta (98%) over a vitreous carbon substrate (2%). Ta has been used in clinical applications for many decades as pacemaker electrodes, foil and mesh for nerve repair, and radiopaque bone markers due to its excellent ductility, toughness, corrosion resistance, and in vivo bioactivity [96]. There has been renewed interest in using Ta for orthopedic and dental applications as an implant coating because of its good apposition to human bone [18,97,98]. The cultivation of mesenchymal stem cells on Ta surfaces resulted in a significantly increased mean cellular area and cell alkaline phosphatase activity compared with Ti and chromium surfaces tested [99].

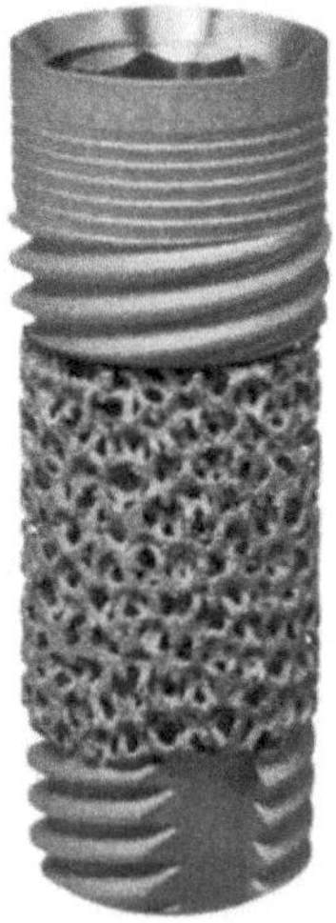

Figure 5.2 *Trabecular Metal* dental implant with a structure and elasticity similar to cancellous bone. This dental implant has been developed by Zimmer Dental Inc., Carlsbad, CA, USA, and consists of a titanium cervical and internal core section (upper section) covered by a *Trabecular Metal* sleeve (middle section) and joined by a titanium apical section (lower section).
Courtesy of Zimmer Dental Inc.

5.3.4 Pore characteristics

Porosity is a morphological property independent of the material and is defined as the percentage of void space in a solid. The porosity of most implants is usually determined to compromise between maintaining the mechanical strength of the implant while still providing adequate pore size for tissue ingrowth. The pores of the scaffold provide the cells with the necessary space to migrate, to form connections, to proliferate, and eventually to differentiate into the needed cell phenotype. Concurrently, the pores within the scaffold provide the space where new bone tissue formation as well as vascularization within this tissue occur.

A large pore size of scaffolds can allow for effective nutrient supply, gas diffusion, and metabolic waste removal but can also lead to low cell attachment and intracellular signaling, while a small pore size can do the opposite [100]. An optimum pore size required for implant fixation remains undefined; however, there is a general consensus that the pore sizes between 100 and 500 μm are necessary for most bone ingrowth settings [101,102]. The minimum pore size for acceptable bone ingrowth has been reported by some researchers to be in the range of 100–150 μm [103,104]. To ensure ingrowth of bone tissue into the pores, the material must have at least 60% porosity [105]. Nevertheless, care should be taken not to adversely affect the mechanical properties of the Ti foam scaffold with increasing the pore size and porosity. Although the growth rate and the formation of new bone increase with pore size [106], when the pore size is increased beyond 1 mm there seems to be an increasing tendency for the formation of fibrous tissue [107]. The results given by Klawitter and Hulbert showed that the pore diameter should be larger than 100 μm in order to ensure blood circulation to the required bone tissue ingrowth [108].

In addition to pore size, it appears that the shape of the pores will also affect the extent of cell ingrowth. Goodman et al. investigated the influence of pore cross-sectional shape on tissue ingrowth [109]. Samples with a round pore demonstrated less bone ingrowth as compared to samples with a square pore. Min et al. showed that the size and shape of the pores do not have a significant effect on the elastic property of CP-Ti as long as the pores are separated from each other [110]. Since bone has very different structures, depending on its function and location, a specific pore shape may not be ideal for all potential uses [111]. More investigations are necessary to further understand the effect of pore shape on bone ingrowth into the porous Ti implants.

Most scaffolds for dental and orthopedic applications are designed to ensure that their internal porous structures are interconnected through channels. The interconnectivity of pores, also termed as permeability, is critical in osteogenesis, the transportation of body fluid, and nutrition. The open and connected pores of the porous scaffolds can provide space and channels for bone ingrowth, which helps bone tissue to infiltrate the scaffold and anchor it into position. In other words, a lack of pore interconnectivity within scaffolds results in poor nutrient and oxygen delivery as well as limited waste removal from the scaffold [112,113]. Reportedly, 50% volume of interconnected pores is enough to significantly increase bone filling [114]. The interconnectivity of pores is increased by increasing the total porosity of the implant (usually for smaller sized pores) or by increasing the size of pores. The precise control of each single pore size and shape as well as the location of pores is very difficult to achieve by traditional manufacturing techniques. With the advent of more modern technologies, pore parameters such as size, density, and geometry are increasingly regulated and modified with greater precision and accuracy [115]. Additive manufacturing (AM) technology has extensively been used to fabricate Ti foam scaffolds with desired pore characteristics. AM has the ability to control matrix architecture such as size, shape, interconnectivity, geometry, and orientation, producing biomimetic structures that vary in design and material composition [97,116,117]. There are several AM techniques that have been utilized for the fabrication of metal foam scaffolds, such as 3D printing, electron beam melting, selective laser melting (SLM), direct metal deposition, selective laser sintering (SLS), and direct metal laser sintering (DMLS) [118].

The innovative aspect of AM is that the information can be modified and/or combined with other information to form complex and irregular geometries [119]. Because the AM method manufactures each implant to order, a customized medical implant with a controlled degree of porosity can be produced to fit the indication and patient. The hierarchical structure capabilities of AM contribute to the development of more optimal bone-ingrowth structures for osseointegration.

Laser sintering is an AM process that builds up parts layer by layer. EOS GmbH has established a safe and effective solution for its customers in the laser sintering of dental prostheses. It uses 3D data on the oral condition of the patient as a basis; this is generated using intraoral scanners or by impression or model scans. Leader Italia and AB Dental are two companies producing dental implants with laser sintering from EOS.

LayerWise is also an innovative company specializing in AM solutions founded in 2008 as a spin-off company from the University of Leuven, with an exclusive focus on metal 3D printing. In 2014, LayerWise was fully acquired by 3D Systems. LayerWise and DentWise (the dental division of LayerWise) developed the capability to produce porous orthopedic and dental scaffolds with optimal repeatability and maximum consistency of their mechanical and physical properties.

5.4 Osseointegration in titanium foam scaffolds

One of the basic requirements of dental implantology is that an implant has to be osseointegrated. The quality of the healing that takes place at the bone–implant interface ensures that a biological interfacial lock occurs, one that is predictably long lasting. The apparent advantages of some materials observed in a laboratory do not necessarily predict their clinical efficacy. In an in vivo model system, the tested materials may not always incorporate into host tissues due to a variety of factors, including lack of fixation, infection, mechanical failure, poor biocompatibility, or undesirable local reactions by the normal host tissue to the implant or implant material [120]. Nevertheless, Ti and some of its alloys have proven their suitability as implant materials in bone surgery over many years in the fields of osteosynthesis, oral implantology, and in certain applications in joint prosthetics. Fig. 5.3 shows new bone formation within the Ti dental implant during the healing period.

Some systematic and local factors that have been associated with the osseointegration of dental implants are as follows [121–123]:

(1) *Material*: It was initially believed that osseointegration is unique to CP-Ti. Further studies revealed that other materials such as zirconium and some ceramics (particularly hydroxyapatite) can also form an intimate bond with bone. However, these materials have not been as extensively studied and developed as CP-Ti for dental implant applications. (2) *Surface composition*: It is thought that CP-Ti owes its ability to form an osseointegrated interface to its native and highly biocompatible

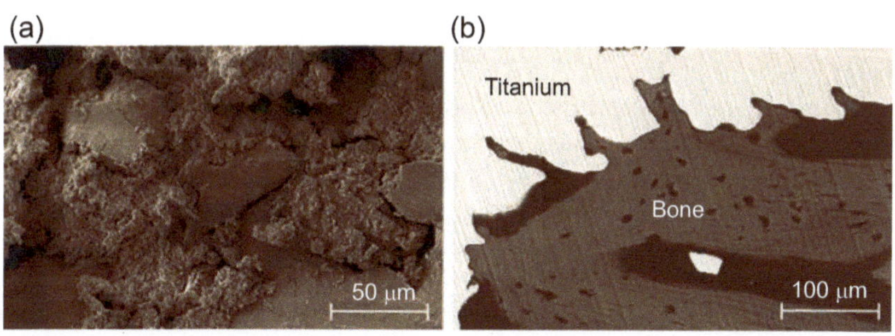

Figure 5.3 Scanning electron microscope (a) secondary electron and (b) backscattered images of new bone formation inside the titanium implant cavities and pores in human after 8 weeks. Courtesy of Leader Italia Srl.

surface oxide, Ti dioxide, which forms spontaneously on its surface. Surface composition can take the form of surface coatings (such as coating with hydroxyapatite), changes in the composition of the implant material by selective surface coping with small quantities of other elements, or the local use of biochemical molecules involved naturally in mediating bone formation, such as bone morphogenic proteins (BMPs). (3) *Heat*: The amount of heat produced by dental implant osteotomy should be carefully controlled by slow drilling speeds and large amounts of coolant. Heating of bone to a temperature in excess of 47°C can result in cell death and denaturation of collagen. Consequently, osseointegration is prevented, and the implant is surrounded by a fibrous capsule. (4) *Contamination*: Contamination of the implant site by organic and inorganic debris can disrupt the osseointegration process. Contamination of the implant site can occur from sources like the air of the operating room, resident bacteria on the patient's skin and body, and chemical reagents and debris from drills. (5) *Initial stability*: It is known that osseointegration is strongly affected by the stability of the implant in its osteotomy site. Osseointegration is more likely to occur when direct contact between the bone and the implant surface is maintained. This property is associated with the quality and geometry of the implant, bone morphology, and bone density. Thus screw-shaped and/or porous implants will be more readily stable than the smooth surfaces with no thread or variation on them. (6) *Bone quality*: It is a function of bone density, anatomy, and volume. It relates to the thickness and density of cortical and cancellous bone and the amount of bone resorption. (7) *Early loading and micromotion*: There is compelling evidence that premature loading and excessive relative movement result in the formation of a fibrous capsule rather than osseointegration. (8) *Occlusal overloads*: It has been shown that excessive mechanical loads on an osseointegrated implant can result in a breakdown of the interface and implant failure. Moreover, the stress distribution of occlusal force through the implant to the surrounding bones can affect the osseointegration process.

One way to physically improve overall osseointegration is to use 3D porous surface implants. The interconnected porosity of foam scaffolds is designed to enhance stability through a high volume of bone ingrowth. Fig. 5.4 illustrates how a porous structure provides sufficient space for bone ingrowth and enhances early osseointegration. As outlined in the previous sections, pore characteristics, including pore size, pore shape, porosity, and pore interconnectivity, have shown their significant influence on osseointegration and the long-term stability of porous implants [124–127]. Rosa and coworkers studied the influence of a porous Ti structure (pore size: 50–400 μm; porosity: 60%) on osseointegration and cell behavior [128]. Osteogenic cells derived from human alveolar bone were cultured on solid Ti, as a control, and porous Ti for periods of up to 17 days. The results indicated that porous Ti is a more appropriate substrate than solid Ti for osteogenic cell adhesion, proliferation, and production of a mineralized matrix. In a similar study, the effects of different thicknesses of a porous Ti coating were examined on osteoblast phenotype expression [129]. The authors observed that the expression of an osteoblast phenotype and the production of a mineralized extracellular matrix were higher on the thicker porous coating (1.5 mm) than its counterparts with porous coatings of 0.5 and 1 mm.

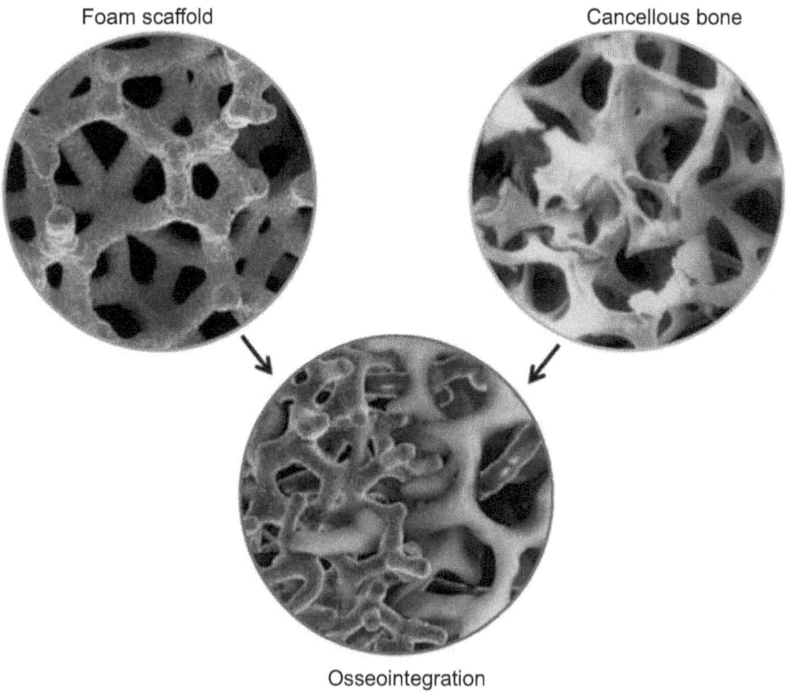

Figure 5.4 Schematic representation of the osseointegration of a foam scaffold. A foam scaffold can provide structural support for the bone ingrowth to achieve durable biological fixation. Courtesy of Zimmer Dental Inc.

Simmons et al. compared the early tissue-healing response and resulting implant stability for two surface designs by characterizing the histological and mechanical properties of the healing tissue around Ti-6Al-4V-sintered, porous-surfaced, and Ti plasma-sprayed implants [130]. The plasma spray-coated design was selected as representative of implants with a textured surface for comparison to the 3D surfaces presented by the sintered surface structure. The pull-out tests and structural assessments indicated significantly higher rates of osseointegration with the porous-surfaced design. Bone ingrowth was observed within the pores of the sintered porous surface layer as early as 8 days after implantation. Increasing the rate of osseointegration is important for increasing the probability of successful implant performance.

5.5 Dental implants with porous titanium coating

All implant materials intended for dental and orthopedic applications must contain complex topographical features. Surface topography and roughness are of the utmost importance for bone bonding and biological fixation of dental and orthopedic implants. Most surface topographical features provide initial stabilization until bone can grow and attach to the implant surface to establish further improvement in implant bonding [131]. Surface modification and coating of dental implants are aimed at creating 3D nano- and microscale porous structures for accelerating and improving bone and implant integration. It has been found that for endosseous screw-shaped implants (threaded implants), regions of high stress concentration develop in the bone during implant loading, especially adjacent to the superior-most threads. As an alternative strategy, porous surface implants have been developed and used for achieving lower peak peri-implant bone stresses that allow efficient force transfer over a greater portion of the bone-interfacing implant surface [132]. Also, for the case of short implants, the porous implant exhibits a more favorable stress distribution in the cancellous bone than a solid implant [133]. In an in vivo study, Story et al. coated cylindrical dental implants with a porous Ti structure and implanted them in canine mandibles and femorals. They found more bone ingrowth for the higher porosity coatings at all time points (14 weeks) in the femorals and at the initial time points (2 and 4 weeks) in the mandibles [134].

A variety of methods have been developed to produce a porous coating on implants, with the specific aim of enhancing osseointegration. More information on these fabrication methods can be found in the literature [20,131]. The fabrication of porous-surfaced Ti and Ti-6Al-4V implants normally involves either plasma-spraying or sintering powders onto a solid substrate [90,135,136]. Porous-surfaced implants fabricated by sintering Ti alloy powders on machined Ti alloy substrates showed remarkable performance as "so-called short ($\leq$7 mm)" implants [132]. The overall porous surface layer was approximately 0.3 mm thick and consisted of two or three layers of sintered Ti-6A1-4V alloy powders securely bonded to the underlying solid substrate. Human clinical and animal studies explored the contribution of these characteristics to two significant features, namely reliable osseointegration of "short" implants and rapid bone ingrowth (osteoconductivity). Porous-surfaced implants of 7, 9, and 12 mm length have also been used with equal success for supporting fixed partial dentures and as free-standing implants [137].

Nevertheless, the commonly used coating methods suffer from some major drawbacks. Defects or failures such as microcracking, poor adhesion between the coatings and substrates, and delamination have been reported in the coating systems [90,138]. Besides, the use of a porous coating does not solve the problem of mechanical mismatch between the implant and the bone. To tackle these problems, the fabrication of fully porous dental implants or implants consisting of monolithic solid cores with a porous surface have been studied and developed. Fig. 5.5 shows two types of Ti foam scaffolds produced by powder metallurgy.

Typically, the biomechanical strength of fully porous dental implants is too low to withstand the occlusal forces that a patient will exert upon them. Therefore an implant with a gradient pore structure was brought into application [139–144]. While the outer porous surface layer provides space for bone ingrowth and mechanical interlocking between the implant and bone, the solid core satisfies the required strengths for

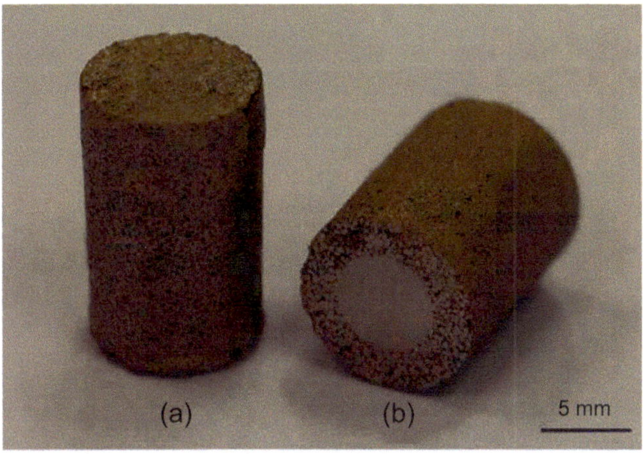

Figure 5.5 Titanium foam scaffold with (a) a fully porous structure and (b) a solid core and porous surface layer. The scaffolds were fabricated by a sintering method using titanium-agglomerated particles to ensure a porous structure with interconnected pores. The solid core was made from elemental titanium powder.

load-bearing applications. Depending on the fabrication method and the final application, porous surface layers are produced, ranging from 10 μm to a few millimeters. In order to obtain an ideal surface for osteoblast cell growth, Kutty et al. manufactured a graded porosity on the surface of a Ti dental implant while maintaining a dense core in a Ti sample via a one-step microwave-processing route [145]. The thickness of the porous region and the pore size were 100−200 μm and 30−100 μm, respectively.

Using the SLM method, it is feasible to join very thin sections (20−60 μm) together. This method permits very complex geometries to be created with a gradient pore structure perpendicular to the long axis of the implant [146]. Traini et al. reported that the rough surface of the Ti-6A1-4V dental implant with a porous surface and a solid inner layer structure favors new bone ingrowth and thus improves the connection strength between the implant and alveolar bone. It was also shown that the elastic modulus of the implant was effectively reduced by the porous surface layer, thereby minimizing the stress shielding between the implant and the human alveolar bone [146]. Since 2009, Leader Italia Srl. has developed a new Ti dental implant using DMLS, as seen in Fig. 5.6. This technique uses a laser as the heating source to sinter powdered material. The combined effects of self-threading fixtures and a porous surface promote attachment and integration of the implant to the bone. A few clinical studies have been conducted on DMLS-produced Ti implants as well as the application of DMLS technology for the fabrication of custom-made implants [147−153]. For instance, Mangano and his coworkers found that the use of four DMLS-produced Ti implants to support bar-retained maxillary overdentures represented a safe and successful procedure, with excellent 3-year survival rates and a low incidence of biological complications [152].

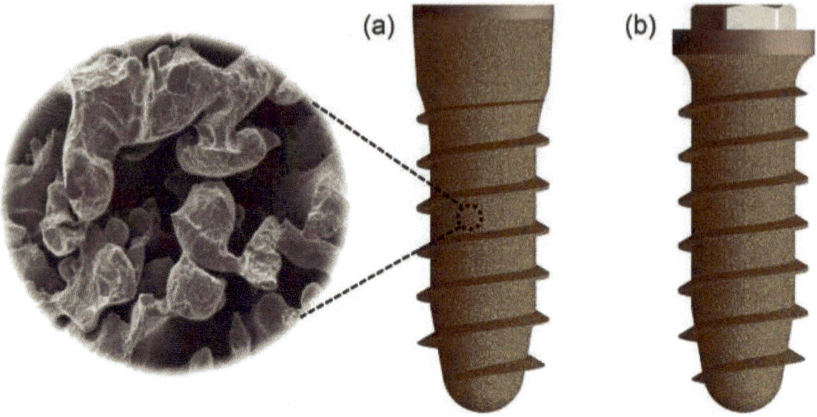

Figure 5.6 Porous titanium dental implant screw, branded as TiXos, with excellent osseointegration characteristics produced by the direct metal laser sintering technique. The implants are supplied with (a) internal hex and (b) external hex, featuring a highly porous surface with interconnected pores.
Courtesy of Leader Italia Srl.

5.6 Dental applications of titanium scaffolds: advancement and challenges

Endosseous dental implants have become a promising treatment in prosthodontics and restorative dentistry since the early 1970s. Despite the myriad of technological advances in the following decades, the potential for clinical failure is a significant concern for both the dentist and the patient. Success rates of endosseous implants depend on the site of the implant, bruxism (grinding of the teeth) or other large occlusal forces, hygiene in the mouth, preoperative or postoperative infection, placement in the bone of inadequate quality or quantity, the clinical status of the patient, the skill and experience of the surgeon, biomechanical elements, and the type and size of implant material. In fact, all of these factors interact and determine success or failure [64,154,155].

Though efforts to improve the osseointegration properties of implants have inspired much of the literature around dental implants for the last 50 years, it becomes apparent that there are numerous known and possibly several unknown factors that need to be considered in the fabrication of dental implants in order to adequately address these needs. For instance, while osseointegration of implants in regions of poor bone quality (i.e., low bone density, in the case of highly cancellous bone, or low vascularity, in the case of primarily cortical bone) or insufficient quantity of bone (in terms of the width or height of the alveolar ridge) remains problematic, new design and/or material innovations need to be explored to further promote osseointegration of dental implants in these areas [1,156,157]. The question is posed as to whether the Ti foam scaffold would potentially be a suitable candidate to address these limitations.

The porous structures of most metallic implants cannot be very well controlled using the conventional production techniques, involving space holder and replication methods [158,159]. These techniques mostly result in porous structures with a certain pore size range, rather than structures with an accurately defined pore size [160−162]. Some of these limitations have been addressed by AM technology that involves creating a reticulated skeleton with deposition of a metal onto the surface [163]. Nevertheless, even the dental implants produced by AM technology may exhibit drawbacks. It has been reported that the dental implants produced by SLS or DMLS exhibit apparent defects, such as rough surface, balling effect, pores and cracks, distortion in threads, etc. From the engineering standpoint, pores and defects are favorable sites for the initiation and propagation of cracks, thereby affecting the mechanical properties of the dental implants under long-term cyclic loading [133]. Engineering pore distributions to match the mechanical properties of bone is commonly accepted to be the next major improvement in the design of open-cell porous scaffolds.

Another problem in dental applications of porous biomaterials is the aggressive chemical environment in the mouth. Unlike most orthopedic surgical sites, the oral cavity is an unsterile environment, which is inhabited by over 500 different bacterial species that favor corrosion. Corrosion can also severely limit the fatigue life and ultimate strength of the material, leading to the mechanical failure of the implant. There is a low but finite prevalence of corrosion-related fractures of implants. Increased surface areas, such as in porous implants, have shown higher corrosion rates when tested in vitro compared to conventional nonporous implants [127,164−166]. On the contrary, Seah et al. reported that in highly porous Ti compacts with an open, interconnected pore morphology, the free flow of species resulted in a material with a high resistance to corrosion [167]. The interactions of the host tissue, saliva, and microorganisms can make it difficult to predict how porous dental implants would react to this complex oral environment [2]. Atomic absorption spectroscopy of blood samples collected from patients with porous-surfaced dental implants during the implantation period of 3 years did not demonstrate any significant increase in retained alloy elements (e.g., Ti, Al, V) [162]. The question of the long-term host response to such implants remains an important issue requiring proper clinical follow-up studies.

Dental implants are subjected to many loading cycles during their lifetime, mainly those produced during mastication. Fatigue may cause dental implants to break, with serious consequences from a clinical standpoint. Thus it is highly important to determine the durability of a dental implant and its components subjected to chewing forces and occlusal loads, especially in the posterior regions of the maxilla and mandible. A major concern with the use of porous implants in highly loaded applications is the effect of the porous structure on fatigue strength [20]. Studies have shown drastic reductions in the fatigue strength of Ti-6Al-4V alloy fabricated as porous coatings on solid core structures [135,168]. Wolfarth and Ducheyne reported that the high cycle fatigue strength of porous coated Ti-6A1-4V alloy is approximately one-third of the solid alloy with a similar shape [138]. This is mostly due to highly stress-concentrated regions at particle substrate neck regions acting as crack initiation sites [169].

The concept of using surface porosity to anchor the implant in position within the surrounding bone has been proven to be clinically successful in the unloaded state.

Young proposed a design and implanting technique using porous Ti as an anchoring site. The post implants showed the development of healthy gingiva, whereas both buried and post implants demonstrated the ability to become firmly anchored by tissue growth into porosity [126,170]. In another study, two types of endosseous dental implants were produced, and their functionality was tested. One type consisted of a porous sintered Ti−30Ta alloy, and the other had a special surface structure consisting of Ti wire loops. The functionality was tested after insertion into an artificial jaw, which had properties corresponding to the natural jaw bone. The elastic properties of both implants were similar to the properties of the bone. In addition, the implants had a safe anchorage bone ingrowth. In animal experiments using the implant with surface loops it was observed that the bone entered the loops and even extremely small surface cavities in the wire loops [171].

The lack of direct contact at the porous surface−bone interface also has an adverse effect on bone ingrowth and the stability of the implant. This apposition is often not achieved because of the design of the implant, relative motion (sometimes called micromotion), or instruments as well as the operative technique [20]. A study by Dalton et al. suggests that gaps greater than 1 mm significantly decrease attachment and bone ingrowth [172].

In order to enhance the communication between cells and to facilitate their organization within the porous scaffold, it is desirable to integrate cell-recognizable ligands and signaling growth factors on the surface of the scaffolds. Indeed, biofactors that influence cell proliferation, differentiation, migration, morphologies, and gene expression can be incorporated in the scaffold design and fabrication to enhance the cell growth rate and direct cell functions [169]. A variety of biomimetic coatings have been found to be helpful for implants. For example, coating implants with BMPs may enhance osseointegration and shorten healing time after implantation, thereby improving implant success rates [173,174].

Kim et al. compared the bone growth into the porous section and biomechanical stability of implants with a 3D porous Ta material in their midsection with a traditional threaded Ti alloy implant system [175]. The implants were placed in the individual mandibles of eight dogs, and the biomechanical stability was assessed for a maximum of 12 weeks. The results exhibited the same degree of stability for both series of implants.

5.7 Conclusion and future trends

New materials, designs, and techniques have been developed for dental restorations and implants. The principal research efforts have been aimed at reducing the treatment time, either by decreasing the time necessary for osseointegration or through more immediate loading of the implant. For this reason, special attention is given to the manufacturing of implants that closely mimic the architecture and properties of the surrounding alveolar bone of the maxilla and mandible.

The interest in using porous scaffolds for dental applications has been gaining momentum and continues to be the hot spot of clinical research in the 21st century. The focus, thereby, has mainly been on applications that involve bone ingrowth into the porous Ti scaffolds with a fully porous structure or with a solid core and porous surface/coating. For load-bearing dental implants, Ti and its alloys have so far shown the greatest potential as the basis for such scaffolds, due to their excellent corrosion resistance, biocompatibility, and high degree of strength-to-weight ratio.

Significant progress has been made to fabricate various porous Ti scaffolds by using different techniques. Some of these techniques allow for greater control of pore architecture and porosity within scaffolds. The macro and microstructure of porous scaffolds, such as pore size, pore shape, porosity, and pore interconnectivity, affect osteogenic cell adhesion, migration, ingrowth, and the production of a mineralized matrix. However, engineering porous scaffolds with ideal pore characteristics for hard tissue engineering applications remains a complex and challenging process. In addition, most of the available techniques for the fabrication of porous scaffolds are unable to serve as reliable methods for the further development of reproducible porous scaffolds. Ongoing and future research will continue to develop new techniques to control the pore characteristics of scaffolds and generate dental implants containing gradients of pore size and porosity for the regeneration of craniofacial bone.

It is only recently that researchers have begun to understand the combination of parameters that need to be addressed in the successful implementation of porous scaffolds in vivo. A large number of studies have been performed to hasten osseointegration in porous Ti scaffolds and to improve their mechanical properties under occlusal and masticatory forces by altering the surface chemistry, introducing new biocompatible alloys, designs, and pore characteristics, or impregnating surface coatings with bone growth factors such as BMPs. It is thus envisaged that the breakthroughs and developments in manufacturing methods, micro- and nanoengineering, metallurgy, and biology will lay the foundations for more advanced and functional Ti foam scaffolds for dental applications.

Acknowledgments

I would like to thank Dr. Carina Freitas for her support and kind assistance during the preparation of this chapter. I would also like to acknowledge Dr. Keivan Nazari for supplying me with the photo of Ti foam scaffolds.

References

[1] Gupta S. Oral and maxillofacial devices. In: Pruitt LA, Chakravartula AM, editors. Mechanics of biomaterials: fundamental principles for implant design. Cambridge, UK: Cambridge University Press; 2011. p. 505−59.

[2] Bencharit S, Byrd WC, Altarawneh S, Hosseini B, Leong A, Reside G, et al. Development and applications of porous tantalum trabecular metal-enhanced titanium dental implants. Clin Implant Dent Relat Res 2014;16:817−26.

[3] Brennan M, Houston F, O'Sullivan M, O'Connell B. Demographics of implant placement and complications of a patient subgroup in a dental hospital population. J Irish Dent Assoc 2009;56:85–92.
[4] Misch CE. Dental implant prosthetics. 2nd ed. St. Louis, Missouri: Elsevier-Mosby; 2014.
[5] Cherchève R. Les implants endo-osseux. Paris: Maloine; 1962.
[6] Cherchève R. The philosophies which governed the origin, development and present-day use of endosseous dental implants. J Oral Implant Transpl Surg 1966;12:28–34.
[7] McCabe JF, Walls AWG. Applied dental materials. 9th ed. Oxford, UK: Blackwell Publishing; 2008.
[8] Brånemark PI, Adell R, Breine U, Hansson BO, Lindström J, Ohlsson A. Intra-osseous anchorage of dental prostheses. I. Experimental studies. Scand J Plast Reconstr Surg 1969;3:81–100.
[9] Brånemark PI, Hansson BO, Adell R, Breine U, Lindström J, Hallén O, et al. Osseointegrated implants in the treatment of the edentulous jaw. Experience from a 10-year period. Scand J Plast Reconstr Surg 1977;16:1–132.
[10] Brånemark PI. Introduction to osseointegration. In: Brånemark PI, Zarb GA, Albrektsson T, editors. Tissue-integrated prosthesis: osseointegration in clinical dentistry. Chicago: Quintessence; 1985. p. 11–76.
[11] Bornstein MM, Valderrama P, Jones AA, Wilson TG, Seibl R, Cochran DL. Bone apposition around two different sandblasted and acid-etched titanium implant surfaces: a histomorphometric study in canine mandibles. Clin Oral Implants Res 2008;19:233–41.
[12] Cho SA, Park KT. The removal torque of titanium screw inserted in rabbit tibia treated by dual acid etching. Biomaterials 2003;24:3611–7.
[13] Degidi M, Nardi D, Piattelli A. 10-year follow-up of immediately loaded implants with TiUnite porous anodized surface. Clin Implant Dent Relat Res 2012;14:828–38.
[14] Mendes VC, Moineddin R, Davies JE. The effect of discrete calcium phosphate nanocrystals on bone-bonding to titanium surfaces. Biomaterials 2007;28:4748–55.
[15] Rupp F, Scheideler L, Olshanska N, de Wild M, Wieland M, Geis-Gerstorfer J. Enhancing surface free energy and hydrophilicity through chemical modification of microstructured titanium implant surfaces. J Biomed Mater Res A 2006;76:323–34.
[16] MacDonald DE, Rapuano BE, Deo N, Stranick M, Somasundaran P, Boskey AL. Thermal and chemical modification of titanium-aluminum-vanadium implant materials: effects on surface properties, glycoprotein adsorption, and MG63 cell attachment. Biomaterials 2004;25:3135–46.
[17] Chen L. Finite element analysis of the stress on the implant-bone interface of dental implants with different structures. In: Ebrahimi F, editor. Finite element analysis – new trends and developments. InTech; 2012. p. 55–76.
[18] Helsen JA, Missirlis Y. Biomaterials: a Tantalus experience. Heidelberg: Springer-Verlag; 2010.
[19] Schiefer H, Bram M, Buchkremer HP, Stöver D. Mechanical examinations on dental implants with porous titanium coating. J Mater Sci Mater Med 2009;20:1763–70.
[20] Ryan G, Pandit A, Apatsidis DP. Fabrication methods of porous metals for use in orthopaedic applications. Biomaterials 2006;27:2651–70.
[21] Wen CE, Yamada Y, Shimojima K, Chino Y, Asahina T, Mabuchi M. Processing and mechanical properties of autogenous titanium implant materials. J Mater Sci Mater Med 2002;13:397–401.
[22] Bansiddhi A, Dunand DC. Titanium and NiTi foams for bone replacement. In: Mallick K, editor. Bone substitute biomaterials. Elsevier; 2014.

[23] Haeri M, Jon Goldberg A. Mimicking dentin structure: bio-inspired scaffolds for dental tissue engineering. Mater Today 2014;17:518–9.
[24] Ring ME. A thousand years of dental implants: a definitive history – part 1. Compend Contin Educ Dent 1995;16. 1060, 1062, 1064 passim.
[25] von Fraunhofer JA. Dental materials at a glance. 2nd ed. Oxford, UK: Wiley-Blackwell; 2013.
[26] Ring ME. A thousand years of dental implants: a definitive history – part 2. Compend Contin Educ Dent 1995;16. 1132, 1134, 1136 passim.
[27] Alla RK, Ginjupalli K, Upadhya N, Shammas M, Ravi RK, Sekhar R. Surface roughness of implants: a review. Trends Biomater Artif Organs 2011;25:112–8.
[28] Anusavice K. Phillips' science of dental materials. 12th ed. Missouri: Saunders-Elsevier St. Louis; 2013.
[29] Venable CS, Stuck WG, Beach A. The effects on bone of the presence of metals, based upon electrolysis. Ann Surg 1937;105:917.
[30] Venable CS. Osteosynthesis in the presence of metals. South Med J 1938;31:501.
[31] Collins M, Bassett J, Wen HB, Gervais C, Lomicka M, Papanicolaou S. Trabecular metal™ dental implants: overview of design and developmental research. Zimmer Dental Inc.; 2012. p. 1–8.
[32] Lang NP, Matinlinna JP. Titanium in implant dentistry. In: Matinlinna JP, editor. Handbook of oral biomaterials. Pan Stanford Publishing; 2014. p. 339–58.
[33] A.D.A.C.o.S. Affairs, Titanium applications in dentistry. J Am Dent Assoc 2003;134: 347–9.
[34] McCracken M. Dental implant materials: commercially pure titanium and titanium alloys. J Prosthodont 1999;8:40–3.
[35] Muddugangadhar BC, Amarnath GS, Tripathi S, Dikshit S, Divya MS. Biomaterials for dental implants: an overview. Int J Oral Implantol Clin Res 2011;2:13–24.
[36] Hirschhorn JS, Mcbeath AA, Dustoor MR. Porous titanium surgical implant materials. J Biomed Mater Res Symp 1971;1:49–67.
[37] C.o.D.M. Dental association, instruments and equipment, dental endosseous implants. J Am Dent Assoc 1986;113:949–50.
[38] C.o.D.M. Dental association, instruments and equipment. J Am Dent Assoc 1996;129: 1238–9.
[39] Niinomi M. Recent research and development in titanium alloys for biomedical applications and healthcare goods. Sci Technol Adv Mater 2003;4:445–54.
[40] Ozaki T, Matsumoto H, Watanabe S, Hanada S. Beta Ti alloys with low Young's modulus. Mater Trans 2004;45:2776–9.
[41] Eisenbarth E, Velten D, Müller M, Thull R, Breme J. Biocompatibility of beta-stabilizing elements of titanium alloys. Biomaterials 2004;25:5705–13.
[42] Niinomi M, Nakai M, Hieda J. Development of new metallic alloys for biomedical applications. Acta Biomater 2012;8:3888–903.
[43] Sista S, Nouri A, Li Y, Wen C, Hodgson PD, Pande G. Cell biological responses of osteoblasts on anodized nanotubular surface of a titanium-zirconium alloy. J Biomed Mater Res A 2013;101:3416–30.
[44] Berner S, Dard M, Gottlow J, Molenberg A, Wieland M. Titanium-zirconium: a novel material for dental implants. Eur Cells Mater 2009;17(Suppl. 1):16.
[45] Akahori T, Niinomi M, Suzuki A. Improvement of mechanical properties of dental cast Ti-6Al-7Nb by thermochemical processing. Metall Mater Trans A 2002;33:503–10.
[46] Choubey A, Basu B, Balasubramaniam R. Tribological behaviour of Ti-based alloys in simulated body fluid solution at fretting contacts. Mater Sci Eng A 2004;379:234–9.

[47] Parr GR, Gardner LK, Toth RW. Titanium: the mystery metal of implant dentistry. Dental materials aspects. J Prosthet Dent 1985;54:410–4.
[48] Duerig TW, Melton KN, Stockel D, Wayman CM. Engineering aspects of shape memory alloys. London: Butterworth-Heinemann; 1990.
[49] Miyazaki S. Medical and dental applications of shape memory alloys. In: Otṣuka K, Wayman CM, editors. Shape memory materials. Cambridge University Press; 1998. p. 267–81.
[50] Farzin-nia F, Yoneyama T. Orthodontic devices using Ti–Ni shape memory alloys. In: Yoneyama T, Miyazaki S, editors. Shape memory alloys for biomedical applications. Cambridge, UK.: Woodhead Publishing; 2009. p. 257–96.
[51] Fukuyo S, Suzuki Y, Sairenji E. Shape memory implants. In: Duerig TW, Melton KN, Stockel D, Wayman CM, editors. Engineering aspects of shape memory alloys. Butterworth-Heinemann; 1990. p. 470–6.
[52] Pautke C, Kolk A, Brokate M, Wehrstedt JC, Kneissl F, Miethke T, et al. Development of novel implant abutments using the shape memory alloy nitinol: preliminary results. Int J Oral Maxillofac Implants 2009;24:477–83.
[53] Biesiekierski A, Wang J, Gepreel MA, Wen C. A new look at biomedical Ti-based shape memory alloys. Acta Biomater 2012;8:1661–9.
[54] Wen CE, Xiong JY, Li YC, Hodgson PD. Porous shape memory alloy scaffolds for biomedical applications: a review. Physica Scripta 2010:1–8. 014070.
[55] Takahashi E, Sakurai T, Watanabe S, Masahashi N, Hanada S. Effect of heat treatment and Sn content on superelasticity in biocompatible TiNbSn alloys. Mater Trans 2002;43: 2978–83.
[56] Bansiddhi A, Dunand DC. Shape-memory NiTi foams produced by replication of NaCl space-holders. Acta Biomater 2008;4:1996–2007.
[57] Bansiddhi A, Dunand DC. Shape-memory NiTi foams produced by solid-state replication with NaF. Intermetallics 2007;15:1612–22.
[58] Köhl M, Habijan T, Bram M, Buchkremer HP, Stöver D, Köller M. Powder metallurgical near-net-shape fabrication of porous NiTi shape memory alloys for use as long-term implants by the combination of the metal injection molding process with the space-holder technique. Adv Eng Mater 2009;11:959–68.
[59] Li DS, Zhang YP, Eggeler G, Zhang XP. High porosity and high-strength porous NiTi shape memory alloys with controllable pore characteristics. J Alloys Compd 2009;470: 1–5.
[60] Dunand DC, Mari D, Bourke MAM, Roberts JA. NiTi and NiTi-TiC composites: Part IV. Neutron diffraction study of twinning and shape-memory recovery. Metall Mater Trans A 1996;27:2820–36.
[61] Gibson LJ, Ashby MF. Cellular solids: structure and properties. 2nd ed. UK: Cambridge University Press; 1997.
[62] Gotman I, Ben-David D, Unger RE, Böse T, Gutmanas EY, Kirkpatrick CJ. Mesenchymal stem cell proliferation and differentiation on load-bearing trabecular Nitinol scaffolds. Acta Biomater 2013;9:8440–8.
[63] Liu X, Wu S, Yeung KW, Chan YL, Hu T, Xu Z, et al. Relationship between osseointegration and superelastic biomechanics in porous NiTi scaffolds. Biomaterials 2011;32: 330–8.
[64] Porter JA, von Fraunhofer JA. Success or failure of dental implants? A literature review with treatment considerations. Gen Dent 2005;53:423–32.
[65] Misch CE. Dental implant prosthetics. St. Louis, Missouri: Elsevier-Mosby; 2015.

[66] Deporter D, Ogiso B, Sohn DS, Ruljancich K, Pharoah M. Ultrashort sintered porous-surfaced dental implants used to replace posterior teeth. J Periodontol 2008;79:1280–6.
[67] el Askary AS, Meffert RM, Griffin T. Why do dental implants fail? Part I. Implant Dent 1999;8:173–85.
[68] Snauwaert K, Duyck J, van Steenberghe D, Quirynen M, Naert I. Time dependent failure rate and marginal bone loss of implant supported prostheses: a 15-year follow-up study. Clin Oral Investig 2000;4:13–20.
[69] Gealh WC, Mazzo V, Barbi F, Camarini ET. Osseointegrated implant fracture: causes and treatment. J Oral Implantol 2011;37:499–503.
[70] Palmer RM, Howe LC, Palmer PJ. Implants in clinical dentistry. New York: Informa Healthcare; 2012.
[71] Abuhussein H, Pagni G, Rebaudi A, Wang HL. The effect of thread pattern upon implant osseointegration. Clin Oral Implants Res 2010;21:129–36.
[72] Orsini E, Giavaresi G, Trirè A, Ottani V, Salgarello S. Dental implant thread pitch and its influence on the osseointegration process: an in vivo comparison study. Int J Oral Maxillofac Implants 2012;27:383–92.
[73] Noorthoek DR. Macroscopic and microscopic dental implant design: a review of the literature. University of Florida; 2013.
[74] Williams DF. Definitions in biomaterials. In: Proceedings of a consensus conference of the European Society for Biomaterials (ESB). Amsterdam: Elsevier; 1987.
[75] Williams DF. On the mechanisms of biocompatibility. Biomaterials 2008;29:2941–53.
[76] Schmalz G. Determination of biocompatibility. In: Schmalz G, Arenholt-Bindslev D, editors. Biocompatibility of dental materials. Berlin: Springer-Verlag; 2009. p. 13–43.
[77] Elias CN. Factors affecting the success of dental implants. In: Turkyilmaz I, editor. Implant dentistry – a rapidly evolving practice. Rijeka, Croatia: InTech; 2011. p. 319–64.
[78] Karande TS, Agrawal CM. Functions and requirements of synthetic scaffolds in tissue engineering. In: Laurencin CT, Nair LS, editors. Nanotechnology and tissue engineering: the scaffold. Boca Raton, FL: CRC Press; 2008. p. 53–86.
[79] Elshahawy W, Watanabe I. Biocompatibility of dental alloys used in dental fixed prosthodontics. Tanta Dent J 2014;11:150–9.
[80] Rao S, Ushida T, Tateishi T, Okazaki Y, Asao S. Effect of Ti, Al, and V ions on the relative growth rate of fibroblasts (L929) and osteoblasts (MC3T3-E1) cells. Biomed Mater Eng 1996;6:79–86.
[81] Walker PR, LeBlanc J, Sikorska M. Effects of aluminum and other cations on the structure of brain and liver chromatin. Biochemistry 1989;28:3911–5.
[82] Brunette DM, Tengvall P, Textor M, Thomsen P. Titanium in medicine. Heidelberg: Springer Verlag; 2001.
[83] Arenholt-Bindslev D, Bleeg H. Characterization of two types of human oral fibroblast with a potential application to cellular toxicity studies: tooth pulp fibroblasts and buccal mucosa fibroblasts. Int Endod J 1990;23:84–91.
[84] de Souza Costa CA, Hebling J, Scheffel DL, Soares DG, Basso FG, Ribeiro AP. Methods to evaluate and strategies to improve the biocompatibility of dental materials and operative techniques. Dent Mater 2014;30:769–84.
[85] Schmalz G. Concepts in biocompatibility testing of dental restorative materials. Clin Oral Investig 1997;1:154–62.
[86] Klötzer WT, Langeland K. Testing of materials and methods for crown and bridge prosthesis on animals. Schweiz Monatsschr Zahnheilkd 1973;83:163–244.

[87] Okeson JP. Management of temporomandibular disorders and occlusion. 6th ed. St. Louis, Missouri: Mosby Elsevier; 2008.
[88] Howell AH, Manley RS. An electronic strain gauge for measuring oral forces. J Dent Res 1948;27:705–12.
[89] Eckert SE, Salinas TJ. Implant fractures: etiology, prevention, and treatment. In: Froum SJ, editor. Dental implant complications. Wiley-Blackwell; 2010. p. 100–9.
[90] Asaoka K, Kuwayama N, Okuno O, Miura I. Mechanical properties and biomechanical compatibility of porous titanium for dental implants. J Biomed Mater Res 1985;19: 699–713.
[91] Nouri A, Chen XB, Li YC, Yamada Y, Hodgson PD, Wen CE. Synthesis of Ti-Sn-Nb alloy by powder metallurgy. Mater Sci Eng A 2008;485:562–70.
[92] Nouri A, Hodgson PD, Wen CE. Effect of process control agent on the porous structure and mechanical properties of a biomedical Ti-Sn-Nb alloy produced by powder metallurgy. Acta Biomater 2010;6:1630–9.
[93] An YH. Mechanical properties of bone. In: An YH, Draughn RA, editors. Mechanical testing of bone and the bone–implant interface. Boca Raton, Florida: CRC Press; 2000. p. 41–63.
[94] Bose S, Roy M, Bandyopadhyay A. Recent advances in bone tissue engineering scaffolds. Trends Biotechnol 2012;30:546–54.
[95] Bencharit S, Byrd WC, Hosseini B. Immediate placement of a porous-tantalum, trabecular metal-enhanced titanium dental implant with demineralized bone matrix into a socket with deficient buccal bone: a clinical report. J Prosthet Dent 2015;113:262–9.
[96] Balla VK, Bose S, Davies NM, Bandyopadhyay A. Tantalum-a bioactive metal for implants. JOM 2010;62:61–4.
[97] Wauthle R, van der Stok J, Amin Yavari S, Van Humbeeck J, Kruth JP, Zadpoor AA, et al. Additively manufactured porous tantalum implants. Acta Biomater 2015;14:217–25.
[98] Hanzlik JA, Day JS. Bone ingrowth in well-fixed retrieved porous tantalum implants. J Arthroplasty 2013;28:922–7.
[99] Stiehler M, Lind M, Mygind T, Baatrup A, Dolatshahi-Pirouz A, Li H, et al. Morphology, proliferation, and osteogenic differentiation of mesenchymal stem cells cultured on titanium, tantalum, and chromium surfaces. J Biomed Mater Res A 2008;86:448–58.
[100] Annabi N. Porous biomaterials. In: Ramalingam M, Tiwari A, Ramakrishna S, Kobayashi H, editors. Integrated biomaterials for biomedical technology. Scrivener Publishing LLC; 2012. p. 35–66.
[101] Muschler GF, Nakamoto C, Griffith LG. Engineering principles of clinical cell-based tissue engineering. J Bone Joint Surg (American) 2004;86:1541–58.
[102] Cameron HU, Pilliar RM, Macnab I. The rate of bone ingrowth into porous metal. J Biomed Mater Res 1976;10:295–302.
[103] Pilliar RM. P/M processing of surgical implants: sintered porous surfaces for tissue-to-implant fixation. Int J Powder Metall 1998;34:33–45.
[104] Bobyn JD, Pilliar RM, Cameron HU, Weatherly GC. The optimum pore size for the fixation of porous-surfaced metal implants by the ingrowth of bone. Clin Orthop Relat Res 1980;150:263–70.
[105] Bram M, Schiefer H, Bogdanski D, Köller M, Buchkremer HP, Stöver D. Implant surgery: how bone bonds to PM titanium. Metal Powder Rep 2006;61:26–31.
[106] Linxi Z, Quanzhan Y, Guirong Z, Fangxin Z, Gang S, Bo Y. Additive manufacturing technologies of porous metal implants. China Foundry 2014;11:322–31.
[107] Bobyn JD, Miller J. Features of biologically fixed devices. In: Simon S, editor. Orthopaedic basic science. Chicago: American Academy of Orthopaedic Surgeons; 1994. p. 613–6.

[108] Klawitter JJ, Hulbert SF. Application of porous ceramics for the attachment of load bearing internal orthopedic applications. J Biomed Mater Res A 1971;5:161–229.
[109] Goodman S, Toksvig-Larsen S, Aspenberg P. Ingrowth of bone into pores in titanium chambers implanted in rabbits: effect of pore cross-sectional shape in the presence of dynamic shear. J Biomed Mater Res 1993;27:247–53.
[110] Min SY, Kim Y, Lee TK, Seo S, Jung HS, Kim D, et al. The effect of porosity on the elasticity of pure titanium: an atomistic simulation. Met Mater Int 2010;16:421–5.
[111] Oh S, Oh N, Appleford M, Ong JL. Bioceramics for tissue engineering applications – a review. Am J Biochem Biotechnol 2006;2:49–56.
[112] Murphy WL, Dennis RG, Kileny JL, Mooney DJ. Salt fusion: an approach to improve pore interconnectivity within tissue engineering scaffolds. Tissue Eng 2002;8: 43–52.
[113] Truscello S, Kerckhofs G, Van Bael S, Pyka G, Schrooten J, Van Oosterwyck H. Prediction of permeability of regular scaffolds for skeletal tissue engineering: a combined computational and experimental study. Acta Biomater 2012;8:1648–58.
[114] Wazen RM, Lefebvre LP, Baril E, Nanci A. Initial evaluation of bone ingrowth into a novel porous titanium coating. J Biomed Mater Res B 2010;94:64–71.
[115] Barbas A, Bonnet AS, Lipinski P, Pesci R, Dubois G. Development and mechanical characterization of porous titanium bone substitutes. J Mech Behav Biomed Mater 2012; 9:34–44.
[116] Ryan GE, Pandit AS, Apatsidis DP. Porous titanium scaffolds fabricated using a rapid prototyping and powder metallurgy technique. Biomaterials 2008;29:3625–35.
[117] El-Hajje A, Kolos EC, Wang JK, Maleksaeedi S, He Z, Wiria FE, et al. Physical and mechanical characterisation of 3D-printed porous titanium for biomedical applications. J Mater Sci Mater Med 2014;25:2471–80.
[118] Vlasea M, Basalah A, Azhari A, Kandel R, Toyserkani E. Additive manufacturing for bone load bearing applications. In: Zhang LG, Fisher JP, Leong KW, editors. 3D bio-printing and nanotechnology in tissue engineering and regenerative medicine. Academic Press-Elsevier; 2015. p. 231–63.
[119] Gibson I, Rosen D, Stucker B. Additive manufacturing technologies: 3D printing, rapid prototyping and direct digital manufacturing. 2nd ed. New York, USA: Springer; 2015.
[120] Lewallen EA, Riester SM, Bonin CA, Kremers HM, Dudakovic A, Kakar S, et al. Biological strategies for improved osseointegration and osteoinduction of porous metal orthopedic implants. Tissue Eng B 2014;00:1–13.
[121] Hobkirk JA, Watson RM, Searson LJJ. Introducing dental implants. Churchill Livingstone; 2003.
[122] Sones AD. Complications with osseointegrated implants. J Prosthet Dent 1989;62: 581–5.
[123] van Steenberghe D. A retrospective multicenter evaluation of the survival rate of osseointegrated fixtures supporting fixed partial prostheses in the treatment of partial edentulism. J Prosthet Dent 1989;61:217–23.
[124] Bauer S, Schmuki P, von der Mark K, Park J. Engineering biocompatible implant surfaces: part I: materials and surfaces. Prog Mater Sci 2013;58:261–326.
[125] Dabrowski B, Swieszkowski W, Godlinski D, Kurzydlowski KJ. Highly porous titanium scaffolds for orthopaedic applications. J Biomed Mater Res B: Appl Biomater 2010;95: 53–61.
[126] Young FA. Porous titanium dental implants. J Biomed Mater Res 1974;8:401–7.
[127] Mour M, Das D, Winkler T, Hoenig E, Mielke G, Morlock MM, et al. Advances in porous biomaterials for dental and orthopaedic applications. Materials 2010;3:2947–74.

[128] Rosa AL, Crippa GE, de Oliveira PT, Taba MJ, Lefebvre LP, Beloti MM. Human alveolar bone cell proliferation, expression of osteoblastic phenotype, and matrix mineralization on porous titanium produced by powder metallurgy. Clin Oral Implants Res 2009;20: 472–81.

[129] Canabarro A, Crippa GE, Shirozaki MU, Sampaio EM, Lefebvre LP, De Oliveira PT, et al. Effect of porous titanium coating thickness on in vitro osteoblast phenotype expression. J Osseointegration 2011;1:17–23.

[130] Simmons CA, Valiquette N, Pilliar RM. Osseointegration of sintered porous-surfaced and plasma spray-coated implants: an animal model study of early postimplantation healing response and mechanical stability. J Biomed Mater Res 1999;47:127–38.

[131] Nouri A, Wen C. Introduction to surface coating and modification for metallic biomaterials. In: Wen C, editor. Surface coating and modification of metallic biomaterials. Cambridge, UK: Woodhead Publishing; 2015. p. 3–60.

[132] Pilliar RM. Implant surface design and local stress fields—effects on peri-implant bone formation and retention with "short" porous-surfaces implants. In: Jokstad A, editor. Osseointegration and dental implants. Wiley-Blackwell; 2008. p. 230–7.

[133] Chen J, Chen X, Zhang X, Eichstädt O, Du R, Deng F, et al. Computer-aided design and manufacturing of dental implants with irregular geometries. In: Natal Jorge RM, Reis Campos JC, Vaz MAP, Santos SM, Tavares JMRS, editors. Biodental engineering III. London, UK: CRC Press; 2014. p. 51–6.

[134] Story BJ, Wagner WR, Gaisser DM, Cook SD, Rust-Dawicki AM. In vivo performance of a modified CSTi dental implant coating. Int J Oral Maxillofac Implants 1998;13: 749–57.

[135] Yue S, Pilliar RM, Weatherly GC. The fatigue strength of porous-coated Ti-6%Al-4%V implant alloy. J Biomed Mater Res 1984;18:1043–58.

[136] Pilliar RM. Porous-surfaced metallic implants for orthopaedic applications. J Biomed Mater Res 1987;21:1–33.

[137] Rokni S, Todescan R, Watson P, Pharoah M, Adegbembo AO, Deporter D. An assessment of crown-to-root ratios with short sintered porous-surfaced implants supporting prostheses in partially edentulous patients. Int J Oral Maxillofac Implants 2005;20: 69–76.

[138] Wolfarth D, Ducheyne P. Effect of a change in interfacial geometry on the fatigue strength of porous-coated Ti-6A1-4V. J Biomed Mater Res 1994;28:417–25.

[139] Wen CE, Yamada Y, Nouri A, Hodgson PD. Porous titanium with porosity gradients for biomedical applications. Mater Sci Forum 2007;539–543:720–5.

[140] Dewidar MM, Lim JK. Properties of solid core and porous surface Ti–6Al–4V implants manufactured by powder metallurgy. J Alloys Compd 2008;454:442–6.

[141] Miao X, Sun D. Graded/gradient porous biomaterials. Materials 2010;3:26–47.

[142] Vasconcellos LM, Leite DO, Oliveira FN, Carvalho YR, Cairo CA. Evaluation of bone ingrowth into porous titanium implant: histomorphometric analysis in rabbits. Braz Oral Res 2010;24:399–405.

[143] Zhang YP, Li DS, Zhang XP. Gradient porosity and large pore size NiTi shape memory alloys. Scr Mater 2007;57:1020–3.

[144] Kutty MG, Bhaduri S, Jokisaari JR, Bhaduri SB. Development of gradient porosities in Ti dental implant. Ceram Eng Sci Proc 2001;22:587–92.

[145] Kutty MG, Bhaduri S, Bhaduri SB. Gradient surface porosity in titanium dental implants: relation between processing parameters and microstructure. J Mater Sci Mater Med 2004; 15:145–50.

[146] Traini T, Mangano C, Sammons RL, Mangano F, Macchi A, Piattelli A. Direct laser metal sintering as a new approach to fabrication of an isoelastic functionally graded material for manufacture of porous titanium dental implants. Dent Mater 2008;24:1525–33.
[147] Mangano C, Mangano F, Shibli JA, Luongo G, De Franco M, Briguglio F, et al. Prospective clinical evaluation of 201 direct laser metal forming implants: results from a 1-year multicenter study. Lasers Med Sci 2012;27:181–9.
[148] Mangano C, Mangano FG, Shibli JA, Ricci M, Perrotti V, d'Avila S, et al. Immediate loading of mandibular overdentures supported by unsplinted direct laser metal-forming implants: results from a 1-year prospective study. J Periodontol 2012;83:70–8.
[149] Mangano F, Pozzi-Taubert S, Zecca PA, Luongo G, Sammons RL, Mangano C. Immediate restoration of fixed partial prostheses supported by one-piece narrow-diameter selective laser sintering implants: a 2-year prospective study in the posterior jaws of 16 patients. Implant Dent 2013;22:388–93.
[150] Figliuzzi M, Mangano F, Mangano C. A novel root analogue dental implant using CT scan and CAD/CAM: selective laser melting technology. Int J Oral Maxillofac Surg 2012; 41:858–62.
[151] Mangano FG, De Franco M, Caprioglio A, Macchi A, Piattelli A, Mangano C. Immediate, non-submerged, root-analogue direct laser metal sintering (DLMS) implants: a 1-year prospective study on 15 patients. Lasers Med Sci 2014;29:1321–8.
[152] Mangano F, Luongo F, Shibli JA, Anil S, Mangano C. Maxillary overdentures supported by four splinted direct metal laser sintering implants: a 3-year prospective clinical study. Int J Dent 2014;2014:1–9.
[153] Shibli JA, Mangano C, Mangano F, Brasil O, Lins B, Cozzolino F, et al. Histomorphometric evaluation of direct laser metal forming (DLMF) implant surface in the type IV bone: a controlled study in human jaw. POSEIDO 2013;1:45–52.
[154] Park JM, Kim HJ, Park EJ, Kim MR, Kim SJ. Three dimensional finite element analysis of the stress distribution around the mandibular posterior implant during non-working movement according to the amount of cantilever. J Adv Prosthodont 2014;6:361–71.
[155] Tagger Green N, Machtei EE, Horwitz J, Peled M. Fracture of dental implants: literature review and report of a case. Implant Dent 2002;11:137–43.
[156] Simon Z, Watson PA. Biomimetic dental implants-new ways to enhance osseointegration. J Can Dent Assoc 2002;68:286–8.
[157] Adell R, Eriksson B, Lekholm U, Brånemark PI, Jemt T. Long-term follow-up study of osseointegrated implants in the treatment of totally edentulous jaws. Int J Oral Maxillofac Implants 1990;5:347–59.
[158] Bram M, Stiller C, Buchkremer HP, Stöver D, Baur H. High-porosity titanium, stainless steel, and superalloy parts. Adv Eng Mater 2000;2:196–9.
[159] Nouri A, Chen XB, Hodgson PD, Wen CE. Preparation and characterisation of new titanium based alloys for orthopaedic and dental applications. Adv Mater Res 2007;15–17: 71–6.
[160] Nouri A. Novel metal structures through powder metallurgy for biomedical applications. Victoria, Australia: Institute for Technology Research and Innovation, Deakin University; 2008.
[161] Esen Z. Production and characterization of porous titanium alloys. Ankara: The Graduate School of Natural and Applied Sciences, Middle East Technical University; 2007.
[162] Li JP. Porous titanium for biomedical applications: development, characterization and biological evaluation. Enschede, The Netherlands: Institute for Biomedical Technology, University of Twente; 2007.

[163] Murr LE, Gaytan SM, Medina F, Lopez H, Martinez E, Machado BI, et al. Next-generation biomedical implants using additive manufacturing of complex, cellular and functional mesh arrays. Philos Trans R Soc 2010;368:1999–2032.

[164] Li YH, Rao GB, Rong LJ, Li YY. The influence of porosity on corrosion characteristics of porous NiTi alloy in simulated body fluid. Mater Lett 2002;57:448–51.

[165] Seah KHW, Thampuran R, Chen X, Teoh SH. A comparison between the corrosion behaviour of sintered and unsintered porous titanium. Corros Sci 1995;37:1333–40.

[166] Ducheyne P. In vitro corrosion study of porous metal fibre coatings for bone ingrowth. Biomaterials 1983;4:185–9.

[167] Seah KHW, Thampuran R, Teoh SH. The influence of pore morphology on corrosion. Corros Sci 1998;40:547–56.

[168] Kohn DH, Ducheyne P. A parametric study of the factors affecting the fatigue strength of porous coated Ti-6Al-4V implant alloy. J Biomed Mater Res 1990;24:1483–501.

[169] Matassi F, Botti A, Sirleo L, Carulli C, Innocenti M. Porous metal for orthopedics implants. Clin Cases Miner Bone Metab 2013;10:111–5.

[170] Young FA, Keller JC. Porous titanium dental implants in primates and humans. Eng Med 1984;13:203–6.

[171] Breme J, Biehl V, Schulte W, d'Hoedt B, Donath K. Development and functionality of isoelastic dental implants of titanium alloys. Biomaterials 1993;14:887–92.

[172] Dalton JE, Cook SD, Thomas KA, Kay JF. The effect of operative fit and hydroxyapatite coating on the mechanical and biological response to porous implants. J Bone Joint Surg (American) 1995;77:97–110.

[173] Bessho K, Carnes DL, Cavin R, Chen HY, Ong JL. BMP stimulation of bone response adjacent to titanium implants in vivo. Clin Oral Implants Res 1999;10:212–8.

[174] Zhou F, Nutt SR, Bampton CC, Lavernia EJ. Nanostructure in an Al-Mg-Sc alloy processed by low-energy ball milling at cryogenic temperature. Metall Mater Trans A 2003; 34:1985–92.

[175] Kim DG, Huja SS, Tee BC, Larsen PE, Kennedy KS, Chien HH, et al. Bone ingrowth and initial stability of titanium and porous tantalum dental implants: a pilot canine study. Implant Dent 2013;22:399–405.

Chemical surface modification of a titanium scaffold

6

T. Kokubo, S. Yamaguchi
Chubu University, Kasugai, Aichi, Japan

6.1 Introduction

Titanium (Ti) scaffolds are believed to have great potential in hard tissue engineering. The most important property of the Ti scaffolds in their applications to hard tissue engineering is their compatibility with bone tissue, including the much sought feature of bone-bonding bioactivity.

Therefore various kinds of surface modifications of Ti scaffolds have been attempted for various purposes, including improving their compatibility with living bone and stable fixation to bone tissue.

Among them, chemical treatment by soaking in an aqueous solution under normal pressure and subsequent heat treatment at a moderate temperature under air with normal pressure are not only simple and inexpensive but also can be easily applied uniformly even to the inner surfaces of medical devices of complex shape. They were reviewed by the present authors elsewhere [1]. Among them, the simple chemical and heat treatments, which can effectively induce bone-bonding ability, osteoconductivity, and osteoinductivity of a Ti scaffold, are described in the present chapter.

6.2 Methods of chemical and heat treatments

6.2.1 NaOH and heat treatments

Among the chemical and heat treatments hitherto proposed, NaOH and heat treatments [2] are the simplest and most effective methods for conferring a bone-bonding capacity on Ti metal and its alloys.

In this method, Ti metal is typically soaked in a 5 M NaOH solution at 60°C for 24 h and subsequently heat-treated at 600°C for 1 h in air atmosphere. A layer of sodium hydrogen titanate ($Na_xH_{2-x}Ti_yO_{2y+1}$: $0 < x < 2$ and $y = 2$, 3, or 4) in a fibrous form in and on a nanometer scale approximately 1 μm thick is formed on the surface of the Ti metal with the first NaOH treatment. This layer is converted into the layer of sodium titanate ($Na_2Ti_yO_{2y+1}$: $y = 5$, 6, etc.) accompanied by a small amount of rutile upon subsequent heat treatment without an appreciable change in morphology, as shown in Fig. 6.1 [3]. The Na^+ ions released from the sodium titanate in the body play an important role in forming an apatite layer on the Ti metal, which induces the bone-bonding bioactivity, as discussed later.

Metallic Foam Bone. http://dx.doi.org/10.1016/B978-0-08-101289-5.00006-8

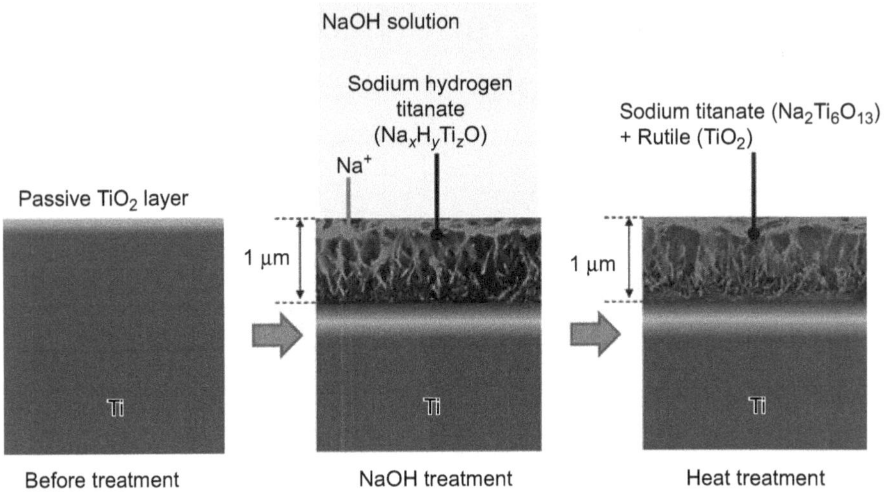

Figure 6.1 Structural change of surface of titanium metal by NaOH and heat treatments. Reproduced from Yamaguchi S, Takadama H, Matsushita T, Nakamura T, Kokubo T. Cross-sectional analysis of the surface ceramic layer developed on Ti metal by NaOH-heat treatment and soaking in SBF. J Ceram Soc Jpn 2009;117:1126–30.

Conventional Ti-based alloys such as Ti-6Al-4V, Ti-6Al-2Nb-Ta, and Ti-15Mo-5Zr-3Al [2] also form a similar surface layer by the same treatments, since the alloying elements such as Al, V, and Mo are selectively released from their surfaces during the first NaOH treatment [4–6]. However, certain new kinds of Ti-based alloys in the system Ti-Zr-Nb-Ta do not form such layers on their surfaces by the NaOH and heat treatments, since the alloying elements are not easily released during the NaOH treatment [7].

Even a small amount of Ca^{2+} ions contaminated in the NaOH solution tends to replace the Na^+ ions in the sodium hydrogen titanate, inhibiting the release of the Na^+ ions in the living body and suppressing apatite formation. The Ca^{2+} ions are highly contaminating, even in a high purity NaOH reagent [8]. The Na^+ ions in the sodium titanate tend to be released via exchange with the H_3O^+ ions in the humid environment, thus suppressing apatite formation [9].

6.2.2 NaOH, $CaCl_2$, heat, and water treatments

This method was proposed as a way of overcoming the problems of the NaOH and heat treatments described above by slightly modifying them.

In this method, the Ti metal is first soaked in 5 M NaOH solution at 60°C for 24 h. After this treatment, it is soaked in 100 mM $CaCl_2$ solution at 40°C for 24 h and then heat-treated at the same 600°C for 1 h in air. In addition, it is finally soaked in water at 80°C for 24 h [10].

During the second $CaCl_2$ treatment, the Na^+ ions in the sodium hydrogen titanate that formed on the surface of the Ti metal by the first NaOH treatment are completely

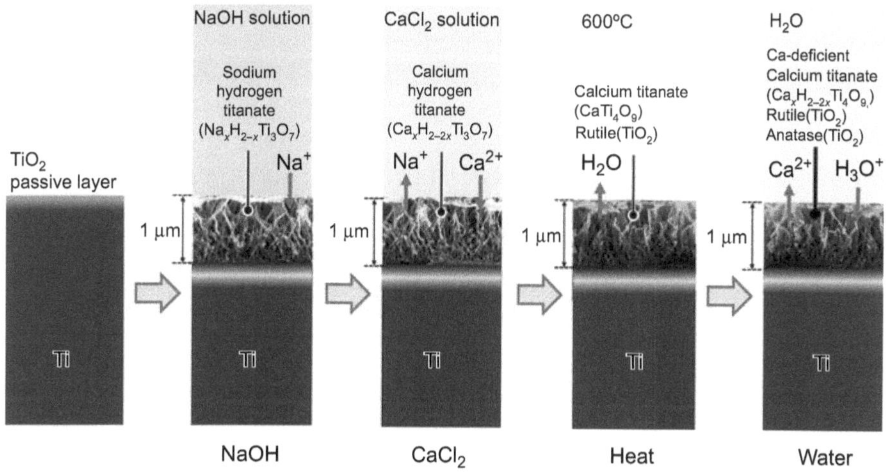

Figure 6.2 Structural change of surface of titanium metal by NaOH, $CaCl_2$, heat, and water treatments.
Reproduced from Yamaguchi S, Takadama H, Matsushita T, Nakamura T, Kokubo T. Apatite-forming ability of Ti-15Zr-4Nb-4Ta alloy induced by calcium solution treatment. J Mater Sci Mater Med 2010;21:439–44.

replaced with the Ca^{2+} ions to form calcium hydrogen titanate. This phase is transformed into calcium titanate by the subsequent heat treatment, and the Ca^{2+} ions in the calcium titanate on the surface of the Ti metal are partially replaced with H_3O^+ ions during the final hot water treatment. As a result, Ca-deficient calcium titanate is formed on the surface of the Ti metal, as shown in Fig. 6.2. The calcium titanate that formed after the heat treatment scarcely releases the Ca^{2+} ions in the body environment, whereas the Ca-deficient calcium titanate formed after the water treatment releases the Ca^{2+} ions, which then play an important role in apatite formation on the Ti metal.

This method is valid not only for the pure Ti metal and conventional Ti-based alloys but also for new kinds of Ti-Zr-Nb-Ta alloys, where the alloying elements tend to suppress the release of the Ca^{2+} ions, since even a small amount of released Ca^{2+} ions is sufficient for apatite formation [11,12]. The Ca^{2+} ions in the Ca-deficient calcium titanate are relatively stable in a humid environment [11].

Various kinds of functional ions such as Mg^{2+} [13], Zn^{2+} [14], Sr^{2+} [15], and Ag^+ [16] can be introduced to the Ca-deficient titanate by adding them into the second $CaCl_2$ solution or final hot water treatment. These ions are released in the living body to promote bone growth as well as prevent infection.

6.2.3 H_2SO_4/HCl and heat treatments

The methods described above are comprised of a heat treatment after an alkali or alkaline earth aqueous solution treatment. In contrast, the present method uses a heat

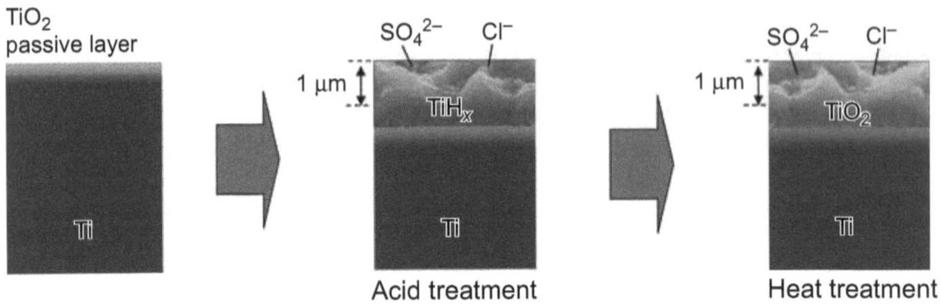

Figure 6.3 Structural change of surface of titanium metal by acid and heat treatments.

treatment after an acid solution treatment. In this method, the Ti metal is typically soaked in 66.3%H_2SO_4/10.6%HCl = 1/1 mixed acid solution at 70°C for 1 h and subsequently heat-treated at a temperature ranging from 500−650°C for 1 h in air [17]. A layer of Ti hydride (TiH_x, where $0 < x < 2$) of micrometer-scale roughness is formed on the surface of the Ti metal by the first acid treatment and transformed into that of rutile by the subsequent heat treatment without any appreciable change in surface morphology. The acid radicals such as SO_4^{2-} and Cl^- ions are adsorbed on its surface during the first acid treatment and remain even after the subsequent heat treatment, as long as the temperature of the heat treatment is kept lower than 700°C, as shown in Fig. 6.3. The Ti oxide adsorbed with the acid radicals plays an important role in forming the apatite on the Ti metal, as discussed later.

The acid solution can be replaced with various other kinds of acid solutions, such as HNO_3 and HCl [18].

However, this method is not suitable for forming the Ti oxide on most of the Ti-based alloys, since the alloying elements are not easily released from the alloys during the acid treatment and tend to form oxides that are rich in these elements after the subsequent heat treatment. In the case of the Ti-based alloys, the Ti oxide surface layers are formed if they are first subjected to an NaOH treatment to remove the alloying elements and are then subjected to the acid and heat treatments [7].

6.2.4 Various chemical and heat treatments

Heat treatment after alkali or acid treatment was discussed in the above section. In the method described in this section, the Ti metal is heat-treated at 600°C for 1 h after exposure to an HCl or NaOH solution, the pH of which are systematically changed from nearly 0 to 14 at 60°C for 24 h [19].

A layer of Ti hydride of micrometer-scale roughness is formed on the Ti metal after exposure to a solution with a pH less than 0.1, whereas a layer of sodium hydrogen titanate of nanometer-scale roughness is formed after exposure to a solution higher than 13.6 in pH. After the subsequent heat treatment, rutile is formed on the Ti metal for the solutions with a pH less than 12.9, whereas sodium titanate and rutile form for the solutions higher than 13.6 in pH without any appreciable change in the surface morphology, as shown in Fig. 6.4 [19].

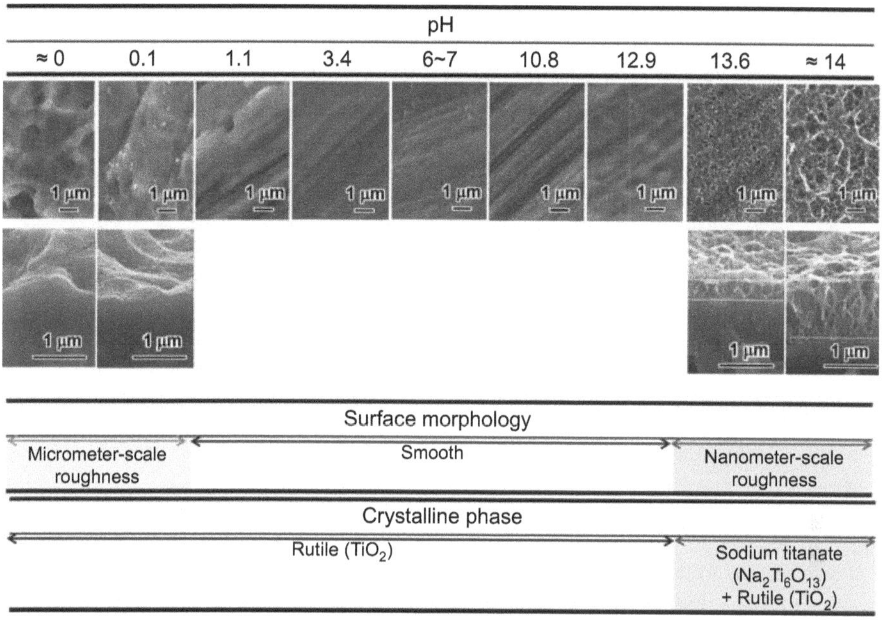

Figure 6.4 Surface structure of titanium metal heat-treated after exposure to solutions with different pHs.
Reproduced from Pattanayak DK, Yamaguchi S, Matsushita T, Nakamura T, Kokubo T. Apatite-forming ability of titanium in terms of pH of the exposed solution. J R Soc Interface 2012;9:2145–55.

The zeta potentials of their surfaces exhibit high positive values for the solutions with a pH less than 1.1, whereas low negative values are exhibited for the solutions higher than 13.6 in pH, as shown in Fig. 6.5 [19].

6.3 Properties of titanium scaffolds subjected to chemical and heat treatments

6.3.1 Apatite-forming ability

It has been shown for various kinds of bone-bonding ceramics such as Bioglass, sintered hydroxyapatite, and glass ceramics A-W that they bond to living bone through an apatite layer that forms on their surfaces in the living body. Furthermore, the apatite that forms on their surfaces in vivo can be reproduced in an acellular simulated body fluid (SBF) with ion concentrations almost equal to those of the human blood plasma [20]. Therefore the bone-bonding capacity of a material can be preliminarily evaluated by examining its apatite formation in SBF.

Ti metal subjected to NaOH and heat treatments to form sodium titanate on its surface produces the apatite on its surface in SBF within 1 day, as shown in Fig. 6.6 [3].

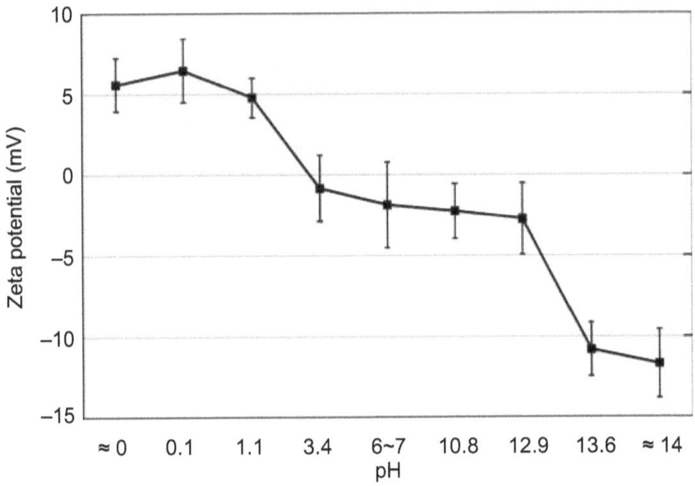

Figure 6.5 Zeta potentials of surface of titanium metal heat-treated after exposure to solutions with different pHs.
Reproduced from Pattanayak DK, Yamaguchi S, Matsushita T, Nakamura T, Kokubo T. Apatite-forming ability of titanium in terms of pH of the exposed solution. J R Soc Interface 2012;9:2145−55.

The conventional Ti-based alloys such as Ti-6Al-4V, Ti-6Al-2Nb-Ta, and Ti-15Mo-5Zr-3Al also form the apatite on their surfaces in SBF after NaOH and heat treatments [2].

The mechanism underlying apatite formation in SBF on the surface of Ti metal subjected to NaOH and heat treatments is schematically shown in Fig. 6.7 [21]. The sodium

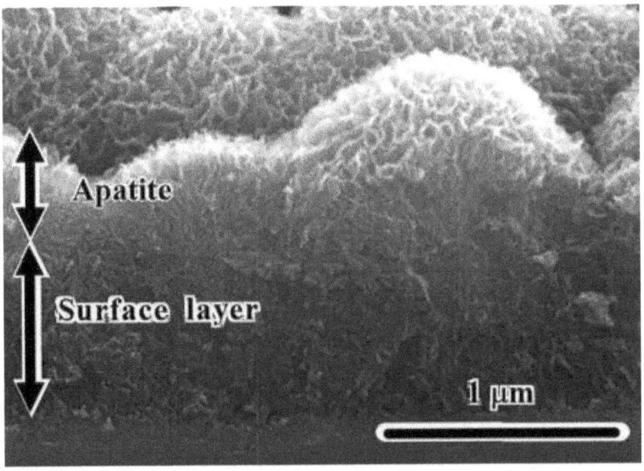

Figure 6.6 Apatite formation in simulated body fluid on titanium metal subjected to NaOH and heat treatments.
Reproduced from Yamaguchi S, Takadama H, Matsushita T, Nakamura T, Kokubo T. Cross-sectional analysis of the surface ceramic layer developed on Ti metal by NaOH-heat treatment and soaking in SBF. J Ceram Soc Jpn 2009;117:1126−30.

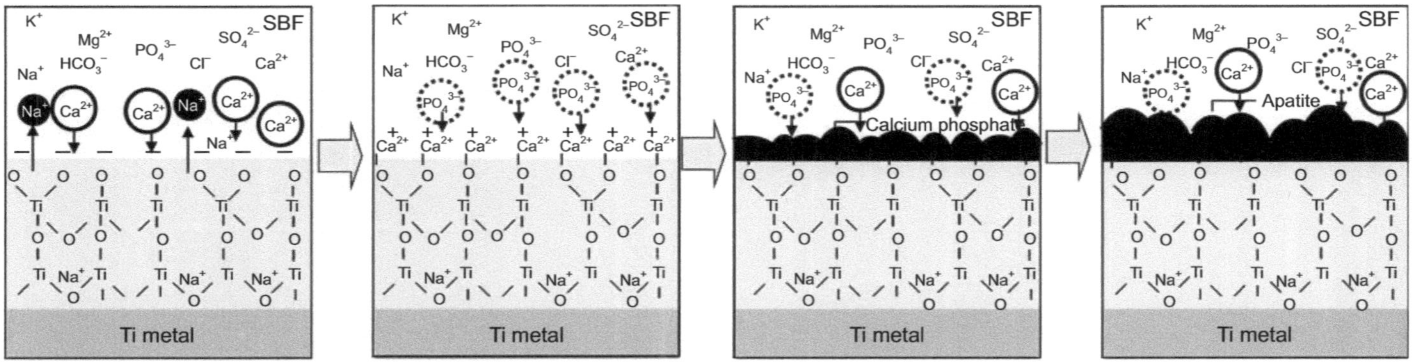

Figure 6.7 Mechanism of apatite formation in simulated body fluid on titanium metal subjected to NaOH and heat treatments. Reproduced from Kim H-M, Himeno T, Kawashita M, Lee J-H, Kokubo T, Nakamura T. Surface potential change in bioactive titanium metal during the process of apatite formation in simulated body fluid. J Biomed Mater Res Part A 2003;67A:1305–09.

titanate on the surface of the Ti metal releases Na^+ ions via exchange with the H_3O^+ ions in SBF to form Ti-OH groups. As a result, the surface is negatively charged so as to be able to combine with the positively charged Ca^{2+} ions in SBF. As the Ca^{2+} ions accumulate, the surface becomes positively charged and is thus able to combine with the negatively charged phosphate ions in SBF, forming an amorphous calcium phosphate. The phase is metastable and eventually transforms into stable crystalline apatite.

When the NaOH solution is contaminated with even a small amount of Ca^{2+} ions, they preferentially enter into the structure of the sodium titanate by replacing the Na^+ ions, preventing apatite formation [8].

In a humid environment, the Na^+ ions in the sodium titanate are easily released via exchange with the H_3O^+ ions of the moisture, hampering its apatite-forming ability in both SBF and the living body [9].

The release of the Na^+ ions in the sodium titanate is suppressed by the presence of alloying elements such as Zr, Nb, and Ta in the structure, thus blocking apatite formation on the Ti metal in SBF and the living body [7].

Ti metal subjected to NaOH, $CaCl_2$, and heat treatments does not form apatite on its surface in SBF after the heat treatment but does form apatite after the subsequent hot water treatment within 3 days, as shown in Fig. 6.8 [10]. This is because the calcium titanate formed by the heat treatment scarcely releases the Ca^{2+} ions in SBF, but the calcium-deficient calcium titanate formed after the subsequent water treatment does easily release them.

The mechanism of apatite formation on Ti metal subjected to NaOH, $CaCl_2$, heat, and water treatments is similar to that of Ti metal subjected to NaOH and heat treatments. The Na^+ ions in the latter case should be replaced with the Ca^{2+} ions in the former.

Various kinds of Ti-based alloys, including both the conventional alloys and the newer Ti-Zr-Nb-Ta alloys, also form apatite on their surfaces in SBF after NaOH,

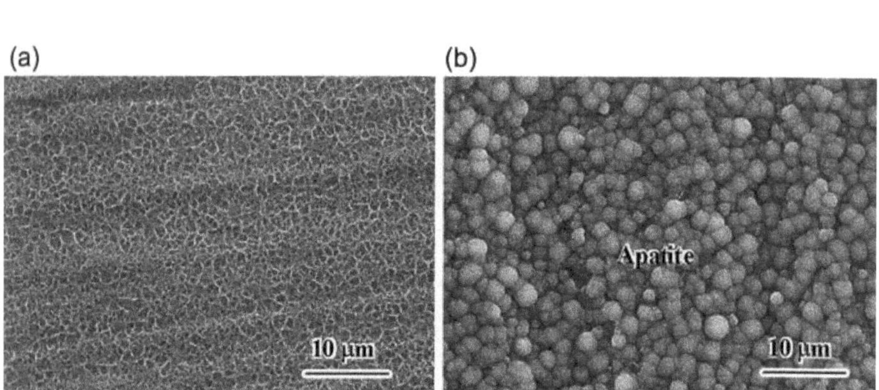

Figure 6.8 Scanning electron microscope pictures of surfaces of titanium metal soaked in simulated body fluid (a) after NaOH, $CaCl_2$, and heat treatments and (b) after the subsequent water treatment.
Reproduced from Kizuki T, Takadama H, Matsushita T, Nakamura T, Kokubo T. Preparation of bioactive Ti metal surface enriched with calcium ions by chemical treatment. Acta Biomater 2010;6:2836–42.

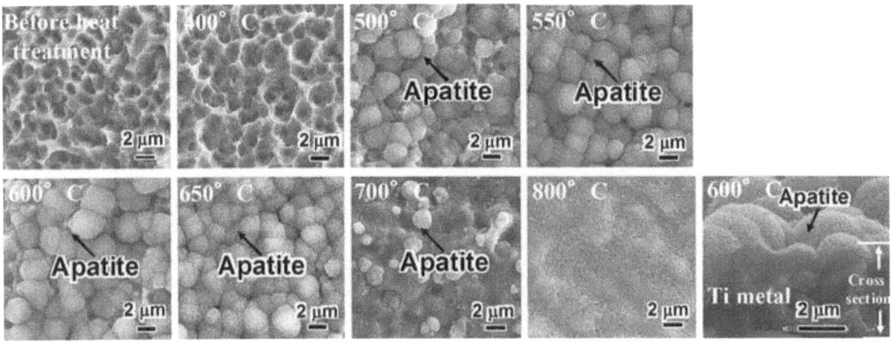

Figure 6.9 Apatite formation in simulated body fluid on titanium metal subjected to acid and heat treatments at various temperatures.
Reproduced from Kokubo T, Pattanayak DK, Yamaguchi S, Takadama H, Matsushita T, Kawai T, et al. Positively charged bioactive charged bioactive Ti metal prepared by simple chemical and heat treatments. J R Soc Interface 2010;7:S503–13.

$CaCl_2$, heat, and water treatments [11,12]. Their apatite-forming abilities are stable, even in a humid environment, since the Ca^{2+} ions in the Ca-deficient calcium titanate are not easily released via exchange with the H_3O^+ ions of the moisture [10]. The Ti metal doped with various ions such as Mg^{2+} [13], Zn^{2+} [14], Sr^{2+} [15], and Ag^+ [16] in their surface calcium titanate layers also form apatite on their surfaces in SBF.

Ti metal subjected to H_2SO_4/HCl and heat treatments forms apatite on its surface in SBF within 1 day when the heat treatment temperature ranges from 500–650°C, as shown in Fig. 6.9 [17].

The mechanism of apatite formation in SBF on the surface of Ti metal subjected to H_2SO_4/HCl and heat treatments is schematically shown in Fig. 6.10 [17]. Ti oxide on the surface of Ti metal subjected to acid and heat treatments exhibits adsorbed acid radicals such as SO_4^{2-} and Cl^- ions. They are dissociated in SBF to create an acidic environment on the TiO_2 layer. The TiO_2 is positively charged in the acidic environment [22] and combines with the negatively charged phosphate ions in SBF. As the phosphate ions accumulate, the negatively charged surface combines with the positively charged Ca^{2+} ions, forming an amorphous calcium phosphate. This phase is metastable and eventually transforms into crystalline apatite.

Apatite formation on Ti metal subjected to acid and heat treatments is stable, even in a humid environment [17].

Ti metal does not form apatite on its surface in SBF in the absence of heat treatment after the acid treatment, as in the case of most dental implants, since its surface is not charged.

Most of the Ti-based alloys subjected to acid and heat treatments do not form apatite on their surfaces in SBF, since the alloying elements tend to form compounds different from TiO_2 on their surfaces after these treatments.

Ti metal heat-treated after exposure to solutions with different pHs forms apatite on its surface in SBF within 1 day when the pH of the solutions are less than 1.1 or higher than 13.8, as shown in Fig. 6.11 [19]. Apatite formation on its surface is attributed to

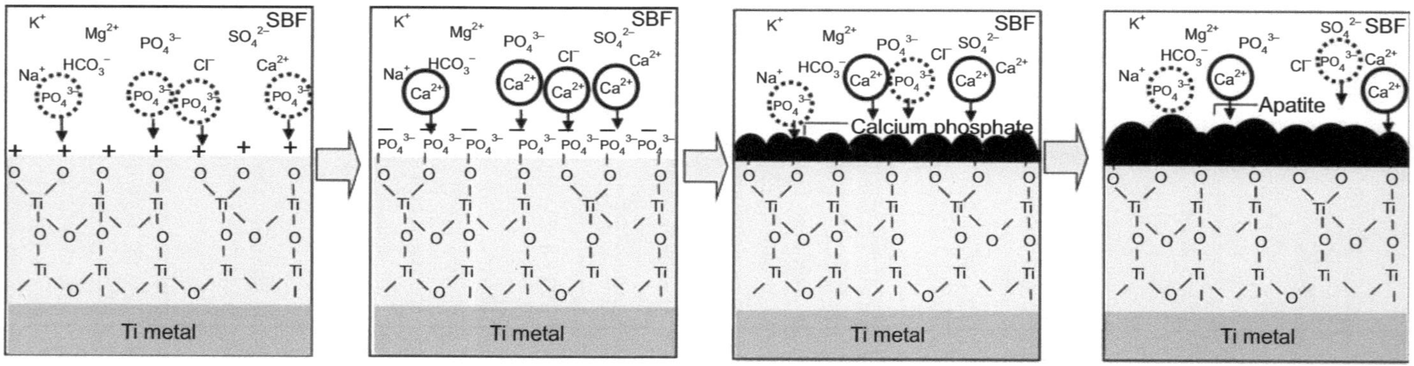

Figure 6.10 Mechanism of apatite formation in simulated body fluid on titanium metal subjected to acid and heat treatments.
Reproduced from Kokubo T, Pattanayak DK, Yamaguchi S, Takadama H, Matsushita T, Kawai T, et al. Positively charged bioactive charged bioactive Ti metal prepared by simple chemical and heat treatments. J R Soc Interface 2010;7:S503–13.

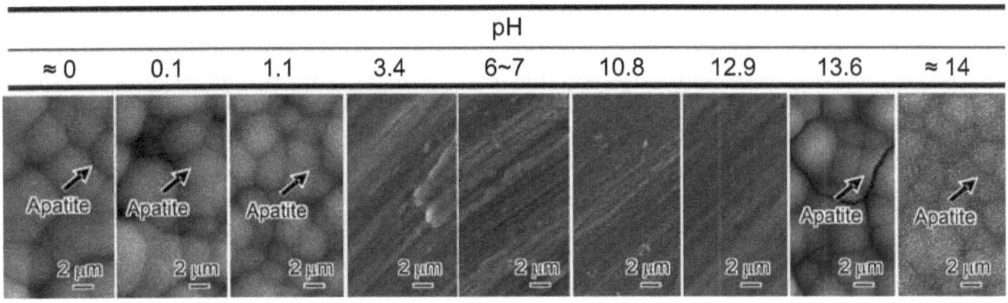

Figure 6.11 Apatite formation in simulated body fluid on titanium metal subjected to heat treatment after exposure to solutions with different pH values.
Reproduced from Pattanayak DK, Yamaguchi S, Matsushita T, Nakamura T, Kokubo T. Apatite-forming ability of titanium in terms of pH of the exposed solution. J R Soc Interface 2012;9:2145–55.

the positive or negative surface charge, in view of the surface structure, as shown in Fig. 6.4 and the zeta potential in Fig. 6.5.

Ti metal does not form apatite on its surface in SBF, even if it is subjected to the heat treatment, insofar as it is not subjected to the preceding acid or alkali treatment, since its surface is neither positively nor negatively charged.

6.3.2 Bone-bonding property

When rectangular specimens were implanted into the tibia of rabbits, Ti metal subjected to NaOH and heat treatments tightly bonded to the living bone through an apatite layer within 8 weeks after implantation without any intervention of fibrous tissue at the interface, as shown in Fig. 6.12 [23]. When tensile stress was applied to the interface, fracture did not occur at the interface but rather in the bone.

Ti-6Al-4V, Ti-6Al-2Nb-Ta, and Ti-15Mo-5Zr-3Al alloys subjected to the same treatments were also confirmed to be tightly bonded to the living bone [24]. When tensile stress was applied to the interface, once again fracture did not occur at the interface but rather in the bone.

Ti-Zr-Nb-Ta alloys, as well as Ti metal subjected to NaOH, $CaCl_2$, heat, and water treatments, were also tightly bonded to the bone without any intervention of fibrous tissue, as shown in Fig. 6.13 [25,26]. Again, when tensile stress was applied to the interface, fracture did not occur at the interface but rather in the bone.

Ti metal subjected to acid and heat treatments bonded to the bone without any intervening fibrous tissue, as shown in Fig. 6.14 [27]. Tensile stress applied to the interface did not result in a fracture at the interface but rather in the bone.

6.3.3 Osteoconductivity and osteoinductivity

Porous Ti metal, which was 40% in porosity and 300–500 μm in pore size, was subjected to NaOH and heat treatments. It was observed to be penetrated with newly

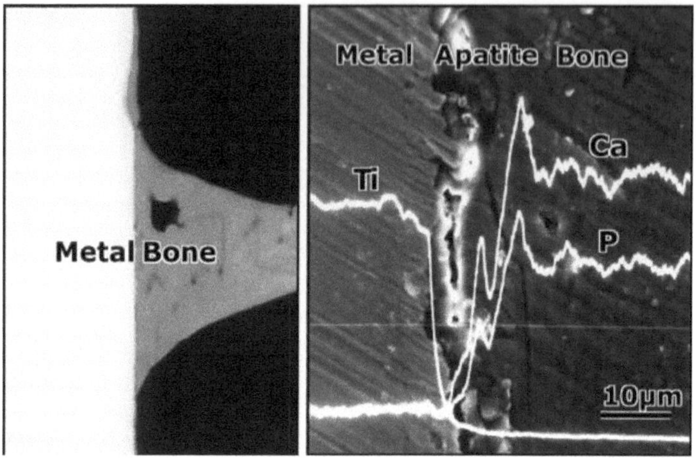

Figure 6.12 Contact microradiograph (left-hand side) and scanning electron microscope picture with energy dispersive X-ray analysis (right-hand side) at the interface of titanium metal subjected to NaOH and heat treatments with neighboring bone, 8 weeks after implantation into rabbit tibia.
Reproduced from Yan W-Q, Nakamura T, Kobayashi M, Kim H-M, Miyaji F, Kokubo T. Bonding of chemically treated titanium implants to bone. J Biomed Mater Res 1997;37: 267–75.

grown bone more deeply, in a larger amount, and with greater affinity than untreated porous Ti metal when implanted into the rabbit femoral condyle [28].

The same porous Ti metal subjected to NaOH and heat treatments was observed to form ectopic bone tissue 12 months after implantation when it was implanted

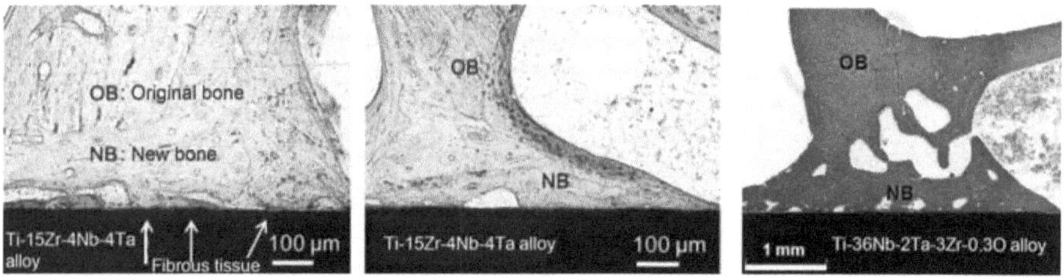

Figure 6.13 Optical micrograph of Ti-Zr-Nb-Ta alloys subjected to NaOH, $CaCl_2$, heat, and water treatments (center and right-hand side) at their interfaces with bone, in comparison with that untreated (left-hand side), 16 weeks after implantation into rabbit tibia.
Reproduced from Fukuda A, Takemoto M, Saito T, Fujibayashi S, Neo M, Yamaguchi S, et al. Bone bonding bioactivity of Ti metal and Ti-Zr-Nb-Ta alloys with Ca ions incorporated on their surfaces by simple chemical and heat treatments. Acta Biomater 2011;7:1379–86; Tanaka M, Takemoto M, Fujibayashi S, Kawai T, Yamaguchi S, Kizuki T, et al. Bone bonding ability of a chemically treated low elastic modulus Ti alloy; gum metal. J Mater Sci Mater Med 2014;25: 635–43.

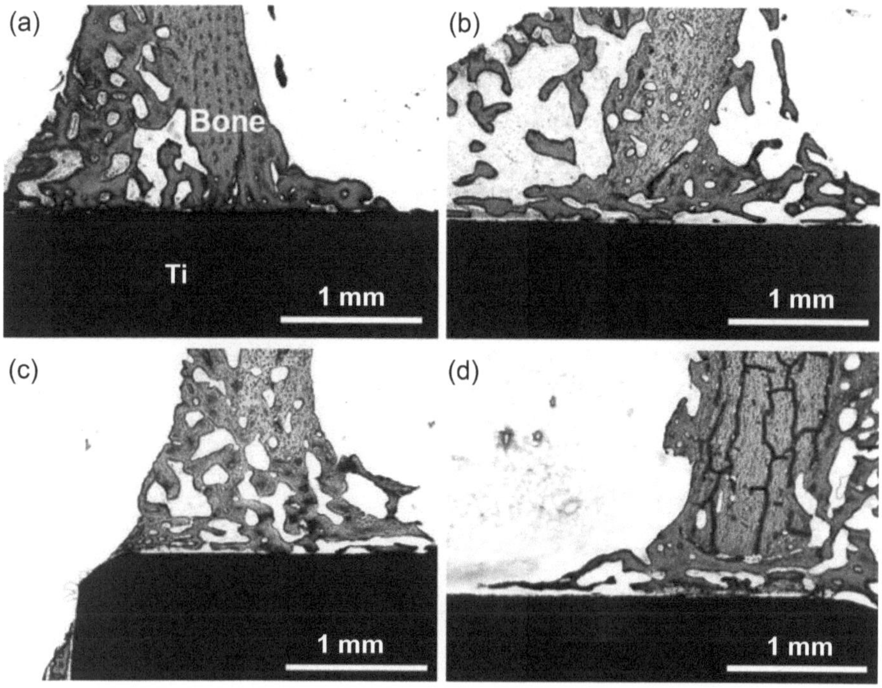

Figure 6.14 Optical micrograph of nondecalcified sections of titanium metals subjected to acid and heat treatments (a) in comparison with those subjected to no treatment (b), only heat treatment (c), and only acid treatment (d), 4 weeks after implantation into rabbit tibia. Reproduced from Kawai T, Takemoto M, Fujibayashi S, Neo M, Akiyama H, Yamaguchi S, et al. Bone-bonding properties of Ti metal subjected to acid and heat treatments. J Mater Sci Mater Med 2012;23:2981–92.

into the muscle of a beagle dog [29]. This kind of ectopic bone formation is called osteoinduction, in contrast with osteoconduction, where bone is formed in bone defects.

Later, it was found that the same porous Ti metal, subjected to HCl treatment after NaOH treatment to remove the Na^+ ions from the Ti metal and finally subjected to heat treatment, is fully penetrated with bone newly grown into the center of the porous structure, as shown in Fig. 6.15, in contrast with untreated porous Ti metal, where no such bone was found. In addition, the same porous Ti metal, Na^+ ions removed, exhibited osteoinduction as early as 3 months after implantation, as shown in Fig. 6.16 [30].

It is assumed that the Na^+ ions released from the wall of the porous body might have an adverse effect on cell activity in the narrow space of the pore by increasing the pH of the local environment. This could inhibit bone formation or growth in the pore, although the released Na^+ ions promote apatite formation on the wall. Ca^{2+} ions released from Ca-deficient calcium titanate might have a similar effect on bone formation in porous Ti metal.

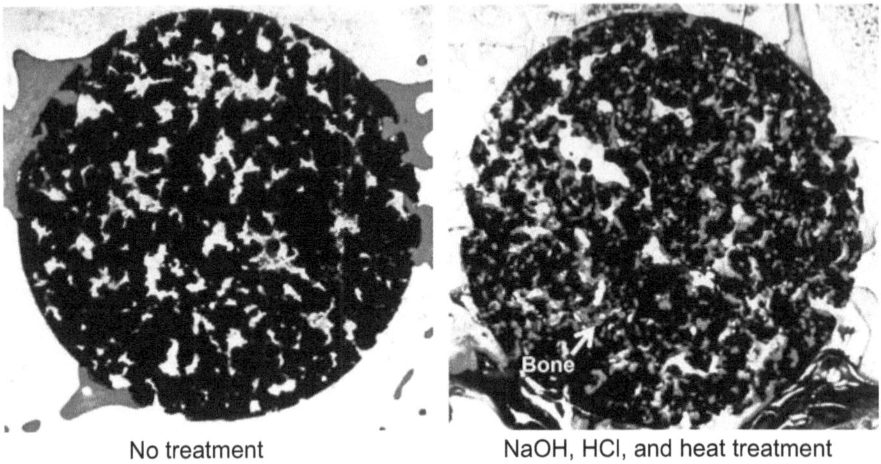

Figure 6.15 Optical micrograph of decalcified sections of porous titanium metal untreated and subjected to NaOH, HCl, and heat treatments, 26 weeks after implantation into rabbit femur. Reproduced from Takemoto M, Fujibayashi S, Neo M, Suzuki J, Kokubo T, Nakamura T. Mechanical properties and osteoconductivity of porous bioactive titanium. Biomaterials 2005; 26:6014–23; Tanaka K, Takemoto M, Fujibayashi S, Kawanabe K, Matsushita T, Kokubo T, et al. Long term study of osteoconductivity of bioactive porous titanium metals: effects of sodium removal by dilute HCl treatment. Key Eng Mater 2009;396–398:353–6.

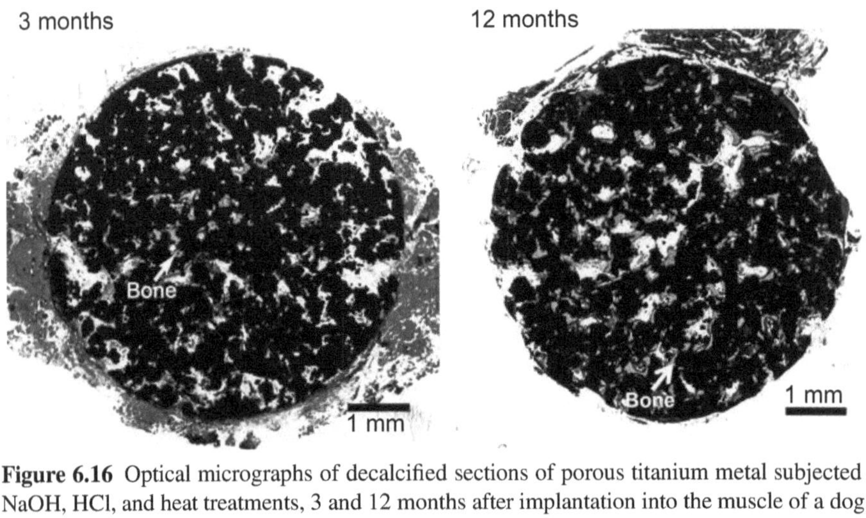

Figure 6.16 Optical micrographs of decalcified sections of porous titanium metal subjected to NaOH, HCl, and heat treatments, 3 and 12 months after implantation into the muscle of a dog. Reproduced from Takemoto M, Fujibayashi S, Neo M, Suzuki J, Matsushita T, Kokubo T, et al. Osteoinductive porous titanium implants: effect of sodium removal by dilute HCl treatment. Biomaterials 2006;27:2682–91.

In contrast, if apatite formation were to be promoted on the pore wall without increasing the pH in the pore, new bone would form and grow along the pore wall. Porous Ti metal that was subjected to HCl treatment after NaOH treatment to remove Na^+ ions and finally subjected to heat treatment indeed exhibited a high degree of osteoinduction as well as osteoconduction.

This is consistent with the result of porous Ti metal subjected to acid and heat treatment to form a Ti oxide free from alkali or alkaline earth ions on its surface. It also exhibited a high degree of osteoinduction [31], as shown in Fig. 6.17, as well as osteoconduction [32].

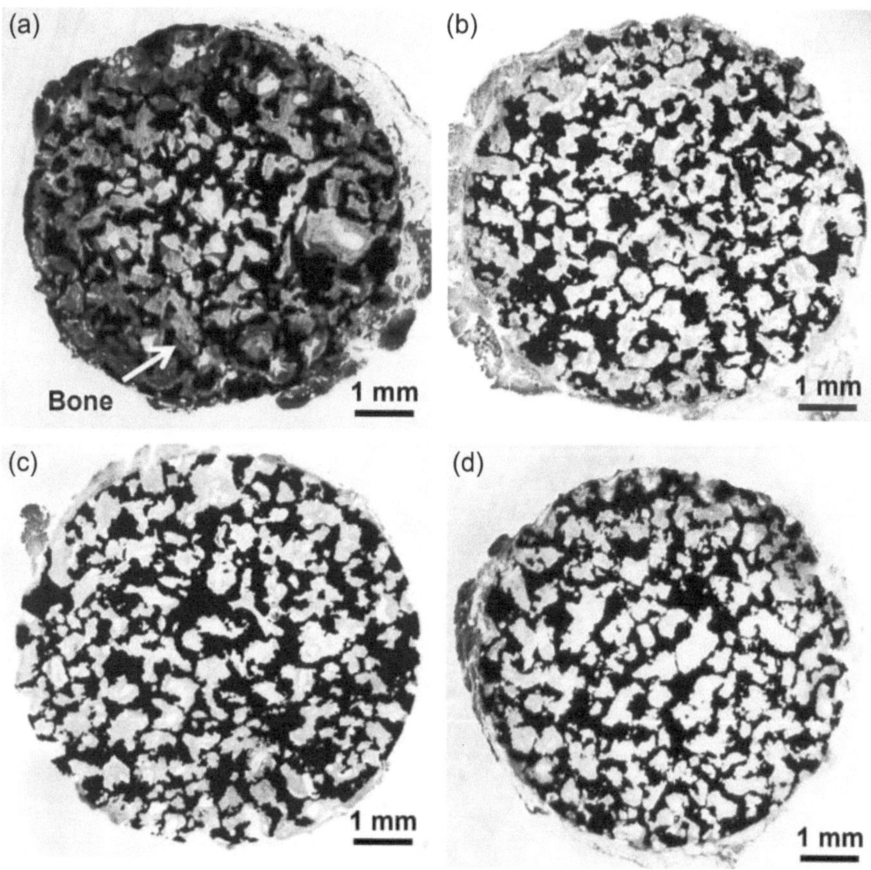

Figure 6.17 Optical micrograph of nondecalcified sections of porous titanium metal subjected to acid and heat treatments (a), in comparison with those subjected to no treatment (b), only heat treatment (c), and only acid treatment (d), 12 months after implantation into muscle of dog.
Reproduced from Kawai T, Takemoto M, Fujibayashi S, Akiyama H, Tanaka S, Yamaguchi S, et al. Osteoinduction on acid and heat treated porous Ti metal samples in canine muscle. PLoS One 2014;9:e88366.

6.4 Clinical application of titanium scaffolds subjected to chemical and heat treatments

Porous Ti metals subjected to chemical and heat treatments to induce bone-bonding property and osteoconductivity as well as osteoinductivity have a variety of useful applications in orthopedic and dental devices.

A porous Ti metal layer was formed on the surface of an artificial total hip joint made of Ti-6Al-2Nb-Ta alloy and subjected to NaOH and heat treatments to induce its bone-bonding property. The resultant product was penetrated into the porous layer by newly grown bone in animal experiments. This kind of bioactive artificial hip joint has been used clinically in Japan since 2007, as shown in Fig. 6.18 [33].

A porous Ti metal subjected to NaOH, HCl, and heat treatments to induce osteoconductivity as well as osteoinductivity was applied to a spinal fusion device in dogs [34]. It was found to be deeply penetrated with newly grown bone and fixed to the surrounding bone. On the basis of this experimental finding in animals, it was clinically applied as a spinal fusion device in five patients in the period November 2008 to June 2009, as shown in Fig. 6.19 [35]. All of the clinical trials were successful.

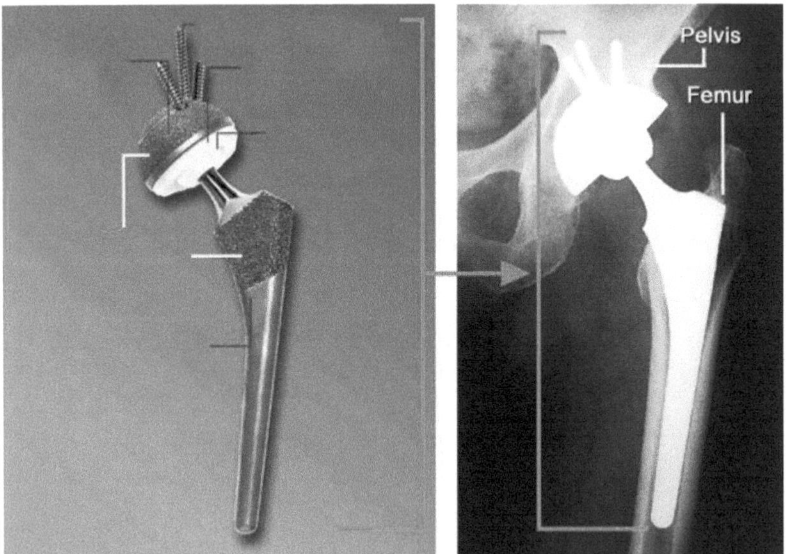

Figure 6.18 Application of porous titanium metal subjected to NaOH and heat treatments to total artificial hip joint.
Modified from Kawanabe K, Ise K, Goto K, Akiyama H, Nakamura T, Kaneuji A, Sugimori T, Matsumoto T. A new cementless total hip arthroplasty with bioactive titanium porous-coating by alkaline and heat treatments: average 4.8-year results. J Biomed Mater Res Part B Appl Biomater 2009;90B:476–81.

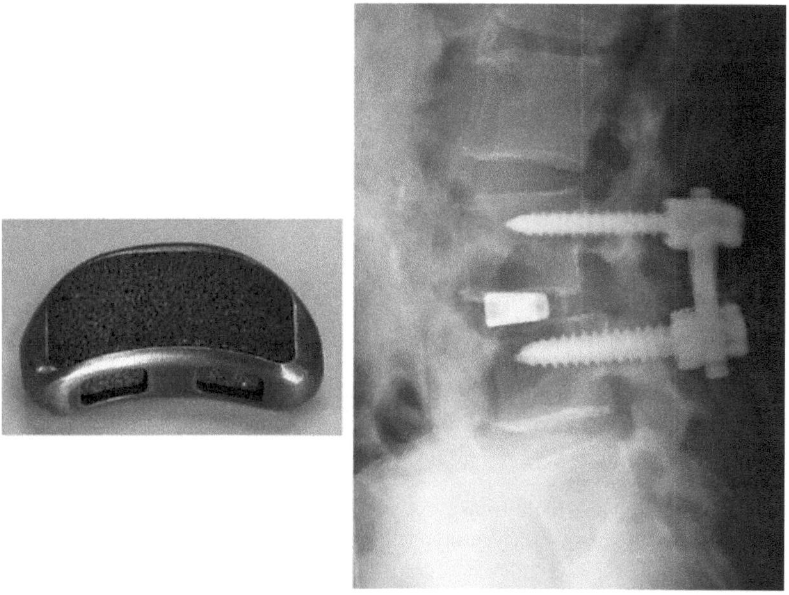

Figure 6.19 Application of porous titanium metal subjected to NaOH, HCl, and heat treatments (left-hand side) to spinal fusion (right-hand side).
Reproduced from Fujibayashi S, Takemoto M, Neo M, Matsushita T, Kokubo T, Doi K, et al. A novel synthetic material for spinal fusion: a prospective clinical trial of porous bioactive titanium metal for lumber interbody fusion. Eur Spine J 2011;20:1486–95.

6.5 Future trends

Ti scaffold subjected to the simple, specific chemical and heat treatments described in this chapter exhibits not only the bone-bonding property but also osteoconductivity and osteoinductivity. Ti metal scaffolds with these unique characteristics are likely to find extensive applications in orthopedic and dental devices in the future.

The details of the structures and properties of this kind of Ti foam are discussed in relation to bone tissue engineering in Chapter 4.

References

[1] Kokubo T, Yamaguchi S. Bioactive titanate layers formed on titanium and its alloys by simple chemical and heat treatments. Open Biomed Eng J 2015;9(Suppl. 1-M2): 13–25.
[2] Kim H-M, Miyaji F, Kokubo T, Nakamura T. Preparation of bioactive Ti and its alloys via simple chemical surface treatment. J Biomed Mater Res 1996;32:409–17.
[3] Yamaguchi S, Takadama H, Matsushita T, Nakamura T, Kokubo T. Cross-sectional analysis of the surface ceramic layer developed on Ti metal by NaOH-heat treatment and soaking in SBF. J Ceram Soc Jpn 2009;117:1126–30.

[4] Kim H-M, Miyaji F, Kokubo T, Nakamura T. Graded surface structure of bioactive titanium prepared by chemical treatment. J Biomed Mater Res 1999;45:100–7.
[5] Kim H-M, Takadama H, Miyaji F, Kokubo T, Nishiguchi S, Nakamura T. Formation of bioactive functionally graded structure on Ti-6Al-4V alloy by chemical surface treatment. J Mater Sci Mater Med 2000;11:555–9.
[6] Kim H-M, Takadama H, Kokubo T, Nishiguchi S, Nakamura T. Formation of bioactive graded surface structure on Ti-15Mo-5Zr-3Al alloys by chemical treatment. Biomaterials 2000;21:353–8.
[7] Yamaguchi S, Takadama H, Matsushita T, Nakamura T, Kokubo T. Preparation of bioactive Ti-15Zr-4Nb-4Ta alloy from HCl and heat treatments after an NaOH treatment. J Biomed Mater Res Part A 2011;97A:135–44.
[8] Kizuki T, Takadama H, Matsushita T, Nakamura T, Kokubo T. Effect of Ca contamination on apatite formation in a Ti metal subjected to NaOH and heat treatments. J Mater Sci Mater Med 2013;24:635–44.
[9] Kawai T, Kizuki T, Takadama H, Matsushita T, Unuma T, Nakamura T, et al. Apatite formation on surface titanate layer with different Na content on Ti metal. J Ceram Soc Jpn 2010;118:19–24.
[10] Kizuki T, Takadama H, Matsushita T, Nakamura T, Kokubo T. Preparation of bioactive Ti metal surface enriched with calcium ions by chemical treatment. Acta Biomater 2010;6: 2836–42.
[11] Yamaguchi S, Takadama H, Matsushita T, Nakamura T, Kokubo T. Apatite-forming ability of Ti-15Zr-4Nb-4Ta alloy induced by calcium solution treatment. J Mater Sci Mater Med 2010;21:439–44.
[12] Yamaguchi S, Kizuki T, Takadama H, Matsushita T, Nakamura T, Kokubo T. Formation of a bioactive calcium titanate layer on gum metal by chemical treatment. J Mater Sci Mater Med 2012;23:873–83.
[13] Yamaguchi S, Matsushita T, Kokubo T. A bioactive Ti metal with a Ca-enriched surface layer releases Mg ions. RSC Adv 2013;3:11274–82.
[14] Yamaguchi S, Matsushita T, Nakamura T, Kokubo T. Bioactive Ti metal with Ca-enriched surface layer able to release Zn ion. Key Eng Mater 2013;529–530:547–52.
[15] Yamaguchi S, Nath S, Matsushita T, Kokubo T. Controlled release of strontium ions from a bioactive Ti metal with a Ca-enriched surface layer. Acta Biomater 2014;10:2282–9.
[16] Kizuki T, Matsushita T, Kokubo T. Antibacterial and bioactive calcium titanate layers formed on Ti metal and its alloys. J Mater Sci Mater Med 2014;25:1737–46.
[17] Kokubo T, Pattanayak DK, Yamaguchi S, Takadama H, Matsushita T, Kawai T, et al. Positively charged bioactive charged bioactive Ti metal prepared by simple chemical and heat treatments. J R Soc Interface 2010;7:S503–13.
[18] Pattanayak DK, Yamaguchi S, Matsushita T, Kokubo T. Nanostructured positively charged bioactive TiO_2 layer formed on Ti metal by NaOH, acid and heat treatments. J Mater Sci Mater Med 2011;22:1803–12.
[19] Pattanayak DK, Yamaguchi S, Matsushita T, Nakamura T, Kokubo T. Apatite-forming ability of titanium in terms of pH of the exposed solution. J R Soc Interface 2012;9: 2145–55.
[20] Kokubo T, Takadama H. How useful is SBF in predicting in vivo bone bioactivity? Biomaterials 2006;15:2907–15.
[21] Kim H-M, Himeno T, Kawashita M, Lee J-H, Kokubo T, Nakamura T. Surface potential change in bioactive titanium metal during the process of apatite formation in simulated body fluid. J Biomed Mater Res Part A 2003;67A:1305–9.

[22] Gold JM, Schmidt M, Steinmann SG. XPS study of amino acid adsorption to titanium surfaces. Helv Phys Acta 1989;62:246–9.
[23] Yan W-Q, Nakamura T, Kobayashi M, Kim H-M, Miyaji F, Kokubo T. Bonding of chemically treated titanium implants to bone. J Biomed Mater Res 1997;37:267–75.
[24] Nishiguchi S, Kato H, Fujita H, Kim H-M, Miyaji F, Kokubo T, et al. Enhancement of bone-bonding strengths of titanium alloy implants by alkali and heat treatments. J Biomed Mater Res (Appl Biomater) 1999;48:689–96.
[25] Fukuda A, Takemoto M, Saito T, Fujibayashi S, Neo M, Yamaguchi S, et al. Bone bonding bioactivity of Ti metal and Ti-Zr-Nb-Ta alloys with Ca ions incorporated on their surfaces by simple chemical and heat treatments. Acta Biomater 2011;7:1379–86.
[26] Tanaka M, Takemoto M, Fujibayashi S, Kawai T, Yamaguchi S, Kizuki T, et al. Bone bonding ability of a chemically treated low elastic modulus Ti alloy; gum metal. J Mater Sci Mater Med 2014;25:635–43.
[27] Kawai T, Takemoto M, Fujibayashi S, Neo M, Akiyama H, Yamaguchi S, et al. Bone-bonding properties of Ti metal subjected to acid and heat treatments. J Mater Sci Mater Med 2012;23:2981–92.
[28] Takemoto M, Fujibayashi S, Neo M, Suzuki J, Kokubo T, Nakamura T. Mechanical properties and osteoconductivity of porous bioactive titanium. Biomaterials 2005;26: 6014–23.
[29] Fujibayashi S, Neo M, Kim H-M, Kokubo T, Nakamura T. Osteoinduction of porous bioactive titanium metal. Biomaterials 2004;25:443–50.
[30] Takemoto M, Fujibayashi S, Neo M, Suzuki J, Matsushita T, Kokubo T, et al. Osteoinductive porous titanium implants: effect of sodium removal by dilute HCl treatment. Biomaterials 2006;27:2682–91.
[31] Kawai T, Takemoto M, Fujibayashi S, Akiyama H, Tanaka S, Yamaguchi S, et al. Osteoinduction on acid and heat treated porous Ti metal samples in canine muscle. PLoS One 2014;9:e88366.
[32] Kawai T, Takemoto M, Fujibayashi S, Akiyama H, Yamaguchi S, Pattanayak DK, et al. Osteoconduction of porous Ti metal enhanced by acid and heat treatments. J Mater Sci Mater Med 2013;24:1701–15.
[33] Kawanabe K, Ise K, Goto K, Akiyama H, Nakamura T, Kaneuji A, et al. A new cementless total hip arthroplasty with bioactive titanium porous-coating by alkaline and heat treatments: average 4.8-year results. J Biomed Mater Res Part B Appl Biomater 2009;90B: 476–81.
[34] Takemoto M, Fujibayashi S, Neo M, So K, Akiyama N, Matsushita T, et al. A porous bioactive titanium implant for spinal interbody fusion: an experimental study using a canine model. J Neurosurg Spine 2007;7:435–43.
[35] Fujibayashi S, Takemoto M, Neo M, Matsushita T, Kokubo T, Doi K, et al. A novel synthetic material for spinal fusion: a prospective clinical trial of porous bioactive titanium metal for lumber interbody fusion. Eur Spine J 2011;20:1486–95.

Nanotopography and surface chemistry of TiO_2–ZrO_2–$ZrTiO_4$ nanotubular surfaces and the influence on their bioactivity and cell responses

7

S. Minagar[1], J. Lin[2,3], Y. Li[4], C.C. Berndt[1,5], C. Wen[1,4]
[1]Swinburne University of Technology, Hawthorn, Victoria, Australia; [2]Zhejiang Industry & Trade Vocational College, Wenzhou, Zhejiang, China; [3]Jilin University, Changchun, Jilin, China; [4]RMIT University, Melbourne, Victoria, Australia; [5]Stony Brook University, Stony Brook, NY, United States

7.1 Introduction

Mineralized collagen fibrils are the basic building blocks of bone [1]. The plate-shaped carbonated apatite or dahllite ($Ca_5 \cdot (PO_4 \cdot CO_3)_3(OH)$) stands in a framework of these collagen fibrils [1,2]. Although dahllite displays a hexagonal crystal symmetry, the crystals of bone are plate-shaped, probably because the plate-shaped octacalcium phosphate is a transition phase. The average length and width of this crystal are 50×25 nm, respectively, with a thickness of 1.5–4 nm [1].

The organized structure of bone has two major functions: a mechanical function and a metabolic function. The metabolic function of bone serves as a reservoir for calcium and phosphate [2]. For example, the remodeling process in hard tissue, which is guided by bone cells and proteins, can also occur on surfaces of bioactive implants by the biomineralization of apatite [3]. Bioactive implant materials can be mineralized into apatite by means of body fluid (in vivo) or simulated body fluid (SBF) (in vitro) when there is an interface to integrate spontaneously with living tissue [3]. The mineralization of crystalline apatite occurs due to the electrostatic interaction of the functional groups of the bioactive surface with the calcium and phosphate ions in the fluid through a transition phase of amorphous calcium phosphate [3].

Research has focused on binary and ternary alloys of titanium (Ti) with biocompatible alloying metals such as tantalum, niobium, and zirconium for application as implants [4–11]. Ti50Zr, with a fine martensitic structure, is one of these new biocompatible alloys and, in comparison to commercially pure titanium (CP-Ti), it exhibits 2.5 times higher hardness and ~2.3–3 times higher tensile strength [6]. Anodization is a surface modification method that can improve the biocompatibility and bioactivity of metal implants. A layer of metal oxide nanotubes forms when electrochemical oxidation is

Metallic Foam Bone. http://dx.doi.org/10.1016/B978-0-08-101289-5.00007-X

undertaken in an electrolyte consisting of fluorine ions [12]. Ti dioxide, fabricated both in aqueous and nonaqueous electrolytes, exhibited bioactivity [12–14]. Hydroxyapatite (HA) can be deposited or mineralized on the surface of a metal implant using physical and chemical techniques such as plasma-spray [15], sputtering [16,17], electron-beam physical vapor deposition [18], and electrodeposition [19]. However, a method that is technically simpler, i.e., immersion in an SBF such as Hank's solution [20,21], is also feasible. The Ca/P atomic ratio of the synthetic HA ($Ca_{10}(PO_4)_6(OH)_2$) formed on a nanotubular layer of TiO_2 by using the immersion method [21,22] is 1.67. Although the formation of a nanotubular layer on Ti50Zr alloy [23] and cell adhesion [24] have been reported, the bioactivity of the nanotubular surfaces in terms of inducing HA still needs to be investigated.

In this study, four different nanotubular layers of TiO_2–ZrO_2–$ZrTiO_4$ and TiO_2 were fabricated with different dimensions of inner diameter (D_i), outer diameter (D_o), and wall thickness (W_t). The size distribution of the nanotubes was evaluated using the statistical method of the normal distribution (also called the Gaussian distribution). HA was mineralized on the surface of (1) TiO_2–ZrO_2–$ZrTiO_4$ nanotubes, (2) the anodized surface of Ti50Zr (flat surface), and (3) bare Ti50Zr alloy and compared to (4) TiO_2 nanotubes, (5) the anodized surface of CP-Ti (flat surface), and (6) bare CP-Ti to evaluate their bioactivity. The effect of nanotube size, the roughness, and the surface chemistry of the nanotubular surface on inducing HA mineralization was elucidated. SaOS2 cells were seeded onto the TiO_2–ZrO_2–$ZrTiO_4$ nanotubular surfaces without and with a coating of an HA layer, and the cellular activities were investigated.

7.2 Experiment

Ti50Zr alloy was prepared by casting, and then disc samples of diameter 8 mm and thickness 2 mm were fabricated by electric discharge machining. After polishing to a 1 μm diamond finish, the samples were ultrasonically cleaned for 15 min each in methanol, isopropanol, acetone, and ethanol prior to rinsing with pure water and drying with a nitrogen stream. CP-Ti (Baoji Boxin Metal Materials Co., Ltd.) foils with dimensions of 10 × 10 mm were degreased and washed in the same manner. The cleaned discs and foils were divided into three groups. The first group of samples was used for the fabrication of TiO_2–ZrO_2–$ZrTiO_4$ and TiO_2 nanotubes using a DC power supply with two-electrode configurations in 1 mol/dm^3 $(NH_4)_2SO_4$ and 0.5 wt% NH_4F (Sigma-Aldrich reagent grades) at different applied potentials. The second group of samples was used for the fabrication of compact films of TiO_2–ZrO_2–$ZrTiO_4$ and TiO_2 (without a nanotubular structure) by anodization in 1 mol/dm^3 $(NH_4)_2SO_4$ at 20 V using the same power supply. After anodization the samples were washed with deionized water for 5 min and dried with a nitrogen stream. The third group of samples was studied without any surface modification. Half of the electrochemically produced surface layers were annealed at 500°C for 3 h in air in a muffle furnace (Nabertherm LT15/13/P330) at a heating rate of 2°C/min.

The sample surfaces, after anodization and soaking in a modified SBF (m-SBF) [25], were analyzed with a field-emission scanning electron microscope (FESEM, ZEISS SUPRA 40 VP) equipped with an energy-dispersive X-ray spectrometer (EDS). The crystalline phases were determined by X-ray diffraction (XRD) using Cu Kα incident radiation at 40 kV and 40 mA over a 2θ range from 10−90 degrees at a scanning step size of 0.02 degrees.

The peaks, valleys, and spacing of the surface textures were characterized by the roughness parameters including mean roughness (S_a) and root mean square (RMS) roughness (S_q) [26]. These surface roughness parameters were measured using a 3D profilometer (Bruker, Contour GT-K1, Bruker Pte Ltd., Singapore) coupled with *Surf-Vision* software (Veeco Instruments Inc, Plainview, NY, USA) [26].

The water contact angle measurements were undertaken using a goniometer (NRL C.A. Goniometer, Ramé-hart, Inc., Succasunna, NJ, USA). The surface energy was calculated using the Owens-Wendt method [27], as follows:

$$(1+\cos\theta)\gamma_L = 2\left(\sqrt{\gamma_L^d\gamma_S^d}+\sqrt{\gamma_L^p\gamma_S^p}\right) \tag{7.1}$$

where γ_L indicates the liquid surface tensions (water: 72.8 mJ/m^2, glycerol: 63.4 mJ/m^2) and γ_L^d and γ_S^d are the liquid and solid dispersive components (water: 21.8 mJ/m^2, glycerol: 37.0 mJ/m^2). The variables γ_L^p and γ_S^p indicate the liquid and solid polar components (water: 51.0 mJ/m^2, glycerol: 26.4 mJ/m^2) and γ_S is the sum of γ_S^d and γ_S^p [28].

The samples were soaked in an m-SBF to evaluate in vitro bioactivity through assessing the ability to induce, form, and grow HA. All three groups of Ti50Zr and CP-Ti samples were soaked in m-SBF for 3 weeks. The m-SBF solutions were prepared according to the procedures described in [25] and [29]. The m-SBF with ionic concentrations equal to human blood plasma was prepared by dissolving reagent-grade chemicals with the composition 5.403 g NaCl, 0.504 g $NaHCO_3$, 0.426 g Na_2CO_3, 0.225 g KCl, 0.230 g $K_2HPO_4-3H_2O$, 0.311 g $MgCl_2-6H_2O$, 0.293 g $CaCl_2$, and 0.072 g Na_2SO_4 in 1 L deionized water buffered with 2-(4-(2-hydroxyethyl)-1-piperazinyl) ethane sulfonic acid (HEPES) (17.892 g HEPES dissolved in 100 mL 0.2 M NaOH) and 1 M NaOH at pH 7.4 and 37°C. After immersion, the samples were rinsed with pure water and dried at room temperature.

All samples for the cell culture studies were sterilized in a muffle furnace at 180°C for 3 h. The samples were placed in a well in the cell culture plate. SaOS2 cells (Barwon Biomedical Research, Geelong Hospital, Victoria, Australia) were seeded on the surface of the $TiO_2-ZrO_2-ZrTiO_4$ samples that exhibited different D_i and D_o as well as W_t.

The seeded cell density was 5×10^3 cells per well (over 100 mm^2 area). An MTS assay (a biochemical cell assey used in research) was used to measure the in vitro proliferation of the SaOS2 cells. The cell morphology was observed by means of scanning electron microscopy (SEM) after cell culturing. The cells were dehydrated for the SEM observation by immersion in a buffer solution in which the ethanol concentrations were increased progressively every 10 min to

60%, 70%, 80%, 90%, and 100%. This procedure was followed by chemical drying using hexamethyldisilazane (Sigma-Aldrich, Australia) for 10 min. A gold layer was deposited on the samples prior to SEM observation.

The cell morphology was also observed using confocal microscopy (Leica SP5, Leica Microsystems, Germany). The cell-seeded samples after cell culture were fixed in paraformaldehyde and then permeabilized with Triton-X 100 in phosphate-buffered saline (PBS) (Sigma-Aldrich, Australia). Subsequently, the samples were stained with 1% phalloidin and 40-6-diamidino-2-phenylindole for 40 min at room temperature. Three washes in PBS were executed between each of the steps. The samples were stored in PBS at 4°C when necessary, and the confocal observations were conducted within 1 week of staining. Significant differences in the cell numbers were analyzed using one-way Analysis of variance (ANOVA) ($\rho < 0.05$).

7.3 Results and discussion

7.3.1 Anodization dynamics for the fabrication of TiO_2–ZrO_2–$ZrTiO_4$ nanotubes

Fig. 7.1 shows SEM images of the nanotubular layers that were fabricated on Ti50Zr discs at applied potentials from 20–35 V. Fig. 7.1(a,c,e) and (g) show the as-formed TiO_2–ZrO_2–$ZrTiO_4$ nanotubes, and Fig. 7.1(b,d,f) and (h) show the nanotubes after annealing at 500°C for 3 h. The formation of the TiO_2–ZrO_2–$ZrTiO_4$ nanotubes [23] resulted from oxidation and dissolution of the oxide layer in the presence of fluorine ions.

The TiO_2–ZrO_2–$ZrTiO_4$ nanotubes formed on the Ti50Zr substrate surface during anodization exhibited different morphologies due to the dissimilar microstructural phases of the Ti50Zr substrate. The microstructure of the Ti50Zr alloy has been reported to be a needle-like structure consisting of α and β phases [30]. The growth rates of the nanotubes were reported as 2.5 nm/V for TiO_2 [31] and 2.9 nm/V for ZrO_2 [32]. Therefore an adherent layer of TiO_2–ZrO_2–$ZrTiO_4$ grew on the substrate surface where the ZrO_2 nanotubes showed longer lengths than the TiO_2 nanotubes because of their higher oxidation rate. The standard electrode potentials are $Zr \rightarrow Zr^{4+} = 1.553$ V and $Ti \rightarrow Ti^{4+} = 2.132$ V [33]. The sample surface consisted of two regions during anodization: (1) the substrate and the inner oxide layer that were dense and protective and (2) the outer oxide layer and the electrolyte that were porous. The pores were suitable sites for initiating tube growth since they trapped fluorine ions and enabled the formation of $[TiF_6]^{2-}$ complexes [12] and $[ZrF_6]^{2-}$ [34] at different reaction rates. The difference between the oxidation and dissolution rates of Ti and zirconium caused the formation of different D_i and D_o and W_t of the nanotubes (Table 7.1) as well as varying nanotube lengths that led to different surface roughness values. Figs. 7.2 and 7.3 show the distribution of D_i, D_o, and W_t values as a function of the applied potential. The distribution of nanotube sizes influenced the physical and chemical properties of the nanotubular surface.

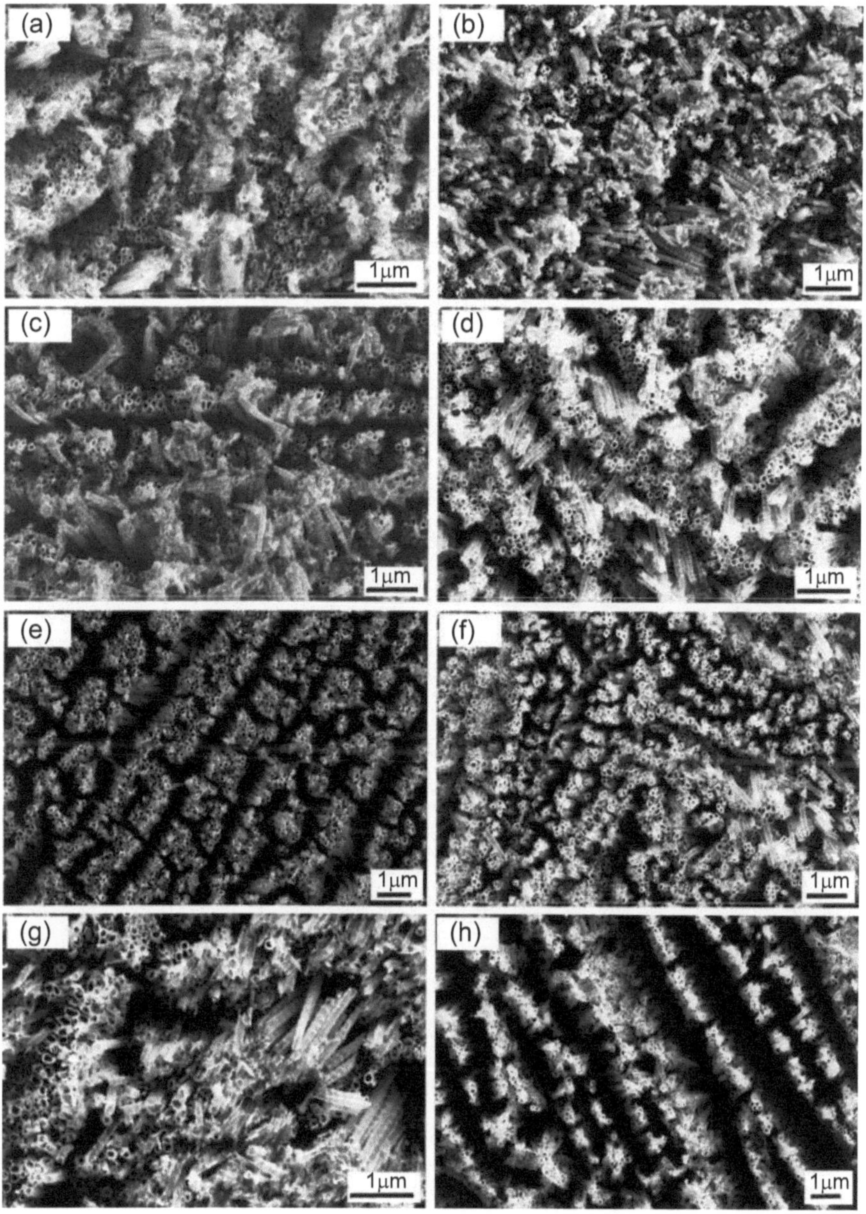

Figure 7.1 Scanning electron microscopy images of nanotubular layers fabricated at (a) 20 V, as-formed; (b) 20 V, annealed; (c) 25 V, as-formed; (d) 25 V, annealed; (e) 30 V, as-formed; (f) 30 V, annealed; (g) 35 V, as-formed; and (h) 35 V, annealed.

Table 7.1 **The distribution of inner diameter (D_i), outer diameter (D_o), and wall thicknesses (W_t) of $TiO_2-ZrO_2-ZrTiO_4$ nanotubes determined by using normal distribution methods**

	As-formed			Annealed		
Applied potential (V)	**D_i (nm)**	**D_o (nm)**	**W_t (nm)**	**D_i (nm)**	**D_o (nm)**	**W_t (nm)**
20	$24 < D_i < 50$	$53 < D_o < 89$	$9 < W_t < 15$	$28 < D_i < 52$	$60 < D_o < 89$	$1 < W_t < 14$
25	$5 < D_i < 82$	$92 < D_o < 126$	$12 < W_t < 25$	$42 < D_i < 76$	$85 < D_o < 120$	$1 < W_t < 8$
30	$56 < D_i < 97$	$96 < D_o < 142$	$13 < W_t < 15$	$41 < D_i < 88$	$91 < D_o < 144$	$1 < W_t < 23$
35	$61 < D_i < 101$	$106 < D_o < 157$	$16 < W_t < 27$	$56 < D_i < 108$	$111 < D_o < 161$	$1 < W_t < 25$

Note: Each graph indicates 300 measurements.

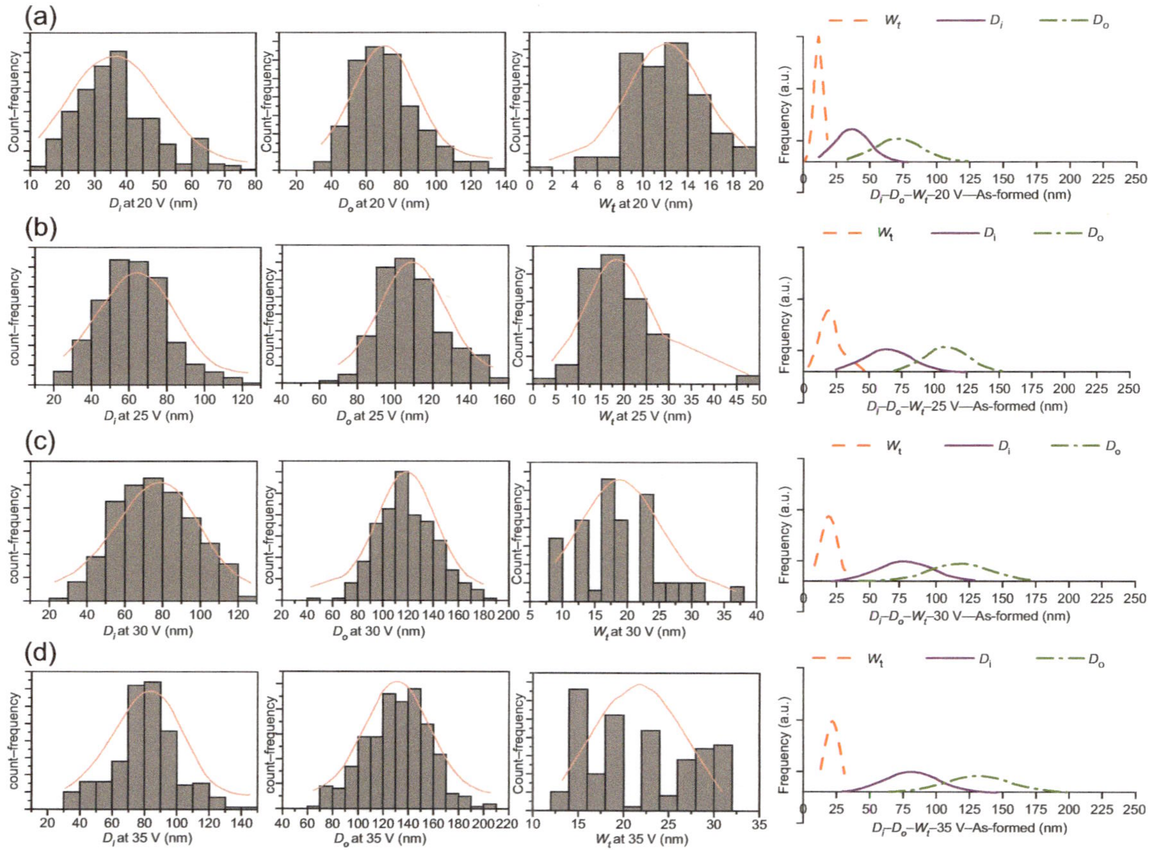

Figure 7.2 Histograms and distribution functions of inner diameter (D_i), outer diameter (D_o), and wall thicknesses (W_t) of as-formed $TiO_2-ZrO_2-ZrTiO_4$ nanotubes fabricated at (a) 20 V, (b) 25 V, (c) 30 V, and (d) 35 V. Note: Each graph indicates 300 measurements.

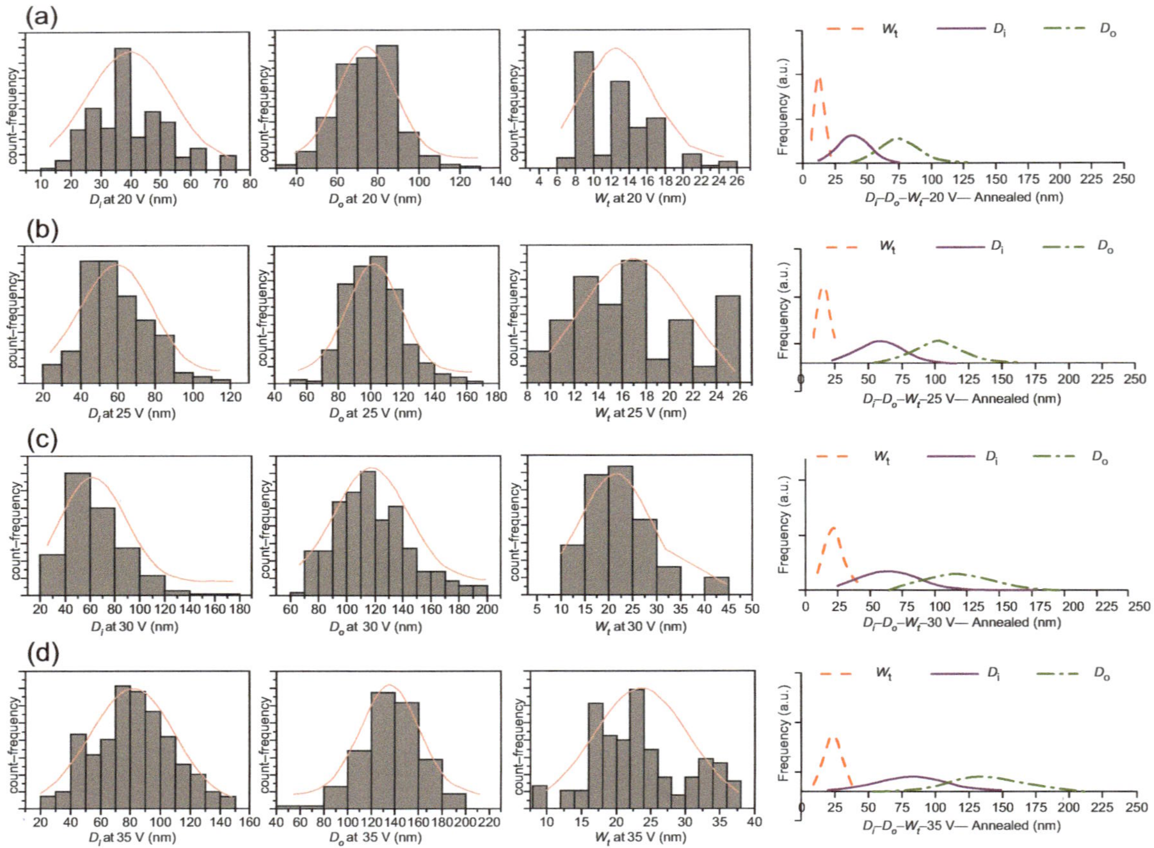

Figure 7.3 Histograms and distribution functions of inner diameter (D_i), outer diameter (D_o), and wall thicknesses (W_t) of annealed TiO_2–ZrO_2–$ZrTiO_4$ nanotubes fabricated at (a) 20 V, (b) 25 V, (c) 30 V, and (d) 35 V. Note: Each graph indicates 300 measurements.

7.3.2 Physical and chemical characteristics of TiO_2–ZrO_2–$ZrTiO_4$ nanotubular layers

The S_a and the water contact angle of the nanotubular surfaces as a function of the applied potential of the as-formed and annealed TiO_2–ZrO_2–$ZrTiO_4$ and TiO_2 nanotubes anodized on Ti50Zr and CP-Ti are presented in Fig. 7.4. The mean S_a of as-formed TiO_2–ZrO_2–$ZrTiO_4$ nanotubular surfaces decreased with an increase in the applied potential. On the contrary, the S_a of the annealed TiO_2–ZrO_2–$ZrTiO_4$ nanotubular surfaces slightly increased with increasing applied potential, and the annealed nanotubular surfaces were smoother than the as-formed nanotubular surfaces. The same trend was observed for TiO_2 nanotubes, although they revealed lower roughness amplitude parameters. After annealing, the S_a of the TiO_2 nanotubes slightly increased or remained constant.

The water contact angle of TiO_2–ZrO_2–$ZrTiO_4$ nanotubes decreased with an increase of D_i for either the as-formed or annealed nanotubes. The values of the water contact angle on the surface of TiO_2–ZrO_2–$ZrTiO_4$ after annealing were lower than those of the as-formed nanotubes. The nanotubular layer of TiO_2–ZrO_2–$ZrTiO_4$ anodized at almost all the applied potentials exhibited superhydrophilic properties ($\theta_W < 10$ degrees) except for the as-formed TiO_2–ZrO_2–$ZrTiO_4$ nanotubes fabricated at an applied potential of 20 V with $D_i = 37$ nm that exhibited hydrophilic properties. The water contact angle of TiO_2 nanotubes decreased with an increase of D_i either for as-formed or annealed nanotubes, and they revealed lower values after annealing.

The TiO_2 nanotubular layer anodized at all the applied potentials exhibited hydrophilic properties. The flat surface and bare metal surfaces of Ti50Zr and CP-Ti revealed hydrophilic properties with water contact angles that were at least 2 times higher than their nanotubular counterpart layers. It can be seen that the water contact angle increased with an increase of S_a for both the as-formed TiO_2–ZrO_2–$ZrTiO_4$ and TiO_2 nanotubes while it decreased on the annealed nanotubular layer. It can be concluded that increasing D_i and the crystalline phase of the nanotubular layer influenced the hydrophilic properties more than the surface roughness. The surface energy of TiO_2–ZrO_2–$ZrTiO_4$, TiO_2 nanotubes, flat surface, and bare Ti50Zr alloy and CP-Ti are listed in Table 7.2.

7.3.3 Bioactivity of TiO_2–ZrO_2–$ZrTiO_4$ and TiO_2 nanotubes and cell adhesion and spreading on the nanotubular surfaces

A dense and uniform layer of the bone-like apatite was formed on the TiO_2–ZrO_2–$ZrTiO_4$ and TiO_2 nanotubular surfaces after soaking in m-SBF, as shown in Figs. 7.5 and 7.6, respectively. It has been reported that an anatase or a rutile structure of TiO_2 nanotubes were more favorable for apatite formation than an amorphous structure [22,35]. Therefore some samples were annealed at 500°C for 3 h to obtain crystalline phases.

The surfaces of the as-formed and annealed TiO_2–ZrO_2–$ZrTiO_4$, TiO_2 nanotubes, and flat surface were covered by nanobristle spheres (Fig. 7.5(c′)) and a layer of

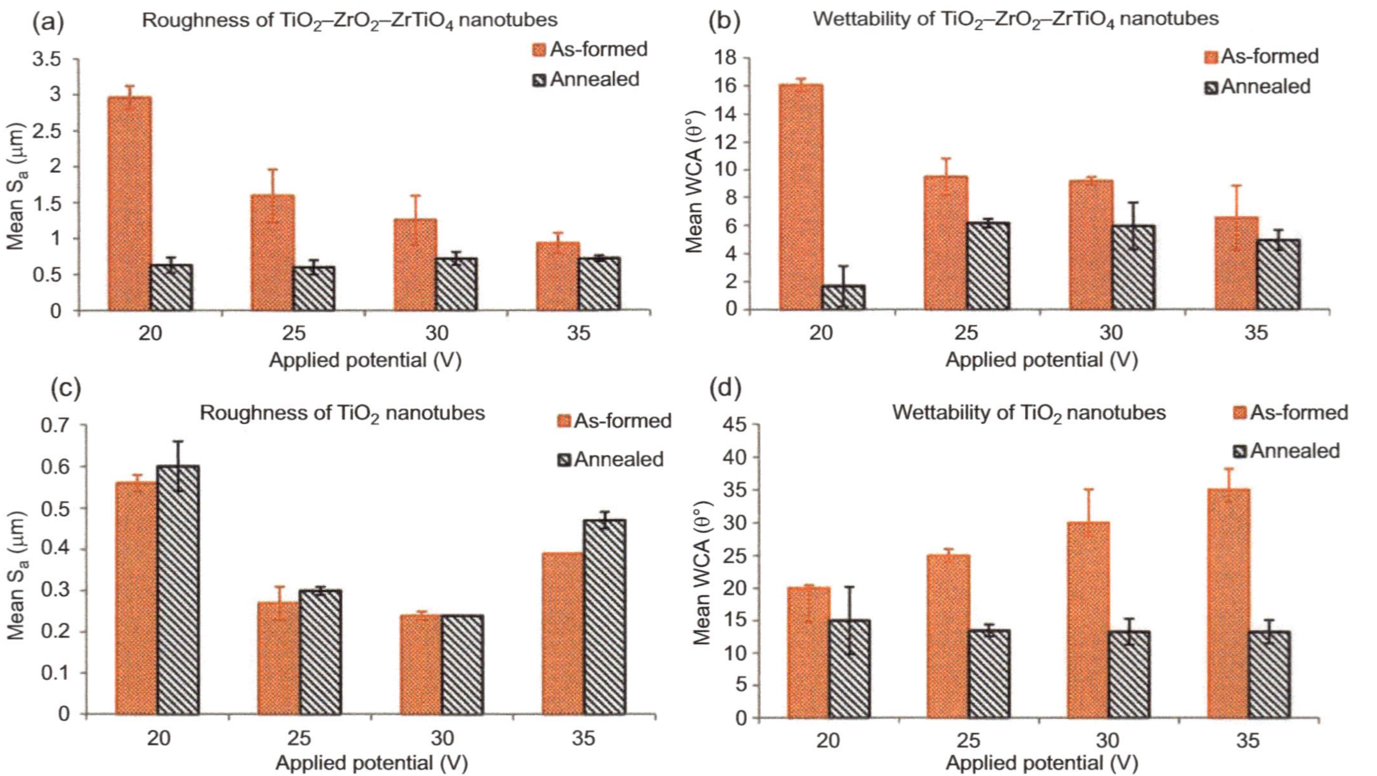

Figure 7.4 (a) The mean roughness (S_a) and (b) the mean water contact angle (WCA) of the as-formed and annealed $TiO_2-ZrO_2-ZrTiO_4$ nanotubular surfaces as a function of the applied potential; (c) the S_a and (d) the WCA of the as-formed and annealed TiO_2 nanotubular surfaces as a function of the applied potential. Note: Each data point is an average of three measurements.

Table 7.2 Calculated surface energy of TiO_2–ZrO_2–$ZrTiO_4$ nanotubular surfaces fabricated on Ti50Zr and TiO_2 nanotubular surfaces on CP-Ti

Anodization conditions		As-formed				Annealed			
		Contact angle (θ)	γ_s^d (mJ/m^2)	γ_s^p (mJ/m^2)	$\gamma_s = \gamma_s^d + \gamma_s^p$ (mJ/m^2)	Contact angle (θ)	γ_s^d (mJ/m^2)	γ_s^p (mJ/m^2)	$\gamma_s = \gamma_s^d + \gamma_s^p$ (mJ/m^2)
20 V	Ti50Zr	20.50 ± 0.4	15.98	52.67	68.65	2.7 ± 0.2	14.93	58.71	73.64
	CP-Ti	28.7 ± 10.1	22.45	41.87	64.32	22.5 ± 4.8	12.95	55.56	68.51
25 V	Ti50Zr	9.5 ± 1.3	15.01	57.63	72.64	6.1 ± 0.3	14.69	58.66	73.35
	CP-Ti	30.0 ± 1.0	18.14	45.24	63.38	13.5 ± 0.9	9.25	65.04	74.29
30 V	Ti50Zr	9.2 ± 0.3	15.45	57.13	72.58	5.9 ± 1.7	15.22	58.00	73.22
	CP-Ti	25.3 ± 5.1	13.98	52.69	66.68	13.3 ± 2.0	13.33	58.83	72.16
35 V	Ti50Zr	6.5 ± 2.3	14.05	59.45	73.50	4.9 ± 0.7	14.20	59.47	73.67
	CP-Ti	18 ± 3	13.62	56.74	70.36	13.3 ± 1.8	10.16	63.57	73.73
Anodized in $(NH_4)_2SO_4$	Ti50Zr	47.7 ± 1.5	0.19	67.89	68.09	20.7 ± 1.5	3.59	74.42	78.01
	CP-Ti	64.8 ± 3.8	7.29	30.25	37.54	47.2 ± 1.2	26.36	27.1	53.46
Bare metal	Ti50Zr	42.2 ± 1.8	14.56	40.68	55.24	–	–	–	–
	CP-Ti	54.5 ± 4.7	15.37	30.17	45.55	–	–	–	–

Note: Each data point is an average of three measurements.

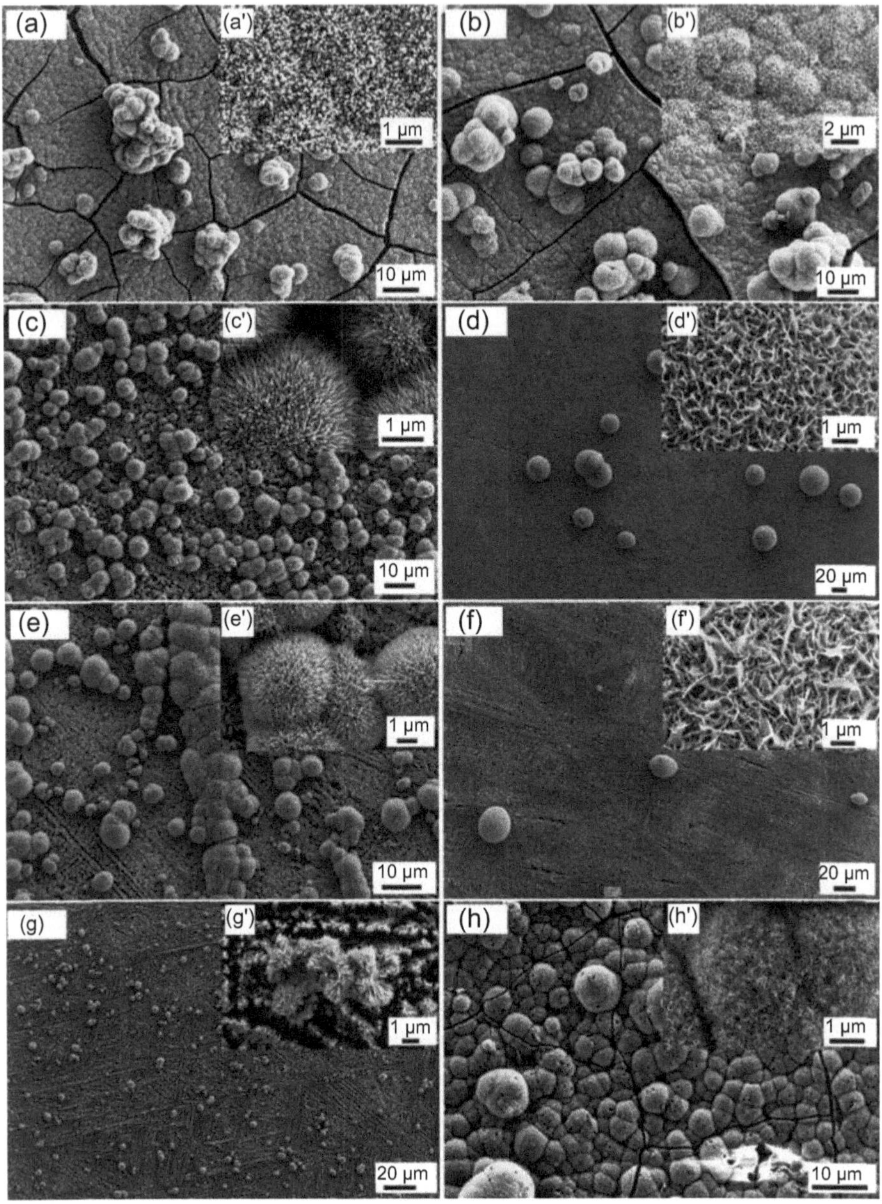

Figure 7.5 Mineralization of hydroxyapatite on the nanotubular surface of $TiO_2-ZrO_2-ZrTiO_4$ fabricated at: (a and a′) 20 V ($D_i = 37$ nm): as-formed; (b and b′) 20 V ($D_i = 40$ nm): annealed; (c and c′) 25 V ($D_i = 64$ nm): as-formed; (d and d′) 25 V ($D_i = 59$ nm): annealed; (e and e′) 30 V ($D_i = 76$ nm): as-formed; (f and f′) 30 V ($D_i = 64$ nm): annealed; (g and g′) 35 V ($D_i = 81$ nm): as-formed; and (h and h′) 35 V ($D_i = 82$ nm): annealed.

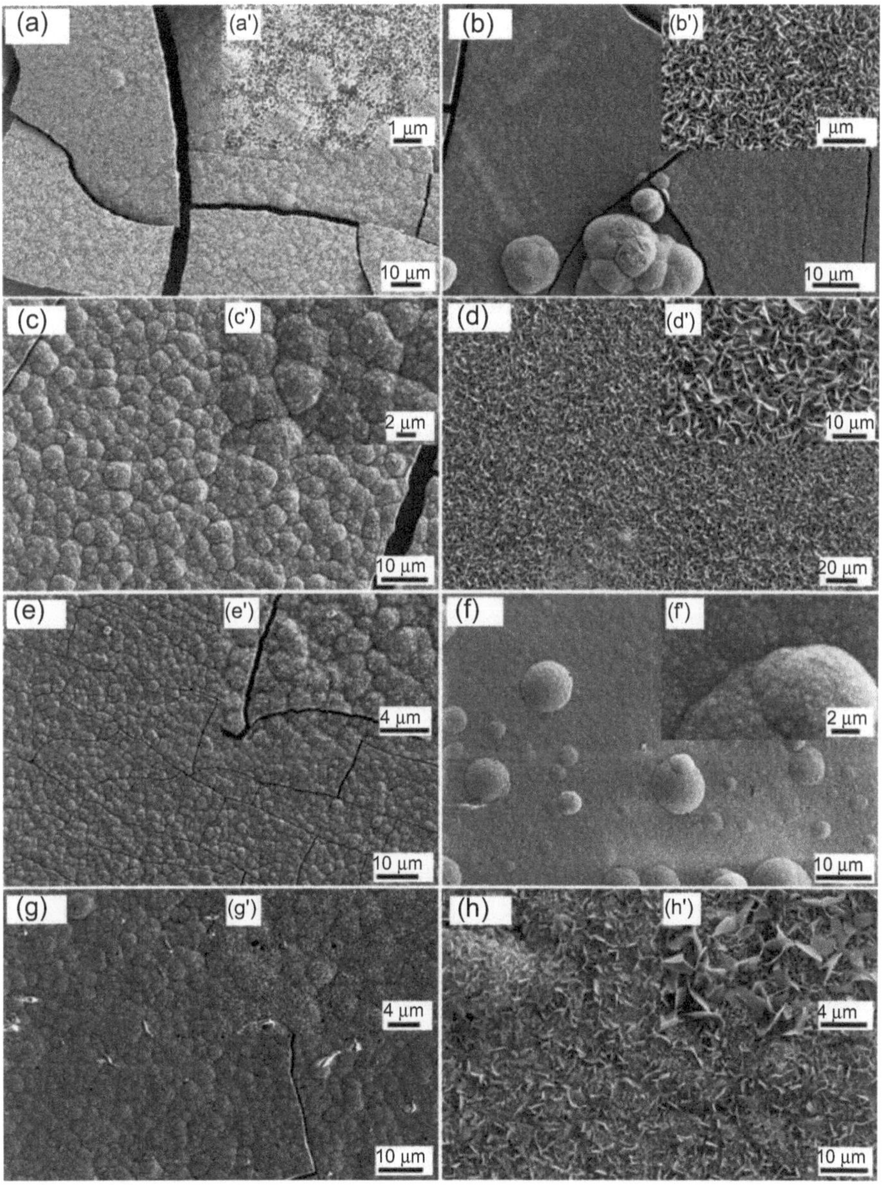

Figure 7.6 Mineralization of hydroxyapatite on the nanotubular surface of TiO_2 fabricated at: (a and a′) 20 V ($D_i = 43$ nm): as-formed; (b and b′) 20 V ($D_i = 51$ nm): annealed; (c and c′) 25 V ($D_i = 52$ nm): as-formed; (d and d′) 25 V ($D_i = 45$ nm): annealed; (e and e′) 30 V ($D_i = 65$ nm): as-formed: (f and f′) 30 V ($D_i = 53$ nm): annealed; (g and g′) 35 V ($D_i = 68$ nm): as-formed; and (h and h′) 35 V ($D_i = 63$ nm): annealed.

nanoflakes (Figs. 7.5(d′) and 7.6(d′)) after 3 weeks of immersion in m-SBF, respectively. However, no HA precipitation was observed on bare metal samples after 3 weeks of immersion or on the flat surface within 3 weeks of immersion in m-SBF.

The EDS spectra of the abovementioned samples detected Ca, P, and O peaks, which are the essential constituents of HA, after immersion in m-SBF for 3 weeks. The XRD patterns of the $TiO_2-ZrO_2-ZrTiO_4$ and TiO_2 nanotubes before and after immersion in m-SBF are shown in Fig. 7.7. The annealed specimen revealed the anatase peak of titania and the orthorhombic phase for a mixture of titania, zirconia, and zirconium titanate prior to immersion in m-SBF. After immersion in m-SBF for 3 weeks, HA peaks appear in the XRD patterns.

Fig. 7.8 shows the atomic percentage of the calcium to phosphate ratio (Ca/P) of HA that was mineralized on the surfaces of the $TiO_2-ZrO_2-ZrTiO_4$ and TiO_2 nanotubes. The Ca/P of HA that precipitated on the nanotubular layer of $TiO_2-ZrO_2-ZrTiO_4$ increased with an increase in W_t for both the as-formed and annealed nanotubes. It can be observed that the Ca/P atomic ratio of HA increased with an increase of S_a for the as-formed $TiO_2-ZrO_2-ZrTiO_4$ nanotubes, but it decreased with an increase of S_a for the annealed samples. On the other hand, the Ca/P ratio increased with a decrease of the water contact angle for both the as-formed and annealed nanotubular layers. The Ca/P atomic ratio increased after annealing for each nanotubular layer fabricated under the same conditions, regardless of the difference in the W_t of the nanotubes.

The Ca/P ratio of HA precipitated on the nanotubular layer of TiO_2 decreased with an increase of W_t for both the as-formed and annealed nanotubes. Increasing S_a of both as-formed and annealed TiO_2 nanotubes resulted in an increase of the Ca/P ratio of HA, although it decreased with a decrease of water contact angle. The Ca/P ratio remained constant after annealing for each nanotubular layer fabricated under the same conditions, regardless of different W_t values.

An HA layer formed on the flat surface of the oxide layer on Ti50Zr and CP-Ti. The measured Ca/P ratios of apatite were (1) 1.27 before and after annealing for Ti50Zr and (2) 1.29 before annealing and 1.22 after annealing for CP-Ti, the values of which were lower than their corresponding nanotubular layers.

The reactions on the surface of the wall of nanotubes subjected to the alkaline aqueous solution of m-SBF are as follows:

$$TiO_2 \cdot nH_2O + OH^- \rightarrow HTiO_3{}^- \cdot nH_2O \quad (7.2)$$

$$ZrO_2 \cdot nH_2O + OH^- \rightarrow HZrO_3{}^- \cdot nH_2O \quad (7.3)$$

$$ZrTiO_4 \cdot nH_2O + OH^- \rightarrow HZrTiO_5{}^- \cdot nH_2O \quad (7.4)$$

The isoelectric point of TiO_2 is reported at a pH of 3.9, and the corresponding value for ZrO_2 is 5.5 [36,37]. Both of these values are lower than the pH of m-SBF (7.4) and indicate the formation of a negative layer of Ti–OH and Zr–OH. The negatively charged surface adsorbs Ca^{2+} by Coulomb forces. A composition of calcium phosphate forms on the positively charged surface (i.e., the Ca-rich layer) due to electrostatic

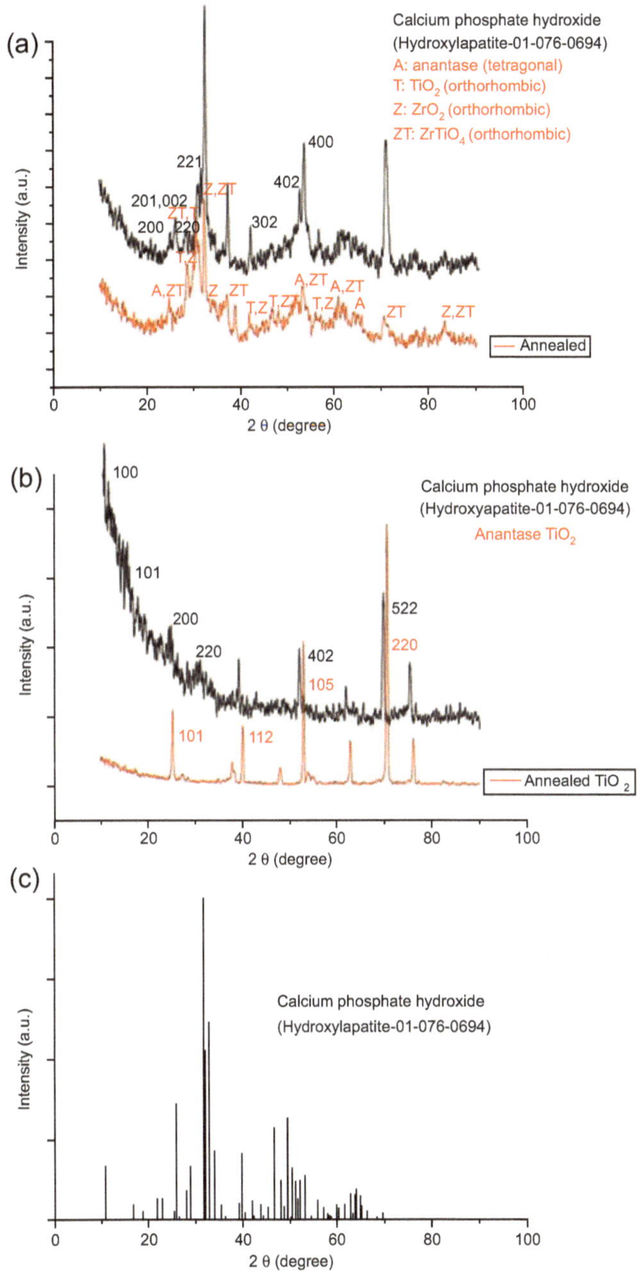

Figure 7.7 X-ray diffraction patterns of: (a) TiO_2–ZrO_2–$ZrTiO_4$ nanotubes anodized at 20 V on Ti50Zr (α and β phases) and annealed at 500°C for 3 h before and after immersion in m-SBF for 3 weeks, showing tetragonal anatase, srilankite (a mixture of orthorhombic TiO_2 and ZrO_2), and orthorhombic $ZrTiO_4$ with mineralized hydroxyapatite; (b) TiO_2 nanotubes anodized at 20 V on CP-Ti (α phase) and annealed at 500°C for 3 h before and after immersion in m-SBF for 3 weeks, showing tetragonal anatase with mineralized hydroxyapatite; and (c) hydroxyapatite.

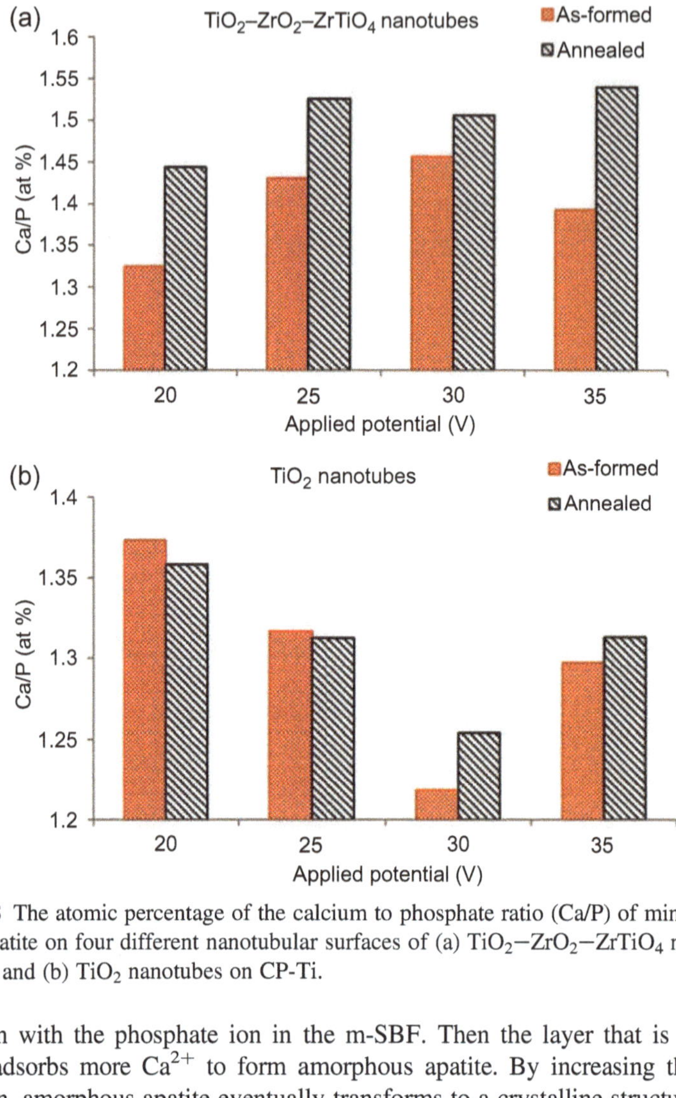

Figure 7.8 The atomic percentage of the calcium to phosphate ratio (Ca/P) of mineralized hydroxyapatite on four different nanotubular surfaces of (a) $TiO_2-ZrO_2-ZrTiO_4$ nanotubes on Ti50Zr and (b) TiO_2 nanotubes on CP-Ti.

interaction with the phosphate ion in the m-SBF. Then the layer that is negatively charged adsorbs more Ca^{2+} to form amorphous apatite. By increasing the time of immersion, amorphous apatite eventually transforms to a crystalline structure that exhibits lower solubility in neutral and basic solutions in comparison to other structural forms of calcium phosphate. Sodium, magnesium, chloride, and carbonate ions may become incorporated into an apatite similar to the composition and structural features of bone mineral since the m-SBF mimics the blood plasma not only in composition but also in concentration [3]. Octacalcium phosphate phase ($Ca_8H_2(PO_4)_6 \cdot 5H_2O$; OCP) is the first formed Ca–P crystal nuclei in the SBF [38]. Thermodynamically, OCP tends to convert to a calcium-deficient HA, although it remains in the apatite lattice with a plate-like morphology.

Consider the observation concerning the change in the Ca/P ratio of HA that is mineralized on the surface of $TiO_2-ZrO_2-ZrTiO_4$ nanotubes. It can be deduced that a direct link exists between W_t and the hydrophilic properties and crystalline phase of nanotubes, rather than the roughness parameters, for inducing the formation and growth of HA on a nanotubular surface. In terms of TiO_2 nanotubes, the hydrophilic properties and roughness parameters revealed a more significant influence on the formation and growth of HA than the W_t and the crystalline phase of the nanotubular layer. The role of morphological features that give rise to high roughness lies in the creation of the initial reaction sites for apatite nucleation and formation.

Figs. 7.9 and 7.10 show the scanning electron microscopy images of SaOS2 cells adhered on the surface of annealed $TiO_2{-}ZrO_2{-}ZrTiO_4$ nanotubes ($D_i = 40$ nm) without and with an HA layer after cell culture for 1 and 7 days, respectively. The HA layer on the nanotubular surface was formed during soaking in m-SBF for 3 weeks, showing a preferred condition for SaOS2 cells to adhere. It can be concluded that changing the chemistry of the surface served the cell to form better contact.

Fig. 7.11 illustrates the percentage of attached cells on a nanotubular surface that was coated with HA formed during soaking in m-SBF in comparison to that of a nanotubular layer without an HA layer with the same D_i. The percentage of total cells was obtained using MTS assay. The percentage of cells attached on the HA-covered nanotubes was $59.7 \pm 13.6\%$, compared to $41.0 \pm 2.6\%$ for the cells attached on the nanotubes without an HA layer. These results revealed the same tendency as those reported previously that indicated that osteoblast proliferation was significantly greater

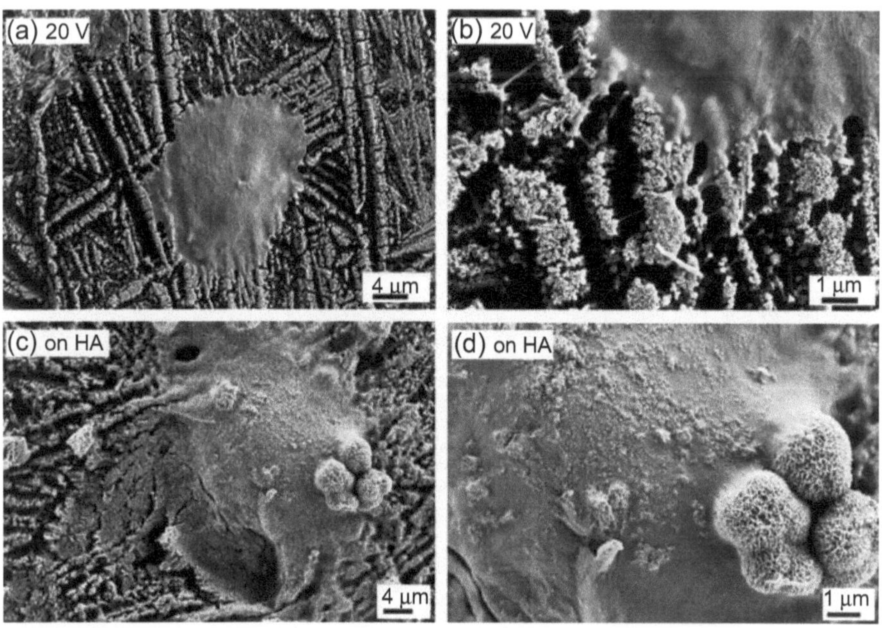

Figure 7.9 Scanning electron microscopy images of SaOS2 cells cultured for 1 day on the $TiO_2{-}ZrO_2{-}ZrTiO_4$ nanotubes ($D_i = 40$ nm): (a) low magnification, (b) higher magnification, (c) with hydroxyapatite coating at low magnification, and (d) with hydroxyapatite coating at high magnification.

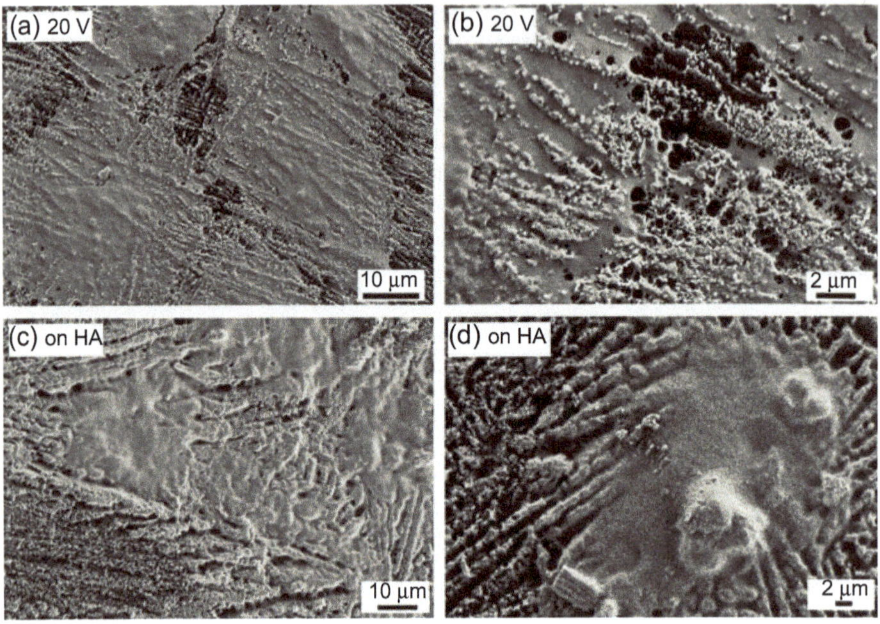

Figure 7.10 Scanning electron microscopy images of SaOS2 cells cultured for 7 days on the TiO_2–ZrO_2–$ZrTiO_4$ nanotubes ($D_i = 40$ nm): (a) low magnification, (b) higher magnification, (c) nanotubes covered with a hydroxyapatite layer at low magnification, and (d) nanotubes covered with a hydroxyapatite layer at high magnification.

on nanophase HA than on conventional formulations of the same ceramic [39]. It has also been reported in a direct comparison that the growth of MG63 osteoblastic cells on an electrodeposited CaP surface was more significant than on an untreated Ti surface [40]. A denser and smaller crystalline size of HA on TiO_2 nanotubes increased the

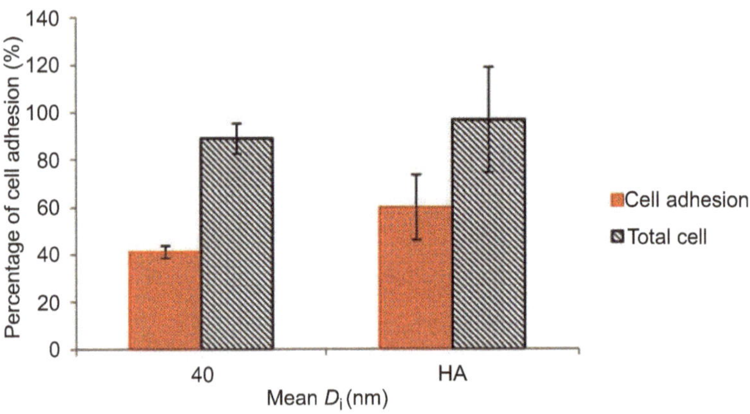

Figure 7.11 The percentage of cells attached to TiO_2–ZrO_2–$ZrTiO_4$ nanotubular surfaces with and without a hydroxyapatite (HA) layer with the same D_i of 40 nm after a 7-days cell culture. Note: Each data point is an average of three measurements.

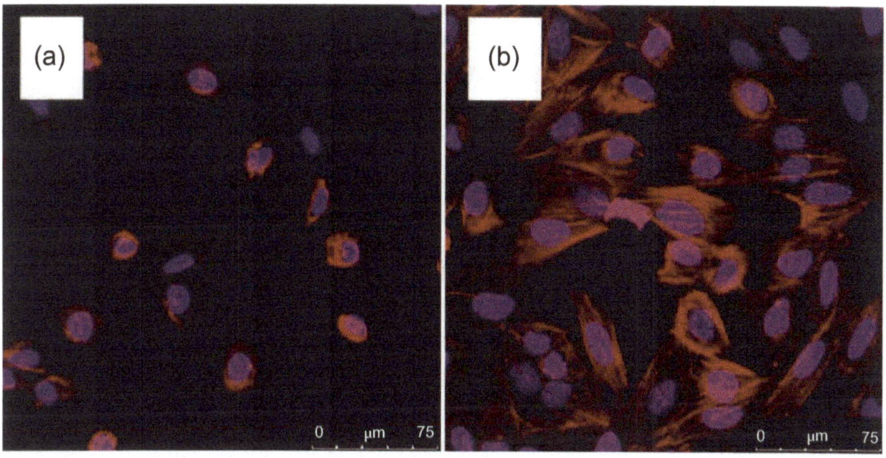

Figure 7.12 Confocal images of stained SaOS2 cells presenting nuclei (blue) and actin stress fibers (red) after 7 days on TiO_2–ZrO_2–$ZrTiO_4$ nanotubes (a) with $D_i = 40$ nm before post-treating and (b) after post-treating with hydroxyapatite.

adhesion of MG63 osteoblastic cells due to the increase in protein activity of such a layer [41]. Fig. 7.12 shows the confocal images of cells grown on the surface of HA-coated TiO_2–ZrO_2–$ZrTiO_4$ nanotubes after a 7-days cell culture.

The length to width ratio (L/W) of the cell nucleus and actin stress fiber on the nanotubular surface was measured by Image-J software using confocal microscopy images after 7 days of cell culture. The L/W ratio of nuclei (~1.5) did not change considerably for the HA-covered TiO_2–ZrO_2–$ZrTiO_4$ nanotubular surface. However, the L/W ratios of the actin stress fibers increased to ~2.2 in comparison with those on the nanotubular layer without an HA coating (~1.5). This result supports the cell response, mentioned previously, with respect to the chemistry changes of the nanotubular layer.

7.4 Conclusions

Nanotubular surfaces of TiO_2–ZrO_2–$ZrTiO_4$ and TiO_2 were fabricated via anodization on Ti50Zr and CP-Ti. The formation of HA on the nanotubular surfaces in comparison to flat anodized surfaces and bare metal surfaces was evaluated. The main conclusions are as follows.

1. The mean D_i and D_o of the nanotubes fabricated on the surfaces of Ti50Zr and CP-Ti increased with an increase in the applied potential from 20 to 25, 30, and 35 V. The mean D_i of TiO_2–ZrO_2–$ZrTiO_4$ nanotubes increased from $D_i = 37$ to 64, 76, and 81 nm, and the mean D_o of TiO_2–ZrO_2–$ZrTiO_4$ nanotubes increased from $D_o = 71$ to 109, 119, and 131 nm, respectively. Similarly, the mean D_i of TiO_2 nanotubes increased from $D_i = 43$ to 52, 65, and 68 nm, and the mean D_o of TiO_2 nanotubes increased from $D_o = 78$ to 102, 108, and 110 nm, respectively.

2. The mean W_t of $TiO_2-ZrO_2-ZrTiO_4$ and TiO_2 nanotubes exhibited a slight increase with an increase in the applied potential from 20 to 35 V, increasing from 12 to 21 nm and 15 to 21 nm, respectively.
3. Annealing of the nanotubes resulted in decreasing D_i and D_o, but unchanged W_t resulted from the changes of the lattice parameters of the phases after annealing.
4. Increasing the applied potential resulted in an increase in D_i of the $TiO_2-ZrO_2-ZrTiO_4$ nanotubes. This led to: (1) decreased roughness parameters of S_a and RMS S_q, (2) increased hydrophilic properties, and (3) increased surface energy of the nanotubular surfaces. After annealing at 500°C for 3 h in air, the mean S_a and S_q of the nanotubular surface decreased, and the hydrophilic properties and surface energy increased. The same tendency was observed for TiO_2 nanotubes anodized on the surface of CP-Ti, although their hydrophilic properties and surface energies were lower than those for $TiO_2-ZrO_2-ZrTiO_4$ nanotubes.
5. The bioactivity of the nanotubular surfaces, that is, their HA formation ability, was influenced by their surface chemistry, chemical potential, hydrophilicity, and nanotopography, which is determined by the crystal structure of the nanotubular phases and the dimensions, including the W_t and length of the nanotubes. These factors contributed to the nucleation and growth of the HA phase.
6. The nanotopography and chemistry of the nanotubular surfaces also affected the Ca/P ratio of the mineralized HA formed during immersion in SBF. The bioactivity of the nanotubular surfaces was clearly enhanced compared with the flat anodized surfaces and the bare metals of Ti50Zr and CP-Ti.
7. The percentage of cells attached to nanotubes covered with HA increased to $59.7 \pm 13.6\%$, in comparison to $41.0 \pm 2.6\%$ for the nanotubular surface without HA coating.

Acknowledgments

SM acknowledges the State Government of Victoria in Australia for supporting and funding this research project through a Victorian International Research Scholarship. The authors acknowledge the financial support for this research by the National Health and Medical Research Council through grant GNT1087290.

References

[1] Weiner S, Wagner HD. The material bone: structure-mechanical function relations. Annu Rev Mater Sci 1998;28:271–98.
[2] Weiner S, Traub W, Wagner HD. Lamellar bone: structure-function relations. J Struct Biol 1999;126:241–55.
[3] Kim H-M, Himeno T, Kawashita M, Kokubo T, Nakamura T. The mechanism of biomineralization of bone-like apatite on synthetic hydroxyapatite: an in vitro assessment. J R Soc Interface 2004;1:17–22.
[4] Okazaki Y, Rao S, Ito Y, Tateishi T. Corrosion resistance, mechanical properties: corrosion fatigue strength and cytocompatibility of new Ti alloys without Al and V. Biomaterials 1998;19:1197–215.
[5] Choe H-C, Saji VS, Ko Y-M. Mechanical properties and corrosion resistance of low rigidity quaternary titanium alloy for biomedical applications. Trans Nonferrous Met Soc China 2009;19:862–5.

[6] Kobayashi E, Matsumoto S, Doi H, Yoneyama T, Hamanaka H. Mechanical properties of the binary titanium-zirconium alloys and their potential for biomedical materials. J Biomed Mater Res 1995;29:943–50.
[7] Fukuda A, Takemoto M, Saito T, Fujibayashi S, Neo M, Yamaguchi S, et al. Bone bonding bioactivity of Ti metal and Ti-Zr-Nb-Ta alloys with Ca ions incorporated on their surfaces by simple chemical and heat treatments. Acta Biomater 2011;7:1379–86.
[8] Nakada H, Numata Y, Sakae T, Okazaki Y, Tanimoto Y, Tamaki H, et al. Comparison of bone mineral density and area of newly formed bone around Ti-15%Zr-4%Nb-4%Ta alloy and Ti-6%A1-4%V alloy implants. J Hard Tissue Biol 2008;17:99–108.
[9] Chen X, Nouri A, Li Y, Lin J, Hodgson PD, Wen C. Effect of surface roughness of Ti, Zr, and TiZr on apatite precipitation from simulated body fluid. Biotech Bioeng 2008;101:378–87.
[10] Sista S, Wen C, Hodgson PD, Pande G. The influence of surface energy of titanium-zirconium alloy on osteoblast cell functions in vitro. J Biomed Mater Res A 2011;97A:27–36.
[11] Michelle Grandin H, Berner S, Dard M. A review of Titanium Zirconium (TiZr) alloys for use in endosseous dental implants. Materials 2012;5:1348–60.
[12] Roy P, Berger S, Schmuki P. TiO_2 nanotubes: synthesis and applications. Angew Chem Int Ed 2011;50:2904–39.
[13] Minagar S, Berndt CC, Wang J, Ivanova E, Wen C. A review of the application of anodization for the fabrication of nanotubes on metal implant surfaces. Acta Biomater 2012;8:2875–88.
[14] Minagar S, Wang J, Berndt CC, Ivanova EP, Wen C. Cell response of anodized nanotubes on titanium and titanium alloys. J Biomed Mater Res A 2013;101A:2726–39.
[15] Khor KA, Dong ZL, Quek CH, Cheang P. Microstructure investigation of plasma sprayed HA/Ti6Al4V composites by TEM. Mater Sci Eng A 2000;281:221–8.
[16] Kim WG, Choe HC. Surface characteristics of hydroxyapatite/titanium composite layer on the Ti-35Ta-xZr surface by RF and DC sputtering. Thin Solid Films 2011;519:7045–9.
[17] Lee K, Choe HC, Kim BH, Ko Y-M. The biocompatibility of HA thin films deposition on anodized titanium alloys. Surf Coat Technol 2010;205:S267–70.
[18] Choe HC. Photofunctionalization of EB-PVD HA-coated nano-pore surface of Ti-30Nb-xZr alloy for dental implants. Surf Coat Technol 2013;228:S470–6.
[19] Ma J, Liang CH, Kong LB, Wang C. Colloidal characterization and electrophoretic deposition of hydroxyapatite on titanium substrate. J Mater Sci Mater Med 2003;14:797–801.
[20] Roguska A, Pisarek M, Andrzejczuk M, Dolata M, Lewandowska M, Janik-Czachor M. Characterization of a calcium phosphate-TiO_2 nanotube composite layer for biomedical applications. Mater Sci Eng C 2011;31:906–14.
[21] Kodama A, Bauer S, Komatsu A, Asoh H, Ono S, Schmuki P. Bioactivation of titanium surfaces using coatings of TiO_2 nanotubes rapidly pre-loaded with synthetic hydroxyapatite. Acta Biomater 2009;5:2322–30.
[22] Kunze J, Muller L, Macak J, Greil P, Schmuki P, Muller F. Time-dependent growth of biomimetic apatite on anodic TiO_2 nanotubes. Electrochim Acta 2008;53:6995–7003.
[23] Minagar S, Berndt CC, Gengenbach T, Wen C. Fabrication and characterization of TiO_2–ZrO_2–$ZrTiO_4$ nanotubes on TiZr alloy manufactured via anodization. J Mater Chem B 2014;2:71–83.
[24] Minagar S, Li Y, Berndt CC, Wen C. The influence of titania–zirconia–zirconium titanate nanotube characteristics on osteoblast cell adhesion. Acta Biomater 2015;12:281–9.

[25] Oyane A, Onuma K, Ito A, Kim H-M, Kokubo T, Nakamura T. Formation and growth of clusters in conventional and new kinds of simulated body fluids. J Biomed Mater Res A 2003;64:339−48.
[26] Gadelmawla ES, Koura MM, Maksoud TMA, Elewa IM, Soliman HH. Roughness parameters. J Mater Process Technol 2002;123:133−45.
[27] Owens DK, Wendt RC. Estimation of the surface free energy of polymers. J Appl Polym Sci 1969;13:1741−7.
[28] Dann JR. Forces involved in the adhesive process. I. Critical surface tensions of polymeric solids as determined with polar liquids. J Colloid Interface Sci 1970;32:302−20.
[29] Kokubo T, Takadama H. How useful is SBF in predicting in vivo bone bioactivity? Biomaterials 2006;27:2907−15.
[30] Kim WG, Choe HC, Ko Y-M, Brantley WA. Electrochemical characteristics of nanotube formed Ti−Zr alloy. Quebec City, QC. 2008. p. 462−5.
[31] Taveira LV, Macák JM, Tsuchiya H, Dick LFP, Schmuki P. Initiation and growth of self-organized TiO_2 nanotubes anodically formed in $NH_4F/(NH_4)_2SO_4$ electrolytes. J Electrochem Soc 2005;152:B405−10.
[32] Madou MJ, Kinoshita K. Electrochemical measurements on metal oxide electrodes-I. Zirconium dioxide. Electrochim Acta 1984;29:411−7.
[33] Shackelford JF, Alexander W. CRC materials science and engineering handbook. CRC Press; 2000 [Chapter 9, Table 309].
[34] Albu SP, Ghicov A, Macak JM, Hahn R, Schmuki P. Self-organized, free-standing TiO_2 nanotube membrane for flow-through photocatalytic applications. Nano Lett 2007;7: 1286−9.
[35] Tsuchiya H, Macak JM, Müller L, Kunze J, Müller F, Greil P, et al. Hydroxyapatite growth on anodic TiO_2 nanotubes. J Biomed Mater Res A 2006;77A:534−41.
[36] Points of zero charge. In: Chemical properties of material surfaces. CRC Press; 2001. p. 731−44.
[37] Surface charging in absence of strongly adsorbing species. In: Chemical properties of material surfaces. CRC Press; 2001. p. 65−309.
[38] Ma Q, Li M, Hu Z, Chen Q, Hu W. Enhancement of the bioactivity of titanium oxide nanotubes by precalcification. Mater Lett 2008;62:3035−8.
[39] Webster TJ, Ergun C, Doremus RH, Siegel RW, Bizios R. Enhanced functions of osteoblasts on nanophase ceramics. Biomaterials 2000;21:1803−10.
[40] Peng P, Kumar S, Voelcker NH, Szili E, Smart RSC, Griesser HJ. Thin calcium phosphate coatings on titanium by electrochemical deposition in modified simulated body fluid. J Biomed Mater Res A 2006;76:347−55.
[41] Narayanan R, Lee H-J, Kwon T-Y, Kim K-H. Anodic TiO_2 nanotubes from stirred baths: hydroxyapatite growth & osteoblast responses. Mater Chem Phys 2011;125:510−7.

Antibacterial design for metal implants

8

L. Ren, K. Yang
Institute of Metal Research, Chinese Academy of Sciences, Shenyang, China

8.1 Introduction

Medical metal materials are an important class of biomaterials owing to their excellent features of high strength and toughness, fatigue resistance, easy processing, etc., which are widely used in clinic. Metal materials are first candidates for those hard tissues repairs in orthopedics and dentistry that require bearing high loading, as well as stents in interventions, and have been used to manufacture various implant devices in these medical areas. Among these, fixation devices for bone fracture, joints, spines, teeth implants, and coronary stents are representatives of high-grade products, varying in different types and specifications. The properties of medical metal materials can be crucial to the performances of these implant devices, even affecting their efficacies for patients. Currently, stainless steels, titanium (Ti) and its alloys, and cobalt-based alloys are the main metal implant materials that are mostly used in clinic, occupying pivotal positions in production and clinical applications of medical metal materials. Biodegradable magnesium (Mg)-based materials are a novel class of medical metal materials that are being developed and have great potential for medical applications.

8.2 Implant-associated bacterial infections

As a common and catastrophic postoperative complication, medical device or implant material-associated bacterial infections, which are also called biomaterial-centered infections, are becoming a severe problem that needs to be solved urgently [1]. Statistics [2] showed that the annual morbidity of the related infections in orthopedics in the United States is about 4.3%. It was reported that half of 2 million cases of nosocomial infections in the United States each year are related to the implants [3], and it costs 7–11 million pounds in the United Kingdom each year for implant-associated infections [4]. According to the data in the Practical Manual of Nosocomial Infection Control, published by the World Health Organization, there are more than 14 million people worldwide suffering pains of nosocomial infections every day, among which 60% are related to the use of medical devices. In a review on infections related to orthopedic implant devices, David et al. pointed out [5] that *Staphylococcus aureus* and *Staphylococcus epidemidis* are the main bacteria causing infections in orthopedics, occupying 34% and 32%, respectively, as shown in Fig. 8.1. A study by Leonhardt

Metallic Foam Bone. http://dx.doi.org/10.1016/B978-0-08-101289-5.00008-1

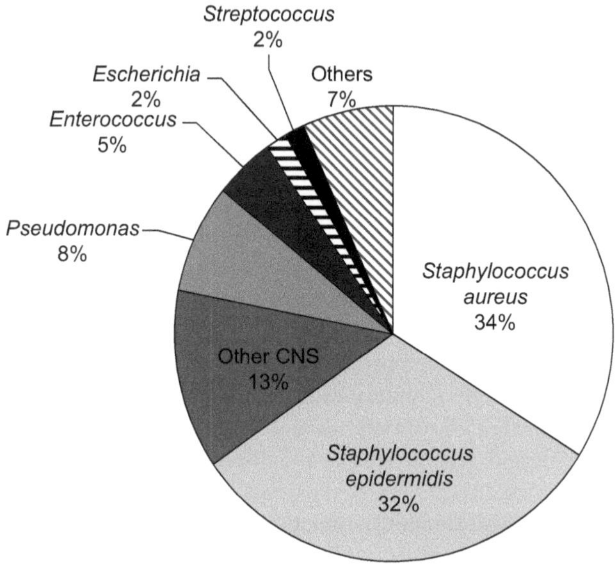

Figure 8.1 Frequency of the main pathogenic species among orthopedic clinical isolates of implant-associated infections [5].

et al. [6] indicated that anaerobic bacteria such as *Streptococcus mutans* and *Porphyromonas gingivalis* are the main bacteria causing infections related to dental implants.

Implant-associated infections are closely related to the bacterial biofilm. The morphology of a bacterial biofilm is shown in Fig. 8.2. The bacterial biofilm is an accumulation of bacterial colonies formed by a single type or multiple types of bacteria in order to adapt to the natural environment. The main composition in the biofilm is the multiglycoprotein complex, which enwraps the bacteria, causes them to adhere to form

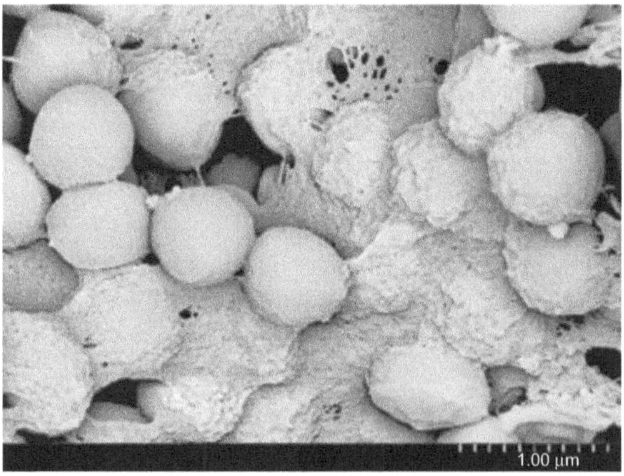

Figure 8.2 Morphology of bacterial biofilm.

a specific structured bacterial complex, and finally irreversibly attaches to the surface of a lesion or implant device [7]. A primary statistic from the National Institute of Health indicated that 80% of bacterial diseases are related to the bacterial biofilm. Bacterial biofilm widely exists in the human body, for instance, in the respiratory tract, as plaque on a tooth, etc., as well as on artificial devices in the body for short- or long-term implantation (catheter, artificial valve, stent, etc.), which has strong antibiotic resistance and immune escape [8].

The employment of antibiotics, ie, the systemic administration of antibiotics orally or by injection, is a standard strategy in clinic to treat infections around the implant. The main shortcoming of this treatment is the difficulty for the antibiotics in reaching a high enough, effective inhibitory concentration against the bacteria around the tissues through the blood circulation. On the other hand, the risk of side effects of the antibiotics is increased. Therefore if the problem of implant-associated infections can be solved by the implant metal material itself, the risk of infections can be effectively reduced, the drug resistance of antibiotics can be avoided, and the side effects of antibiotics due to systemic administration to patients can be decreased, which will promote the effective treatment and prevention of infections around implants and have great clinical value.

8.3 Research and development of antibacterial metals for medical applications

Surface modification, which has been widely used for various metal implants, is an important way for medical metal materials to further enhance their surface properties. Some antibacterial properties can be achieved by using different surface modification methods, such as plasma-spray, magnetron sputtering, ion implantation, and so on, with additions of antibacterial metal elements such as copper (Cu) and silver, nonmetal elements such as fluorine, and antibacterial compounds, including drugs in the coating materials [9–13]. However, although they are feasible in principle, due to the large difference in properties between the coating materials (mostly ceramics and polymers) and the metal matrix there are some shortcomings for surface modifications that largely limit their clinical applications, such as easy dropping off of coatings, difficulty in sustaining antibacterial performance, difficulty in further processing and forming, etc.

If the medical metal materials possess strong antibacterial functions by themselves, the above shortcomings of antibacterial coatings can be overcome, and the relevant metal implants will have steady and durable antibacterial properties, which will be beneficial for avoiding or effectively reducing bacterial infections in clinic with great application value.

8.3.1 Design of antibacterial metals

Research aimed at inhibiting the formation of bacterial biofilm on novel medical metal materials with antibacterial function is an effective way to reduce those bacterial infections. The basic idea for this research is to add the proper amount of antibacterial agent to medical metal materials, making the surfaces of the metals strongly antibacterial. Thus it becomes difficult for bacterial biofilm to form, which can effectively reduce the occurrence of bacterial infections or eliminate them completely [14].

Using Cu ions to kill bacteria has a long history. More than 200 years have passed since Schulthees used Cu sulfate to prevent wheat stinking smut in 1761. In 1885, a Frenchman named Milharde successfully developed an antibacterial agent containing Cu ions, called the Bordeaux mixture, which resolved the crisis of grapes with diseases and insect pests in successive years in chateaus of Bordeaux. Subsequently, there have been a variety of Cu ions containing fungicides, which created a time of Cu ion sterilization application.

Cu is a common alloying element in steels and other alloys. The strength and corrosion resistance of steels can be enhanced and the cold workability of steels can be improved by adding the proper amount of Cu, which creates conditions for the development of medical metal materials with antibacterial functions through Cu alloying. On the other hand, Cu is also an indispensable trace element in the human body, playing many different important biological roles. A deficiency of Cu in the human body may cause anemia, osteoporosis, coronary disease, and other diseases [15,16]. Therefore the physiological characteristics of Cu make Cu-bearing metals a biosafety basis as implant materials.

Various Cu-bearing antibacterial medical metals, including stainless steels, Ti alloys, and cobalt-based alloys, have been newly developed by using the strong and broad-spectrum antibacterial characteristics of Cu ions, which have attractive application prospects. The antibacterial functions possessed by these novel metals are promising for reducing the occurrence of clinical infections. Exciting research progress has been achieved from studies of Cu-bearing antibacterial medical metals.

8.3.2 Antibacterial performance of antibacterial metals

8.3.2.1 Evaluation of antibacterial properties

Staphylococcus aureus (*S. aureus*) and *Escherichia coli (E. coli)*, typical Gram-positive and -negative bacteria, are often used to evaluate the antibacterial properties of antibacterial medical metal materials with the corresponding metal as the comparison. The experimental bacteria, which are recovered before the evaluation test, can be purchased from an officially certified bacteria preservation center. A bacterial suspension with a concentration of $(1.0-10.0) \times 10^5$ cfu/mL is usually prepared for the test.

Co-culture is commonly used to quantitatively evaluate the antibacterial rate of medical metal materials by adding a certain amount of bacterial suspension into a 24-hole plate with samples and keeping it at 37°C for 24 h. After the co-culture with samples, the bacterial suspension is diluted, painted on a solid medium plate, and cultured at 37°C for another 24 h. Then the bacterial colonies on the plate are counted, and the antibacterial rate of the material can be calculated as follows:

$$\text{Antibacterial rate } (\%) = [(A - B)/A] \times 100$$

where A is the number of bacterial colonies on the plate for the comparison metal, and B is the number of bacterial colonies on the plate for the antibacterial metal.

A biofilm can be formed on medical metal materials after they are co-cultured with a bacterial suspension for a period of time. The characteristics of the bacterial biofilm on the surfaces of medical metal materials can be observed and examined by scanning electron microscope (SEM). The bacterial biofilm should be well fixed on the surface of samples before SEM observation, including drying and gold plating.

Fluorescence staining, by which the dead bacteria are stained in red and the live bacteria in green, can be conducted on the bacterial biofilm formed on the surface of samples to further study the survival of bacteria after co-culturing with antibacterial medical metals [17]. Commercial reagent kits for live/dead bacterial staining can be used for such tests. After staining, samples co-cultured with a bacterial suspension can be observed and examined on a laser scanning confocal microscope (LSCM).

Animal tests can be conducted to further verify the *in vivo* antibacterial function of antibacterial medical metals. For example, metal screws that have been dipped in a bacterial suspension for a certain time can be implanted in animal bones or tissues, which can provide direct evidence for clinical applications of such novel medical metal materials.

8.3.2.2 Antibacterial stainless steels

Stainless steels are a class of conventionally used medical metal materials for manufacturing orthopedic and dental implants due to their good mechanical properties, corrosion resistance, fatigue performance, and low cost. 304 and 317L stainless steels, with nominal compositions of low-carbon Fe−18Cr−8Ni (wt%) and ultra-low carbon Fe−18Cr−13Ni−3Mo (wt%), respectively, are two commonly used medical stainless steels in dentistry and orthopedics. Through the addition of proper amounts of Cu in these two steels, two novel stainless steels, 304-Cu and 316L-Cu, have been developed with broad-spectrum antibacterial abilities [18].

A quantitative evaluation of antibacterial rates and observations of bacterial biofilm formation showed that 317L-Cu stainless steel exhibited strong antibacterial functions [18], which has great potential to inhibit postoperative infections. Fig. 8.3 shows that co-cultured with *S. aureus* and *E. coli*, respectively, for different times, the antibacterial rate of 317L-Cu increased in comparison with 317L as the co-culture time extended. It reached 99% after 24 h.

Figs. 8.4 and 8.5 show the SEM images of the formation of bacterial biofilms on 317L and 317L-Cu stainless steels after co-culturing for different times with *S. aureus* and *E. coli*, respectively. It can be seen that biofilms were clearly formed on 317L for both *S. aureus* and *E. coli*, but only a few randomly distributed bacteria, without biofilm, existed on 317L-Cu. LSCM observations by live/dead staining further supported the above mentioned fact that both *S. aureus* and *E. coli* biofilms in green (live bacteria) were formed on the surface of 317L, while mostly dead bacteria in red were formed on the surface of 317L-Cu, as shown in Fig. 8.6.

In order to evaluate the antibacterial function of 317L-Cu stainless steel *in vivo*, screws made of 317L and 317L-Cu stainless steels were implanted into bones of

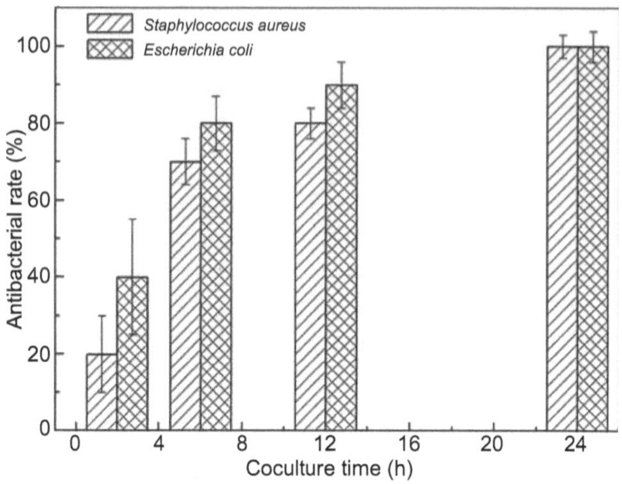

Figure 8.3 Antibacterial rates of 317L-Cu against *Staphylococcus aureus* and *Escherichia coli* after co-culturing with bacteria at 37°C for 2, 6, 12, and 24 h, respectively [18].

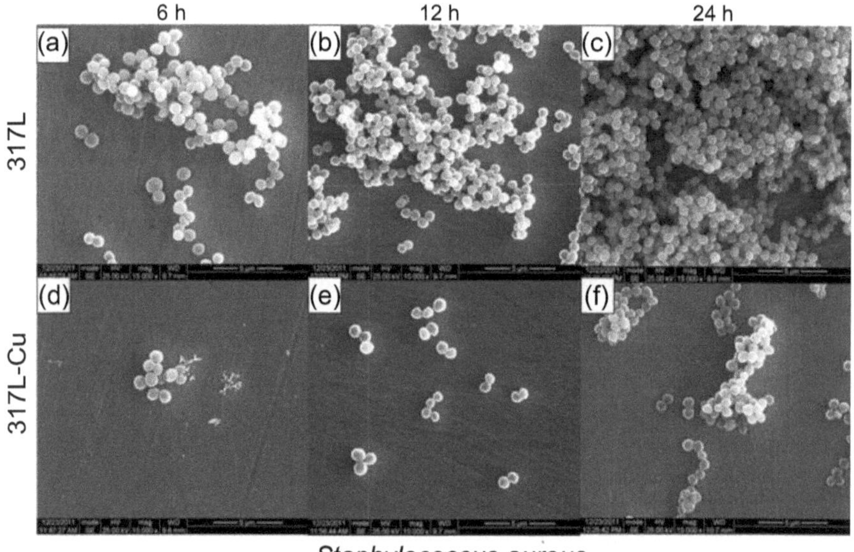

Figure 8.4 Scanning electron microscope images of biofilm formation of *Staphylococcus aureus* on the surfaces of (a–c): 317L and (d–f): 317L-Cu after co-culturing for 6, 12, and 24 h, respectively [18].

rabbits after dipping in *S. aureus* and *E. coli* suspensions, respectively. A histological observation of the bone tissue and a measurement of the amount of bacteria in the bone tissues around the implant indicated that the implantation of 317L-Cu screws exhibited no obvious bone infection, while many inflammatory cells were detected around the

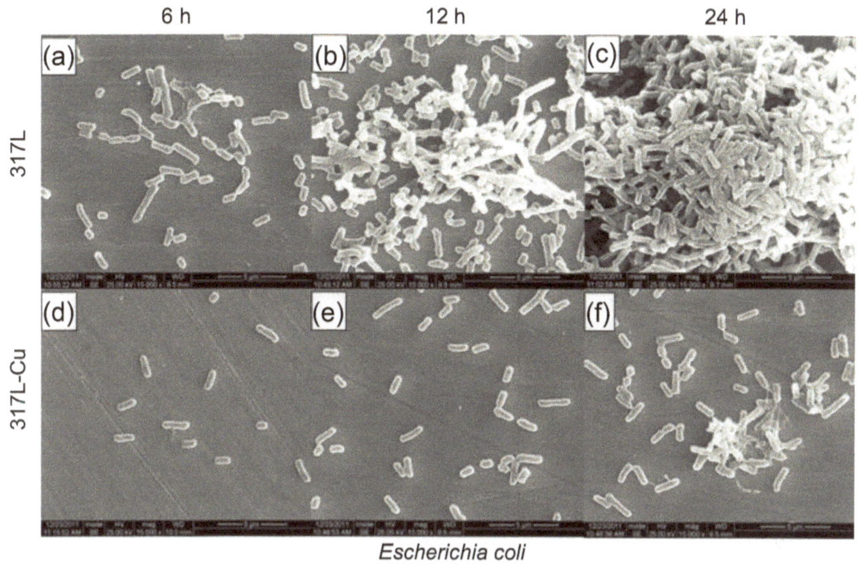

Figure 8.5 Scanning electron microscope images of biofilm formation of *Escherichia coli* on the surfaces of (a–c): 317L and (d–f): 317L-Cu after co-culturing for 6, 12, and 24 h, respectively [18].

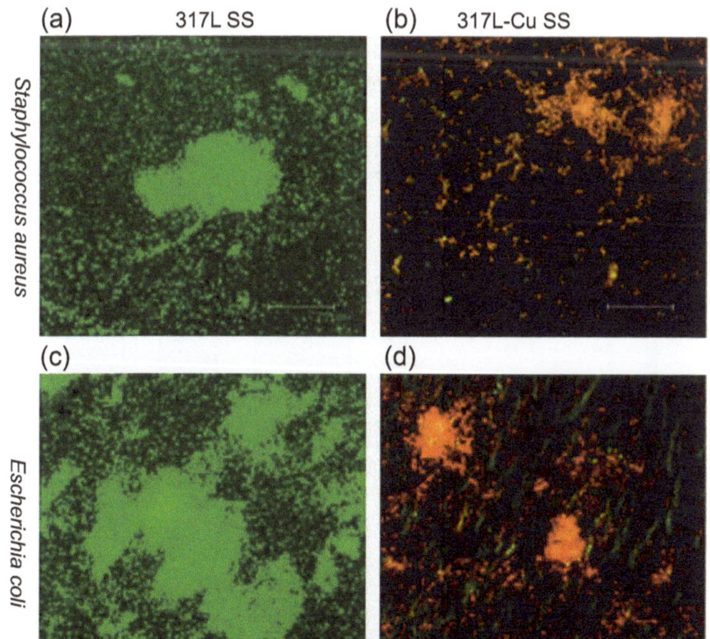

Figure 8.6 Fluorescent images of *Staphylococcus aureus* and *Escherichia coli* co-cultured with 317 and 317-Cu stainless steels at 37°C for 24 h, respectively [18].

317L screw [19]. Therefore it can be concluded that 317L-Cu stainless steel possessed a good antibacterial ability both *in vitro* and *in vivo*.

Since the oral cavity is a place where bacteria easily breed, implants in dentistry can lead to a high risk of infections. Compared with conventional orthodontic 304 stainless steel, the novel 304-Cu stainless steel surface showed less *Porphyromonas gingivalis (P. gingivalis)* [20], which has been regarded as one of the most common bacteria in peri-implants. Co-cultured with *P. gingivalis* for different times, the antibacterial rate of 304-Cu stainless steel increased gradually and reached over 99% after 10 h, as shown in Fig. 8.7. *P. gingivalis* on the surface of 304-Cu appeared to be cracking into pieces, as shown in Fig. 8.8. Therefore 304-Cu stainless steel is a promising candidate for manufacturing microimplants with antibacterial functions in dentistry.

Biosafety is an important issue for the application of novel antibacterial stainless steels. Although Cu is an essential trace element in the human body, excessive Cu will have a certain toxicity to the body. Therefore the Cu ion release from Cu-containing stainless steels needs to be evaluated to provide fundamental biosafety evidence for clinical applications. An *in vitro* experiment showed that the viability of MG63 cells cultured with 317L-Cu stainless steel was not significantly different with the blank control; furthermore, 317L-Cu stainless steel showed an osteoconduction effect with excellent osteoid formation on its surface after implantation [19]. The CCK-8 assay demonstrated that the cytotoxicity to MG63 cells and KB cells of 304-Cu stainless steel was Grade 1, indicating that Cu-containing antibacterial stainless steels should be biosafe [20].

Finally, the mechanical properties and corrosion resistance of Cu-containing antibacterial stainless steels did not change significantly in comparison with conventional stainless steels, indicating that these novel stainless steels will have great potential for applications in stainless steel implants with antiinfection functions.

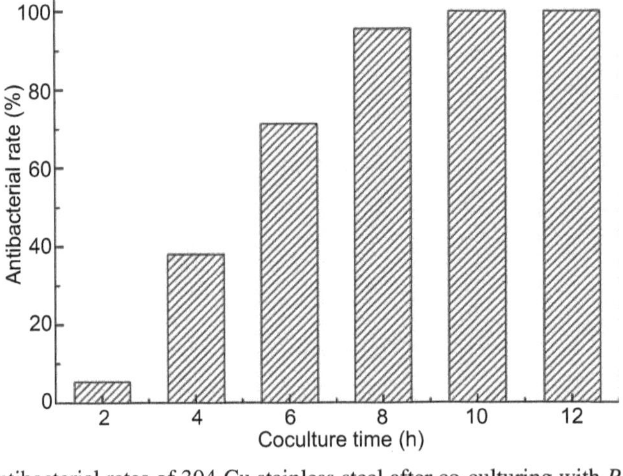

Figure 8.7 Antibacterial rates of 304-Cu stainless steel after co-culturing with *Porphyromonas gingivalis* for different times [20].

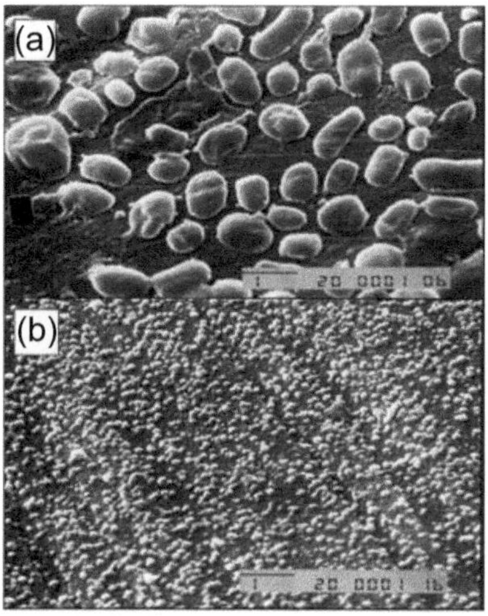

Figure 8.8 Scanning electron microscope morphologies of *Porphyromonas gingivalis* on the surface of (a) 304 and (b) 304-Cu stainless steels after co-culturing for 24 h, respectively.

8.3.2.3 Antibacterial titanium alloys

Ti and its alloys are a class of ideal medical metal materials for orthopedic and dental applications, such as artificial joints, bone fixations, teeth implants, and braces. However, similar to other bioinert metal materials, they do not have antibacterial abilities. Based on the above principle and successful studies on antibacterial stainless steels, the appropriate amount of Cu was added into currently used medically pure Ti and its alloys to develop antibacterial medical Ti alloys, including Ti−Cu and Ti−6Al−4V−Cu alloys [21].

A series of Ti−6Al−4V−xCu (x = 1, 3, 5 wt%) alloys was fabricated by adding different Cu into the commercial medical Ti−6Al−4V alloy in an arc melting furnace. The Ti−6Al−4V−xCu alloy could more effectively kill *E. coli* and *S. aureus* compared with the Ti−6Al−4V alloy, and the antibacterial rate was increased with increase of Cu content in the alloy [21]. Furthermore, the formation of a bacterial biofilm was also inhibited on the Ti−6Al−4V−Cu alloy, as shown in Fig. 8.9. Commercially pure Ti (CP-Ti) is commonly used for teeth implants in dentistry with excellent biocompatibility. A novel Ti−5Cu alloy was developed, which showed that, compared with CP-Ti, the new alloy not only had a higher strength and hardness while maintaining good corrosion resistance, but also possessed a noticeable antibacterial ability against both *E. coli* and *S. aureus*, as shown in Fig. 8.10 [22].

The Ti−6Al−4V−3Cu and Ti−5Cu alloys showed no cytotoxicity to L929 or MC3T3-E1 cells [22,23]. The Ti−5Cu alloy also showed good hemocompatibility with a much lower hemolysis rate. Furthermore, the strength and hardness were increased by more than 20%, and the corrosion resistance was not affected for the two Cu-containing Ti alloys in comparison with conventional alloys. Thus these two novel antibacterial Ti alloys have great potential in orthopedic and dental applications.

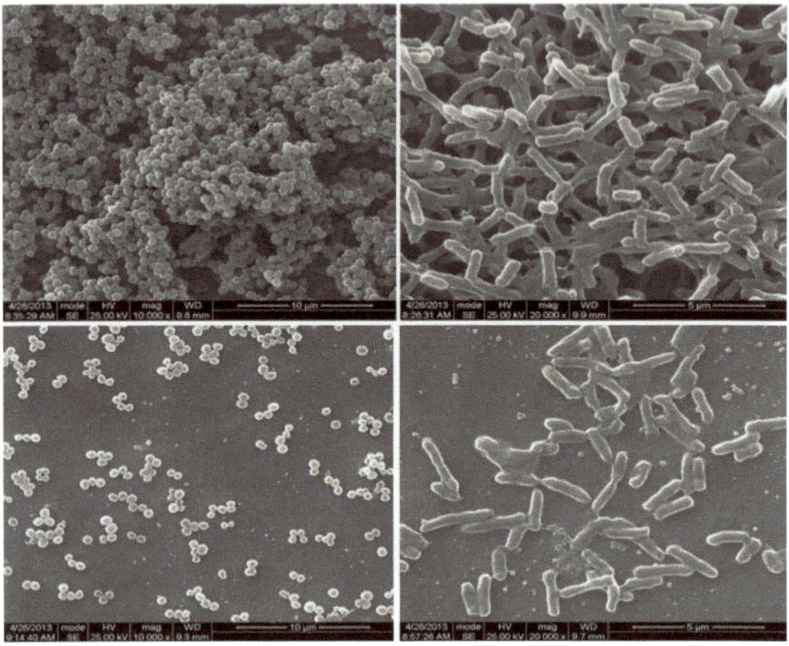

Figure 8.9 Bacterial adhesions on Ti–6Al–4V (upper row) and Ti–6Al–4V–5Cu (bottom row) alloys co-cultured with *Staphylococcus aureus* (left column) and *Escherichia coli* (right column).

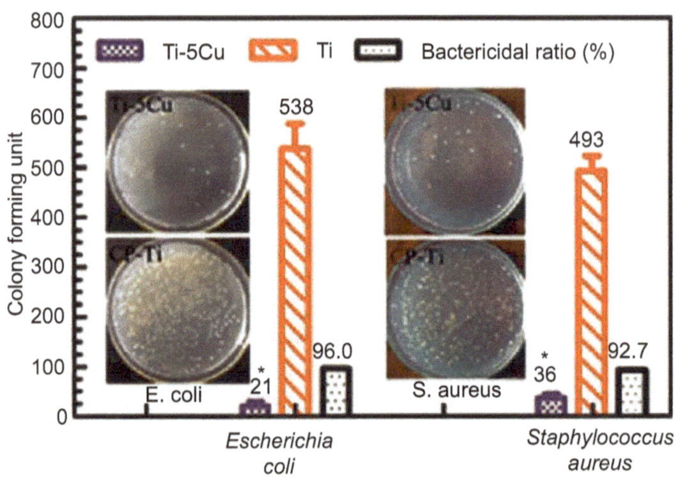

Figure 8.10 Colonization, bactericidal ratio, and representative photo of *Escherichia coli* and *Staphylococcus aureus* after 24 h co-culturing with CP-Ti and a Cu–5Cu alloy [22].

8.3.2.4 Antibacterial cobalt-based alloys

Medical cobalt-based alloys are commonly used in cases where higher strength and hardness are required in orthopedics as well as for dental crowns in dentistry. Based on the composition of currently used alloys, a novel Co—Cr—W—Ni—Cu alloy was fabricated [24]. After co-culturing with *E. coli* or *S. aureus* suspensions for 24 h, the Co—Cr—W—Ni—Cu alloy showed a more powerful antibacterial ability compared with the conventional Co—Cr—W—Ni alloy, and the antibacterial rate of the alloy with a higher Cu content (4.39%) was over 90%. SEM observations revealed that *S. aureus* stacked and formed biofilm on the surface of the Co—Cr—W—Ni alloy, while there were only a few bacteria on the surface of the Co—Cr—W—Ni—Cu alloy, as shown in Fig. 8.11. Thus implant-associated infections are expected to be effectively reduced by using Cu-containing cobalt-based alloy with antibacterial function.

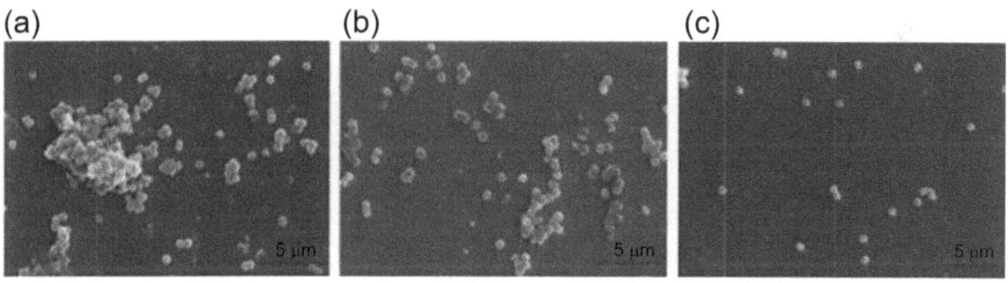

Figure 8.11 Morphologies of *Staphylococcus aureus* on the surfaces of (a) Co—Cr—W—Ni, (b) Co—Cr—W—Ni—2.13% Cu, and (c) Co—Cr—W—Ni—4.39% Cu alloys after co-culturing for 24 h [24].

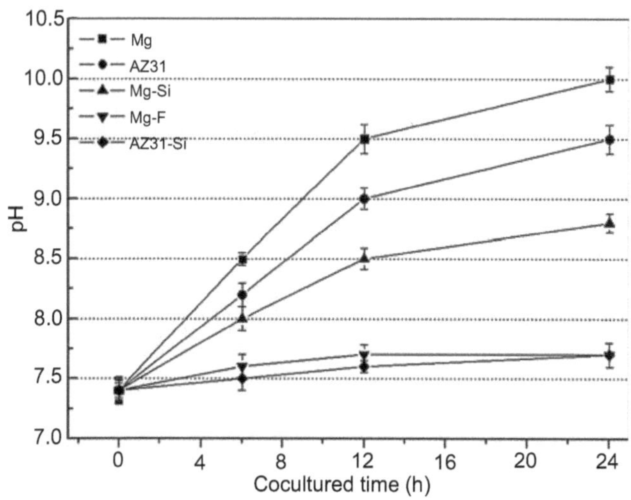

Figure 8.12 pH changes of bacterial suspensions after co-culturing with magnesium-based metals for different times [27].

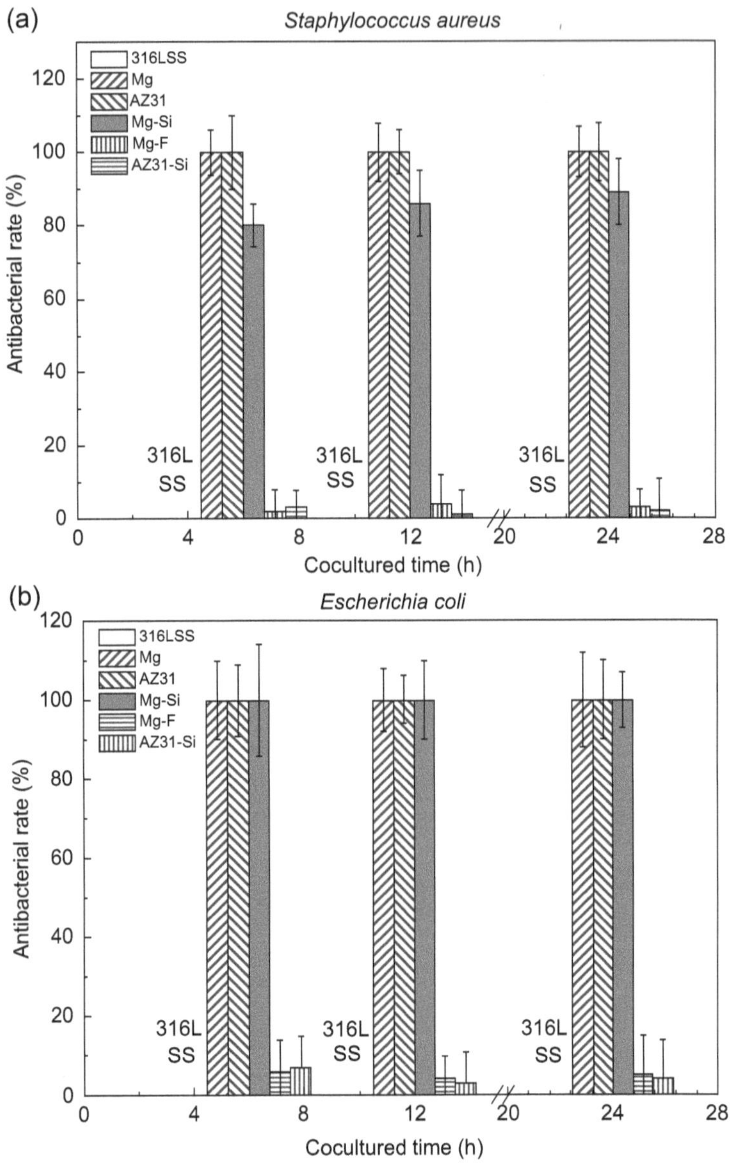

Figure 8.13 Antibacterial rates of magnesium-based metals against (a) *Escherichia coli* and (b) *Staphylococcus aureus*, with 316L stainless steel as a comparison [27].

8.3.2.5 Antibacterial performance of biodegradable magnesium-based metals

Research and development on Mg-based metals have attracted much attention. Mg is an essential element for the human body and easily corrodes in the physiological environment. Due to their low moduli, high specific strength, and especially their biodegradable characteristics, Mg-based metals have a high potential to be used for temporary orthopedic implants and cardiovascular stents. Compared with other types of biodegradable materials, such as polymer or ceramic-based materials, Mg-based metals are more competitive owing to their better mechanical properties and excellent machinability generally featured by metals [25].

The hydroxyl ions produced by Mg degradation in biological environment greatly increase the pH of solution, which can affect the activity of bacteria. Since bacteria usually live in an environment with a pH range of 6.0–8.0, it is hard for them to survive in a higher or lower pH environment. Thus Mg-based metals can kill bacteria effectively during their degradations [26,27]. Pure Mg and AZ31 (Mg–3%Al–1%Zn) showed strong antibacterial abilities against *E. coli* and *S. aureus* with rapidly increased pH values of the bacterial suspensions [27], as shown in Figs. 8.12 and 8.13. However, a surface coating on the Mg-based metal may affect its antibacterial ability due to the inhibitory effect on the pH increase. A porous coating could have a moderate effect on the pH enhancement, still resulting in a relatively strong antibacterial performance, such as the Si-containing micro-arc oxidation-coated pure Mg, denoted as Mg–Si in Figs. 8.12 and 8.13. A dense coating could well protect the Mg-based metal from corrosion, resulting in a much smaller pH enhancement and thus greatly reducing the antibacterial ability, such as the fluoride-coated pure Mg and the Si-containing micro-arc oxidation-coated AZ31 alloy, denoted as Mg–F and AZ31–Si (Figs. 8.12 and 8.13). Thus Mg-based metals will have a new biofunction of being antibacterial in their clinical applications.

8.4 Future prospects

An antibacterial function of medical metal materials has been successfully achieved by properly adding Cu in the currently used medical metals or increasing the alkalinity due to the biodegradation of Mg-based metals. Many metal implants used in orthopedics and dentistry can be newly modified through alloying with Cu to effectively reduce bacterial infections in clinic. The original medical functions of metal implants plus the new antibacterial functions will certainly be beneficial for further improving the medical effect for patients.

References

[1] Stamm WE. Infections related to medical devices. Ann Intern Med 1978;89:764–9.

[2] Zimmerli W, Trampuz A, Ochsner PE. Prosthetic-joint infections. N Engl J Med 2004;351: 1645–54.

[3] Darouiche RO. Treatment of infections associated with surgical implants. N Engl J Med 2004;350:1422–9.

[4] Flock JI, Brennan F. Antibodies that block adherence of to fibronectin. Trends Microbiol 1999;7:140–1.

[5] David C, Lucio M, Renata AC. The significance of infection related to orthopedic devices and issues of antibiotic resistance. Biomaterials 2006;27:2331–9.
[6] Leonhardt A, Berglundh T, Ericsson I, Dahlen G. Putative periodontal and teeth in pathogens on titanium implants and teeth in experimental gingivitis and periodontitis in beagle dogs. Clin Oral Implan Res 1992;3:112–9.
[7] Donlan RM. Biofilms: microbial life on surfaces. Emerg Infect Dis 2002;8:881.
[8] Stewart PS, Costerton JW. Antiblotic resistance of bacteria inbiofilms. Lancet 2001;358: 135–8.
[9] Kazemzadeh-Narbat M, Lai BFL, Ding C, Kizhakkedathu JN, Hancock REW, Wang R. Multilayered coating on titanium for controlled release of antimicrobial peptides for the prevention of implant-associated Infections. Biomaterials 2013;34:5969–77.
[10] Zhong LJ, Pang LQ, Che LM, Wu XE, Chen XD. Nafion coated stainless steel for anti-biofilm application. Colloids Surf B: Biointerfaces 2013;111:252–6.
[11] Popat KC, Eltgroth M, LaTempa TJ, Grimes CA, Desai TA. Titania nanotubes: a novel platform for drug-eluting coatings for medical implants. Small 2007;3:1878–81.
[12] Dong Y, Li X, Tian L, Bell T, Sammons RL, Dong H. Towards long-lasting antibacterial stainless steel surfaces by combining double glow plasma silvering with active screen plasma nitriding. Acta Biomater 2011;7:447–57.
[13] Kalaivani S, Singh K, Ganesanb V, Kannan S. Effect of copper (Cu2+) inclusion on the bioactivity and antibacterial behavior of calcium silicate coatings on titanium metal. J Mater Chem B 2014;2:846–58.
[14] Hetrick EM, Schoenfisch MH. Reducing implant-related infections: active release strategies. Chem Soc Rev 2006;35:780–9.
[15] Shim H, Harris ZL. Genetic defects in copper metabolism. J Nutr 2003;133:1523IS–7IS.
[16] Wapnir RA. Copper absorption and bioavailability. Am J Clin Nutr 1998;67:1054–60.
[17] Sivakumar PM, Iyer G, Natesan L, Doble M. 3′-Hydroxy-4-methoxychalcone as a potential antibacterial coating on polymeric biomaterials. Appl Surf Sci 2010;256:6018–24.
[18] Ren L, Yang K, Guo L, Cai HW. Preliminary study of anti-infective function of a copper-bearing stainless steel. Mat Sci Eng C 2012;32:1204–9.
[19] Cai HW, Guo L, Wang XT, Fu YP, Guan JL, Tan LL, et al. Antibacterial effect of 317L stainless steel contained copper in prevention of implant-related infection in vitro and in vivo. J Mater Sci-Mater Med 2011;22:2525–35.
[20] Zhang D, Ren L, Zhang Y, Xue N, Yang K, Zhong M. Antibacterial activity against Porphyromonas gingivalis and biological characteristics of antibacterial stainless steel. Colloids Surf B: Biointerfaces 2013;105:51.
[21] Ma Z, Ren L, Liu R, Yang K, Zhang Y, Liao Z, et al. Effect of heat treatment on Cu distribution, antibacterial performance and cytotoxicity of Ti–6al–4v–5cu alloy. J Mater Sci Technol 2015;31:723–32.
[22] Ma Z, Li M, Liu R, Ren L, Zhang Y, Pan H, et al. In vitro study on an antibacterial Ti–5Cu alloy for medical application. J Mater Sci-Mater Med 2016;27:91.
[23] Ren L, Ma Z, Li M, Zhang Y, Liu WQ, Liao ZH, et al. Antibacterial properties of Ti-6Al-4V-xCu alloys. J Mater Sci Technol 2014;30:699–705.
[24] Wang S, Yang CG, Ren L, Shen M, Yang K. Study on antibacterial performance of Cu-bearing cobalt-based alloy. Mater Lett 2014;129:88–90.
[25] Witte F. The history of biodegradable magnesium implants: a review,. Acta Biomater 2010;6:1680–92.
[26] Robinson DA, Griffith RW, Shechtman D, Evans RB, Conzemius MG. In vitro antibacterial properties of magnesium metal against *Escherichia coli*, *Pseudomonas aeruginosa* and *Staphylococcus aureus*. Acta Biomater 2010;6:1869–77.
[27] Ren L, Lin X, Tan L, Yang K. Effect of surface coating on antibacterial behavior of magnesium based metals. Mater Lett 2011;65:3509–11.

The bioactivity and bone cell attachment of nanotubular layers anodized in aqueous and nonaqueous electrolytes

9

S. Minagar[1], Y. Li[2], C.C. Berndt[1,3], C. Wen[1,2]
[1]Swinburne University of Technology, Hawthorn, Victoria, Australia; [2]RMIT University, Melbourne, Victoria, Australia; [3]Stony Brook University, Stony Brook, NY, United States

9.1 Introduction

A nanostructure is defined when at least one dimension of a system is less than 100 nm, and such structures have been found to influence the chemical and physical properties of the bulk material [1]. Compared to organic materials, more studies have investigated the nanomorphology of metal oxides on metal surfaces, which have revealed excellent mechanical and chemical properties that may be suitable for biomedical applications [2]. Titanium and some of its alloys are the preferred metal-based biomaterials due to their lower elastic modulus, superior biocompatibility, and better corrosion resistance, which make them the best choice for artificial bones, joints, and dental implants [2].

Surface modifications, including mechanical, physical, and chemical treatments, are essential to convert the neutral oxide layer of an implant to a layer that is more bioactive. Anodic oxidation is a cost-effective, simple, and versatile electrochemical surface treatment that has been used for a decade to fabricate TiO_2 nanotubes on titanium surfaces. Biomedical applications include coatings for improved bioactivity and biocompatibility, drug delivery, and payload release as well as industrial applications in photocatalysis and dark photocatalysis, solar cells, electrochromic devices, and gas–liquid sensing [3]. It has been shown that the chemistry, mechanical properties, and topography of an implant surface affect the cell response such as adhesion, proliferation, shape, migration, survival, and differentiation. Surface chemistry influences surface charges, which enhance protein adsorption [4].

The effect of macro-, micro- and nano-sized topography is related to the roughness amplitude parameter, space and hybrid parameters on the contact mechanism of cells, and cell adhesion [1–5]. Surface chemistry influences adsorption and the rearrangement of proteins that can be defined as short-term adhesion [4]. Surfaces with higher hydrophilic properties, higher surface energy, and functional groups such as OH^- and NH_2^- are the preferred conditions for cell adhesion [4]. TiO_2 nanotubes have been reported to improve surface chemistry, surface topography, the roughness and organization of the surface, and the hydrophilic properties and surface energy [6–8].

Metallic Foam Bone. http://dx.doi.org/10.1016/B978-0-08-101289-5.00009-3

Nanotubular surfaces with a length scale less than 30 nm showed increased cellular activity with a maximum activity at 15 nm [9]. In another study [10], human mesenchymal stem cells adhered and grew on small nanotubes of <50 nm and became elongated and differentiated on larger diameter nanotubes. It is generally thought that cells are forced to adapt under stress by differentiation. Osteoblast cells (MC3T3-E1 mouse) became elongated and adhered more on annealed TiO_2 nanotubes of 100 nm rather than 30–70-nm-diameter nanotubes [11].

Investigation has shown the biocompatibility of the titanium–zirconium alloy (TiZr) [12]. Further, studies were undertaken to fabricate nanotubes on a TiZr surface via anodization and rapid breakdown anodization to enhance its biocompatibility [13–15]. The nanotubular layer exhibited a distribution of nanotubular sizes with different roughness and hydrophilic properties [8]. The MG63 cell line derived from a human osteosarcoma was grown on a nanopatterned scaffold that was fabricated by two-step anodization in a nonaqueous electrolyte [16]. The nanotubular layers fabricated in aqueous and nonaqueous electrolytes exhibited different physical, chemical, and morphological surface properties [8,17,18], which influenced the osteoblast cell adhesion. Therefore it is worthwhile to investigate the processing and characteristics of the two kinds of nanotubular layers.

In this chapter, TiO_2–ZrO_2–$ZrTiO_4$ nanotubular layers were fabricated with average nanotube inner diameters (D_i) of the following: (1) 40 ± 12 nm and (2) 59 ± 17 nm in aqueous electrolyte and (3) 25 ± 5 nm and (4) 45 ± 6 nm in nonaqueous electrolyte, respectively. The roughness, water contact angle, and surface energy of the nanotubular surfaces were characterized, and the hydroxyapatite (HA) mineralization and SaOS2 cell attachment were assessed. The effects of roughness parameters and surface energy of the nanotubular surfaces on the cellular activity are highlighted.

9.2 Experimental

9.2.1 Preparation of the substrate and surface characterization

A Ti50Zr alloy was fabricated by casting 8-mm-diameter rods that were then machined into 2-mm-thick discs by electric discharge machining. The discs were polished to a 1-μm diamond finish. The samples were ultrasonically cleaned for 15 min each in methanol, isopropanol, acetone, and ethanol prior to rinsing with pure water and drying with a nitrogen stream. The cleaned discs were divided into two groups. The first group of samples was used for the fabrication of TiO_2–ZrO_2–$ZrTiO_4$ nanotubes using a DC power supply with two-electrode configurations in 1 M $(NH_4)_2SO_4$ and 0.5 wt% NH_4F (Sigma-Aldrich reagent grades) in an aqueous electrolyte at potentials of 20 and 25 V. The second group of samples was used for the fabrication of the nanotubular layer in a nonaqueous electrolyte composed of 0.5 wt% NH_4F. NH_4F is dissolved in a solution of 5 wt% water in ethylene glycol (Sigma-Aldrich reagent grades) at potentials of 25 and 30 V.

After anodization the first group of samples was washed with deionized water, and the second set of samples was washed with acetone for 5 min. Both sets of samples were then dried under a nitrogen stream. The anodized $TiO_2-ZrO_2-ZrTiO_4$ nanotubes of the second group were posttreated by immersion in 0.5 M HCl at room temperature for 1 min and then rinsed with deionized water for 1 min to dissolve the upper nanoporous layer. Half of the group one samples were annealed at 500°C for 3 h, and half of the second group of samples were annealed at 500 C for 2 h in air in a muffle furnace (Nabertherm LT15/13/P330) at a heating rate of 2°C/min.

The sample surfaces were analyzed after anodization and soaking in a modified simulated body fluid (m-SBF) with a field-emission scanning electron microscope (ZEISS SUPRA 40 VP) equipped with energy-dispersive X-ray spectrometry [19]. The crystalline phases were determined by X-ray diffraction using Cu Kα incident radiation at 40 kV and 40 mA over a 2θ range from 10–90 degrees at a scanning step size of 0.02 degrees.

The roughness parameters, including mean roughness (S_a) and root mean square (RMS) roughness (S_q), were characterized based on the peaks, valleys, and spacing of the surface textures [20]. A 3D profilometer (Bruker, Contour GT-K1; Bruker Pte Ltd, Singapore) coupled with *SurfVision* software (Veeco Instruments Inc.; Plainview, NY, USA) was used for measuring these surface roughness parameters [20].

A goniometer (NRL C.A. Goniometer, Ramé-hart, Inc.; Succasunna, NJ, USA) measured the water contact angle. The Owens-Wendt method was used to calculate surface energy as follows [21]:

$$(1+\cos\theta)\gamma_L = 2\left(\sqrt{\gamma_L^d\gamma_S^d} + \sqrt{\gamma_L^p\gamma_S^p}\right) \tag{9.1}$$

where γ_L indicates the liquid surface tension (water: 72.8 mJ/m^2, glycerol: 63.4 mJ/m^2), and γ_L^d and γ_S^d are the liquid and solid dispersive component (water: 21.8 mJ/m^2, glycerol: 37.0 mJ/m^2). The variables γ_L^p and γ_S^p indicate the liquid and solid polar components (water: 51.0 mJ/m^2, glycerol: 26.4 mJ/m^2), and γ_S is the sum of γ_S^d and γ_S^p [22].

9.2.2 Nanohardness and elasticity measurements

By recording the penetration depth of an indenter into a sample material while the applied load is measured, the areal contact and consequently the hardness of the material can be calculated as well as mechanical properties such as the strain hardening index, fracture toughness, yield strength, and residual stress [23]. The nanomechanical properties of the nanotubular layers such as hardness and elastic modulus were measured by using a nanoindenter (IBIS, Fischer-Cripps Laboratories Pty Ltd, Sydney, Australia) with a three-side pyramidal Berkovich diamond tip that was calibrated against a fused silica standard. The face half-angle of the Berkovich indenter is 65.27–65.3 degrees [23]. Once the maximum prescribed force of 10 mN was reached, loading was stopped, and the load was maintained for 10 s prior to unloading. The data reflects the mean values from multiple indentations, separated by 10-μm intervals that were performed over a 2 × 2 test matrix on each sample. The Oliver-Pharr method [24] was used to calculate the hardness and the elastic modulus. The following equations were used for the calculations [24]:

$$h_c = h_{max} - \varepsilon P_{max}/S \tag{9.2}$$

where ε is a constant of 0.75 that depends on the geometry of the Berkovich indenter, and S is the slope of the unloading curve at the maximum point before the start of unloading. The contact area A is then

$$\mathrm{A} = 24.5h_c^2 \tag{9.3}$$

The hardness is estimated, as below, when the contact area has been determined as above:

$$H = P_{max}/\mathrm{A} \tag{9.4}$$

The relationship between the contact area and the measured unloading stiffness (S) allows the effective elastic modulus (E_{eff}) to be calculated as follows:

$$E_{eff} = S\sqrt{\pi}/2\sqrt{\mathrm{A}} \tag{9.5}$$

The Young's modulus E of a nanotubular layer with Poisson's ratio υ of 0.27 [25] is calculated by

$$1/E_{eff} = \left(1 - \upsilon^2\right)/E + \left(1 - \upsilon_i^2\right)/E_i \tag{9.6}$$

Can we use change to this: where E_i and υ_i are elastic constants, and Poisson's ratio of the indenter is 1.141 and 0.07 GPa, respectively [24].

9.2.3 Assessing hydroxyapatite mineralization and bone cell attachment to nanotubes fabricated in aqueous and nonaqueous electrolytes

The ability to induce, form, and grow HA of the nanotubular surfaces was assessed through soaking the samples in m-SBF for 3 weeks. The procedures for preparing m-SBF have been described previously [19,26]. m-SBF with ionic concentrations equal to human blood plasma was prepared by dissolving reagent-grade chemicals with a composition of 5.403 g NaCl, 0.504 g $NaHCO_3$, 0.426 g Na_2CO_3, 0.225 g KCl, 0.230 g $K_2HPO_4{-}3H_2O$, 0.311 g $MgCl_2{-}6H_2O$, 0.293 g $CaCl_2$, and 0.072 g Na_2SO_4 in 1 L of deionized water that was buffered with 2-(4-(2-hydroxyethyl)-1-piperazinyl) ethane sulfonic acid (HEPES) (17.892 g HEPES dissolved in 100 mL 0.2 M NaOH) and 1 M NaOH at pH 7.4 at 37°C. After immersion, the samples were rinsed by pure water and dried at room temperature.

All samples for the cell culture studies were sterilized in a muffle furnace at 180°C for 3 h. The samples were placed in a 48-well cell culture plate. SaOS2 cells (Barwon

Biomedical Research, Geelong Hospital, Victoria, Australia) were seeded on the surfaces of the TiO_2–ZrO_2–$ZrTiO_4$ nanotubular surface samples that exhibited different inner diameters, outer diameters, and wall thicknesses. The cells were seeded at a density of 5×10^3 cells per well. An MTS assay (a biochemical cell assay used in research) was used to assess the in vitro proliferation of the SaOS2 cells. The cell morphology was observed by means of scanning electron microscopy (SEM) after cell culturing. The cells were dehydrated for the SEM observation by immersion in a buffer solution in which the ethanol concentrations were increased progressively every 10 min to 60%, 70%, 80%, 90%, and 100%. This procedure was followed by chemical drying using hexamethyldisilazane (Sigma-Aldrich, Australia) for 10 min. A gold layer was deposited on the samples prior to SEM observation.

The cell morphology was also observed using confocal microscopy (Leica SP5, Leica Microsystems, Germany). The samples after cell culture tests were fixed in paraformaldehyde and then permeabilized with Triton-X 100 in phosphate-buffered saline (PBS) (Sigma-Aldrich, Australia). Subsequently, the samples were stained with 1% phalloidin and 40-6-diamidino-2-phenylindole for 40 min at room temperature. Three washes in PBS were included between each of the steps. The samples were stored in PBS at 4°C when necessary, and the confocal observations were conducted within 1 week of staining. The significance of any differences in the cell number was analyzed using one-way analysis of variance; ANOVA ($\rho < 0.05$).

9.3 Results and discussion

9.3.1 Formation of TiO_2–ZrO_2–$ZrTiO_4$ nanotubes in aqueous and nonaqueous electrolyte

The initial part of this study investigated the effects of different electrolytes on nanotube size distribution and pattern at a constant F^- concentration in the electrolyte and the two applied potentials. SEM images of the TiO_2–ZrO_2–$ZrTiO_4$ nanotubes fabricated on a Ti50Zr alloy under the applied potentials and in different electrolytes are shown in Fig. 9.1. In this study, the F^- concentration in the electrolyte is denoted as C_{F^-}, the nanotube inner diameter is denoted as D_i, and the outer diameter and wall thickness are denoted as D_o and W_t, respectively. Fig. 9.1(a) and (b) shows the top view of the TiO_2–ZrO_2–$ZrTiO_4$ nanotubes fabricated in 0.5 wt% NH_4F at 20 and 25 V. The top views of TiO_2–ZrO_2–$ZrTiO_4$ fabricated in 0.5 wt % NH_4F in ethylene glycol with 5 wt% water for 90 min at 20 and 30 V are shown in Fig. 9.1(b) and (d).

The mechanism of growing nanotubes on the surface of titanium has been elucidated in prior work [8,17]. In brief, titanium can be passivated when it is exposed to an oxidizing environment or when it is polarized in a standard two- or three-electrode setup of an anodic oxidation cell. If the electrolyte contains fluorine ions, a layer of nanotubes forms instead of the formation of a thick oxide layer. A compact titanium dioxide will be created when the passivating process starts. In the anodizing process, nanotubes start to form via chemical dissolution of the oxide in the presence of fluoride anions, and a competition between oxidation of the metal to TiO_2 and dissolution of TiO_2 to form $[TiF_6]^{2-}$ evolves. When there is an equilibrium between

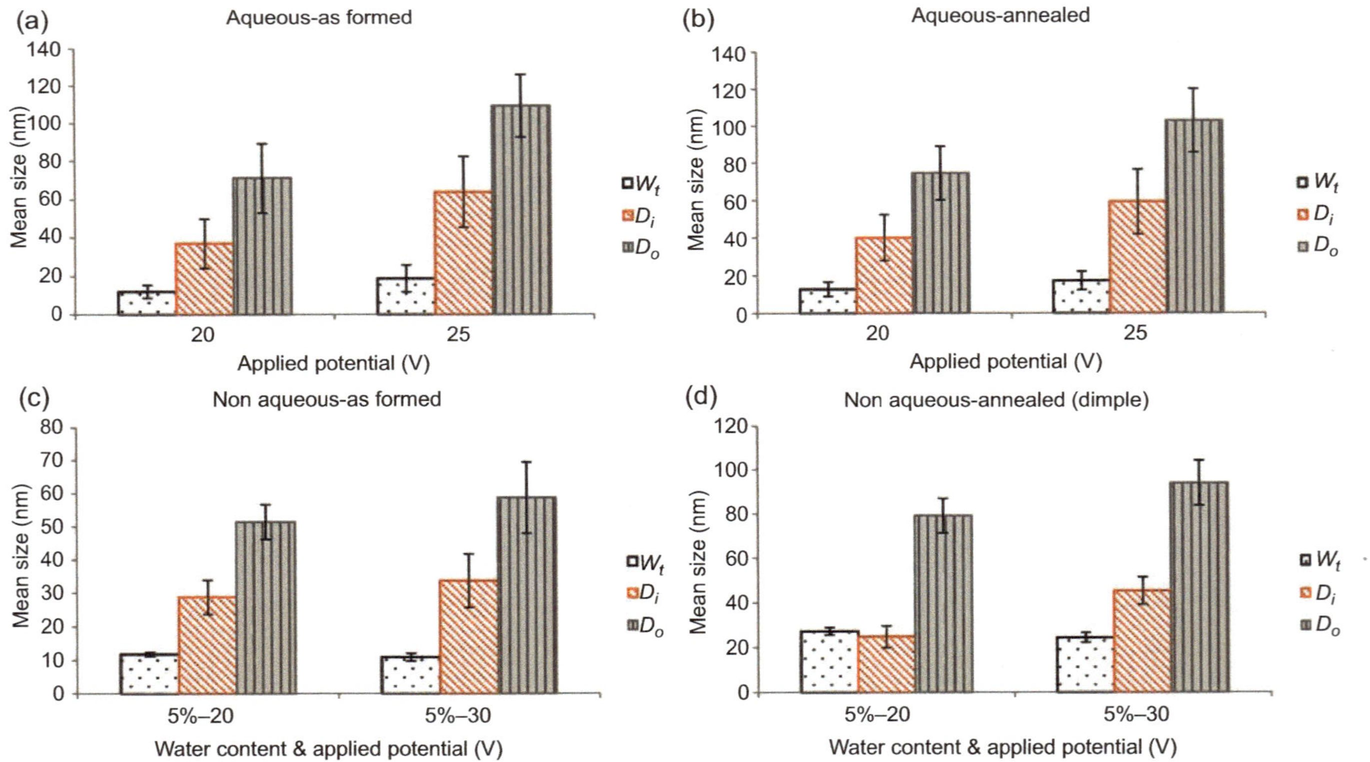

Figure 9.1 Scanning electron microscopy images of nanotubular layers fabricated at (a) 20 V aqueous electrolyte; (b) 5% H_2O, 20 V nonaqueous electrolyte; (c) 25 V aqueous electrolyte; and (d) 5% H_2O, 30 V nonaqueous electrolyte.

oxidation and dissolution, a nanostuctured surface begins to form [5]. In regard to Ti50Zr, the formation of TiO_2–ZrO_2–$ZrTiO_4$ nanotubes is due to oxidation of the alloy to TiO_2, ZrO_2, and $TiZrO_4$ or $ZrTiO_4$ and their subsequent dissolution to form $[TiF_6]^{2-}$ and $[ZrF_6]^{2-}$. The grain structure and needle-like morphology of the underlying alloy influence the orientation and interspace setting of the nanotubes.

Fig. 9.2(a) and (c) shows the nanotubular layers fabricated in aqueous electrolyte after annealing. The nanotubular surface fabricated under nonaqueous electrolyte conditions exhibited cracks in the upper layer after annealing. This upper layer was removed by under ultrasonic conditions to create a dimpled surface that was then subjected to cell culture tests; see Fig. 9.2(b) and (d).

The size distributions of the as-formed and annealed nanotubes fabricated in aqueous and nonaqueous electrolytes were analyzed using normal distribution methods and have been discussed in previous work [8,17,18]. In aqueous electrolyte, increasing the applied potential from 20 to 25 V resulted in a broader distribution of D_i and D_o. That is, either (1) the number of nanotubes with smaller D_i and D_o decreased, or (2) the number of nanotubes with larger D_i and D_o increased due to an increase in the anodic current. The W_t of the nanotubes increased slightly with an increase in the applied potential from 20 to 25 V. Increasing the applied potential from 20 to 30 V during anodization with the same water content in the nonaqueous electrolyte resulted in a broader distribution of D_i and D_o. Thus either (1) the number of nanotubes with smaller D_i and D_o decreased, or (2) the number of nanotubes with larger D_i and D_o

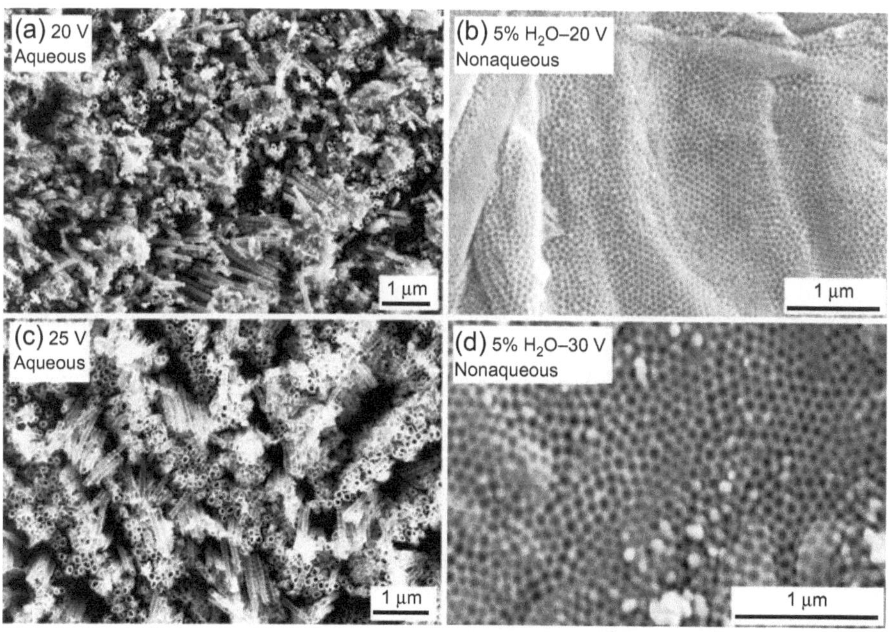

Figure 9.2 Scanning electron microscopy images of annealed nanotubular layers fabricated at (a) 20 V aqueous electrolyte; (b) 5% H_2O, 20 V nonaqueous electrolyte (dimple); (c) 25 V aqueous electrolyte; and (d) 5% H_2O, 30 V nonaqueous electrolyte (dimple).

increased due to the increased anodic current. The extent of increase in the mean W_t was not as great as the mean D_i and D_o. The mean D_i and D_o of nanotubes fabricated in nonaqueous electrolyte were smaller than the mean D_i and D_o of nanotubes fabricated in aqueous electrolyte. Fig. 9.3 shows the mean nanotube size of TiO_2–ZrO_2–$ZrTiO_4$ in aqueous and nonaqueous electrolytes at the two applied potentials.

The amorphous TiO_2–ZrO_2–$ZrTiO_4$ nanotubes fabricated in aqueous electrolyte changed to a mixture of anatase, orthorhombic TiO_2 and ZrO_2, and orthorhombic $ZrTiO_4$, as characterized by X-ray diffraction. The mean D_i increased, the mean D_o decreased, and W_t did not show an obvious change with an increase in applied potential. The amorphous TiO_2–ZrO_2–$ZrTiO_4$ nanotubes fabricated in nonaqueous electrolyte changed to a mixture of tetragonal anatase and rutile, orthorhombic TiO_2 and ZrO_2, and orthorhombic $ZrTiO_4$ after annealing. The mean D_i and D_o and the W_t of the TiO_2–ZrO_2–$ZrTiO_4$ nanotubes increased after annealing.

9.3.2 Surface topography of TiO_2–ZrO_2–$ZrTiO_4$ nanotubes fabricated using aqueous and nonaqueous electrolyte

Three parameters were used to characterize the surface topography of the nanotubular surfaces: amplitude parameters, spacing parameters, and hybrid parameters. The vertical characteristics of surface deviations of nanotubular layers were measured using the amplitude parameter of S_a over the complete 3D surface. The differentiation of peaks, valleys, and the spacing of surface textures are represented by these parameters [20]. The wetting properties of a surface by water, which is its contact angle measured by a goniometer, are used to define the hydrophobicity or hydrophilicity of the surface [27]. They are defined as follows: (1) superhydrophobic: static water contact angle >150 degrees; (2) hydrophobic: water contact angle between 90 and 150 degrees; (3) hydrophilic: water contact angle between 10 and 90 degrees; and (4) superhydrophilic: water contact angle less than 10 degrees [28]. The wettability of a surface is influenced by the type of the material, surface roughness, heterogeneities of the surface, chemical composition, and the presence of any contamination [27].

The S_a and the water contact angle of the surfaces as a function of the electrolyte type and the applied potential of the as-formed and annealed TiO_2–ZrO_2–$ZrTiO_4$ anodized nanotubes are presented in Fig. 9.4.

Increasing the applied potential in the aqueous electrolyte from 20 to 25 V resulted in a decrease in the S_a due to the increased anodic current. Increasing the applied potential from 20 to 30 V in the nonaqueous electrolyte with the same water content resulted in an increase in S_a. The values of S_a of the nanotubular layer of TiO_2–ZrO_2–$ZrTiO_4$ fabricated in aqueous electrolyte were higher than those of the nanotubular layer of TiO_2–ZrO_2–$ZrTiO_4$ anodized in the nonaqueous electrolyte. A direct link was found between the roughness parameter and the wettability or hydrophilic properties of nanotubular layers of TiO_2–ZrO_2–$ZrTiO_4$ fabricated in both aqueous and nonaqueous electrolyte. Increasing the applied potential in the aqueous electrolyte from 20 to 25 V resulted in an increase in the hydrophilic properties of TiO_2–ZrO_2–$ZrTiO_4$ nanotubes. Increasing the applied potential from 20 to 30 V in the nonaqueous electrolyte with the same water content resulted in an increase in the hydrophilic

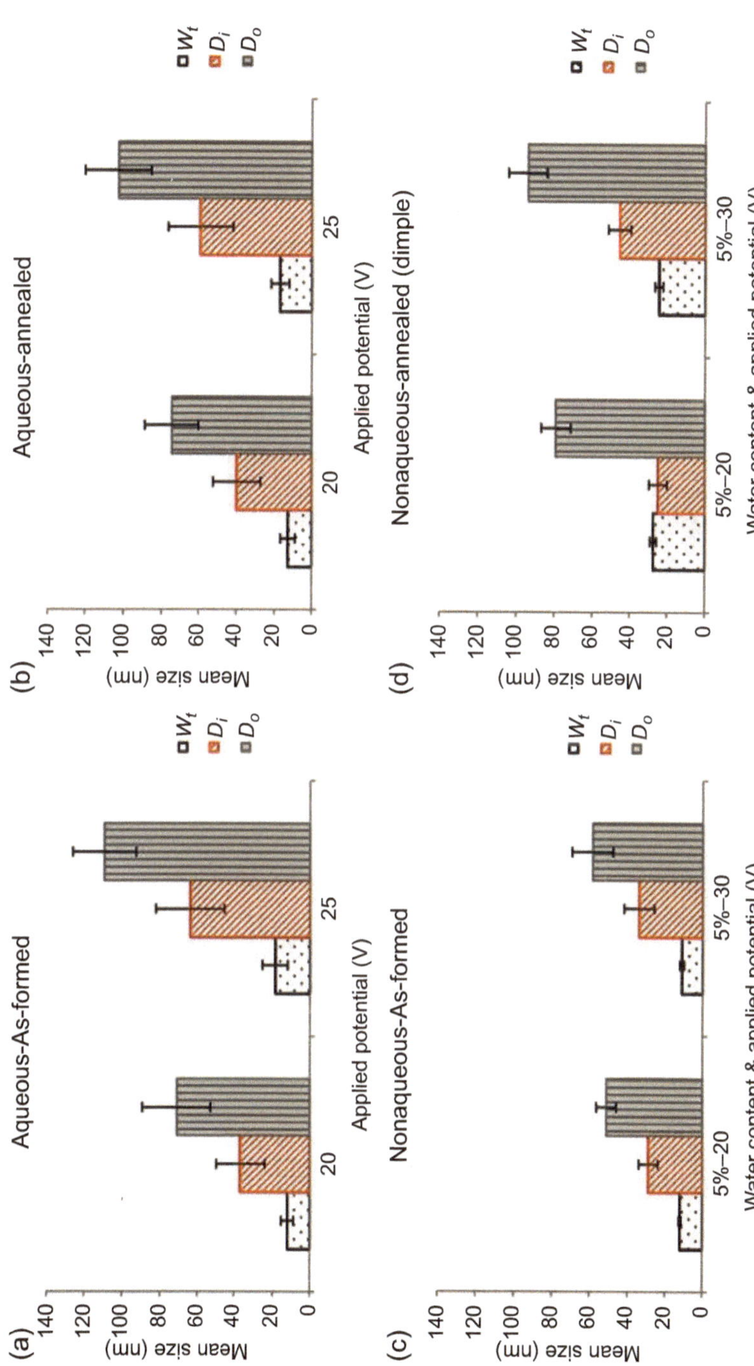

Figure 9.3 Mean nanotube size of TiO_2–ZrO_2–$ZrTiO_4$ as a function of electrolyte type at (a) 20 and 25 V aqueous, as-formed; (b) 20 and 25 V aqueous, annealed; (c) 20 and 30 V nonaqueous, as-formed; and (d) 20 and 30 V nonaqueous, annealed.

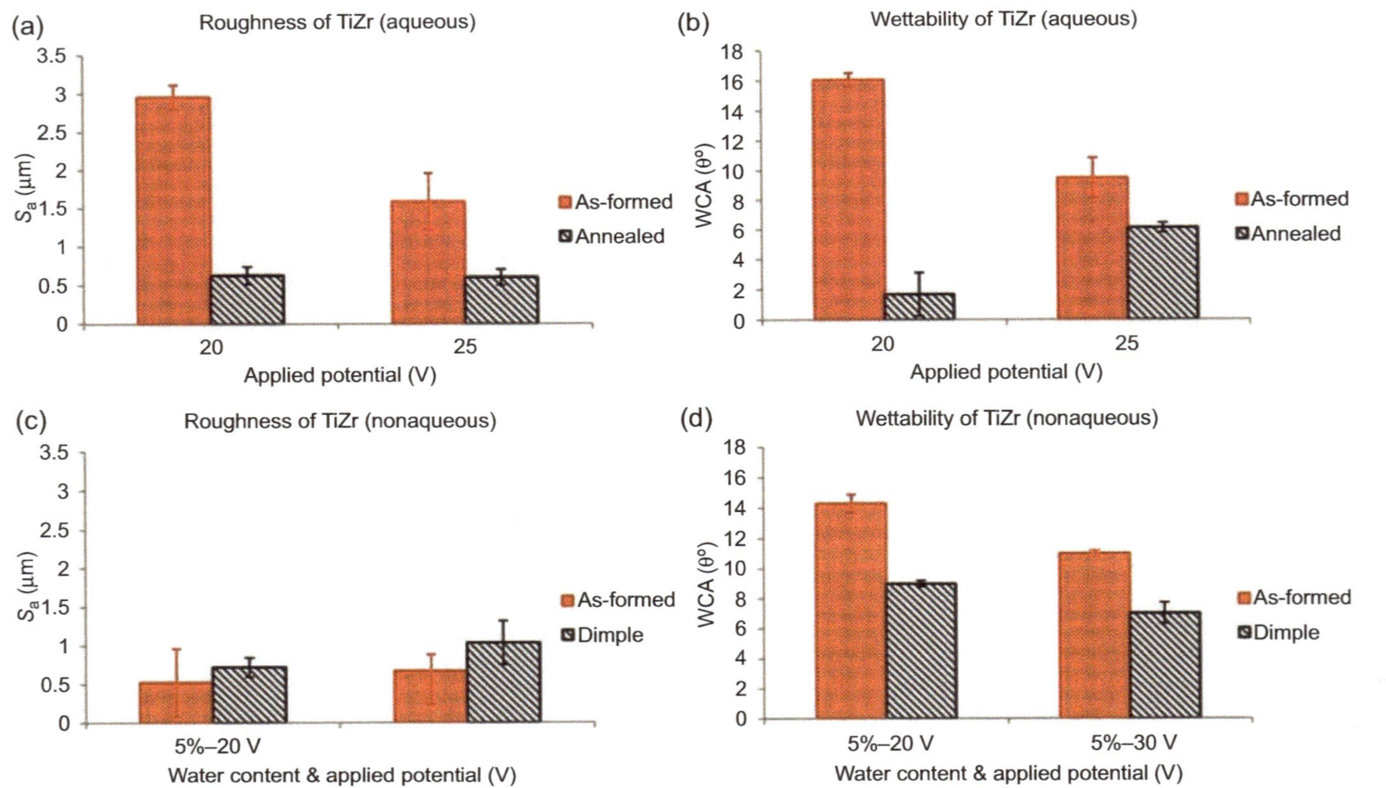

Figure 9.4 (a) The mean roughness (S_a) and (b) the mean water contact angle (WCA) of the as-formed and annealed TiO_2–ZrO_2–$ZrTiO_4$ nanotubular surfaces fabricated in aqueous electrolyte as a function of the applied potential; (c) the mean roughness (S_a); and (d) the mean WCA of the as-formed and annealed TiO_2 nanotubular surfaces fabricated in nonaqueous electrolyte as a function of the applied potential.

properties of $TiO_2-ZrO_2-ZrTiO_4$ nanotubes. The hydrophilic properties of $TiO_2-ZrO_2-ZrTiO_4$ nanotubes fabricated in aqueous electrolyte were higher than those of the $TiO_2-ZrO_2-ZrTiO_4$ nanotubes fabricated in nonaqueous electrolyte, probably because of their different mean D_i and roughness parameters of S_a. The roughness parameters and calculated surface energies of $TiO_2-ZrO_2-ZrTiO_4$ nanotubes fabricated in aqueous and nonaqueous electrolyte are listed in Table 9.1.

There was a direct between the hydrophilic properties and the calculated surface energy of the nanotubular layer of $TiO_2-ZrO_2-ZrTiO_4$ fabricated in aqueous electrolyte. The surface energy of the nanotubular layer increased when the hydrophilic properties increased. Such a link was not observed for the nanotubular layer of $TiO_2-ZrO_2-ZrTiO_4$ fabricated in nonaqueous electrolyte (though residual organic electrolyte may have remained within the nanotubes). The surface energies of the nanotubular layers of $TiO_2-ZrO_2-ZrTiO_4$ fabricated in aqueous electrolyte were almost the same as those of the nanotubular layers of $TiO_2-ZrO_2-ZrTiO_4$ fabricated in nonaqueous electrolyte.

9.3.3 Mechanical properties of $TiO_2-ZrO_2-ZrTiO_4$ nanotubes fabricated in aqueous and nonaqueous electrolyte

The nanomechanical characteristics of the as-formed and annealed $TiO_2-ZrO_2-ZrTiO_4$ nanotubes were measured using nanoindentation to obtain the nanohardness and Young's modulus. Fig. 9.5 shows the curves of the loading–unloading forces with respect to the nanoindentation depths of the as-formed and annealed $TiO_2-ZrO_2-ZrTiO_4$ nanotubes fabricated at different applied potentials in aqueous electrolyte.

The nano Young's modulus and hardness were determined as a function of depth, using the method described in Section 9.2.2. The hardness and elastic modulus were calculated and are presented in Fig. 9.6.

The maximum hardness of the nanotubular layer of $TiO_2-ZrO_2-ZrTiO_4$ anodized in aqueous electrolyte was 211.8 and 336.2 MPa before and after annealing, respectively. These values were lower than the corresponding bare metal, which was measured as 4.38 GPa. The maximum elastic modulus of the nanotubular layer of $TiO_2-ZrO_2-ZrTiO_4$ was 149.9 and 248.7 GPa before and after annealing, respectively, which was higher than the corresponding bare metal, which revealed 102.9 GPa. It can be concluded that the porosity of the nanotubes influenced the hardness, and the ceramic properties of the nanotubular layer influenced the elasticity of the bare metal. By increasing the applied potential and consequently the nanotube size, the hardness and elasticity of nanotubes decreased for as-formed nanotubes and increased for annealed nanotubes.

Nanoindentation was performed to measure the nanohardness and Young's modulus of as-formed and annealed $TiO_2-ZrO_2-ZrTiO_4$ nanotubes fabricated by using nonaqueous electrolyte. Fig. 9.7 shows the loading–unloading forces versus the nanoindentation depths of as-formed and annealed $TiO_2-ZrO_2-ZrTiO_4$ nanotubes fabricated at 5 wt% H_2O nonaqueous electrolyte under two applied potentials.

Table 9.1 Surface index and spacing parameters of annealed and dimpled $TiO_2-ZrO_2-ZrTiO_4$ nanotubular surfaces and their calculated surface energy, fabricated on Ti50Zr

Anodization condition (mean size)	Roughness parameters			Water contact angle (θ)	Surface energy		
	S_m (nm^3/nm^2)	S_c (nm^3/nm^2)	S_v (nm^3/nm^2)		γ_S^d (mJ/m^2)	γ_S^p (mJ/m^2)	$\Gamma_S = \gamma_S^d + \gamma_S^p$ (mJ/m^2)
20 V ($D_i = 40$ nm)	35 ± 9	874 ± 204	124 ± 36	1.7 ± 1.4	15.44	58.10	73.54
25 V ($D_i = 59$ nm)	43 ± 26	1435 ± 223	231 ± 73	6.1 ± 0.3	14.69	58.66	73.35
5 wt% H_2O, 20 V ($D_i = 25$ nm)	62 ± 45	1074 ± 170	81 ± 16	9.0 ± 0.2	13.37	59.91	73.28
5 wt% H_2O, 30 V ($D_i = 45$ nm)	57 ± 28	1581 ± 682	110 ± 40	7.0 ± 0.7	13.85	59.64	73.49

Note: Each data point is an average of three measurements.
Sm, Surface material volume; Sc, Core void volume; Sv, Surface void volume.

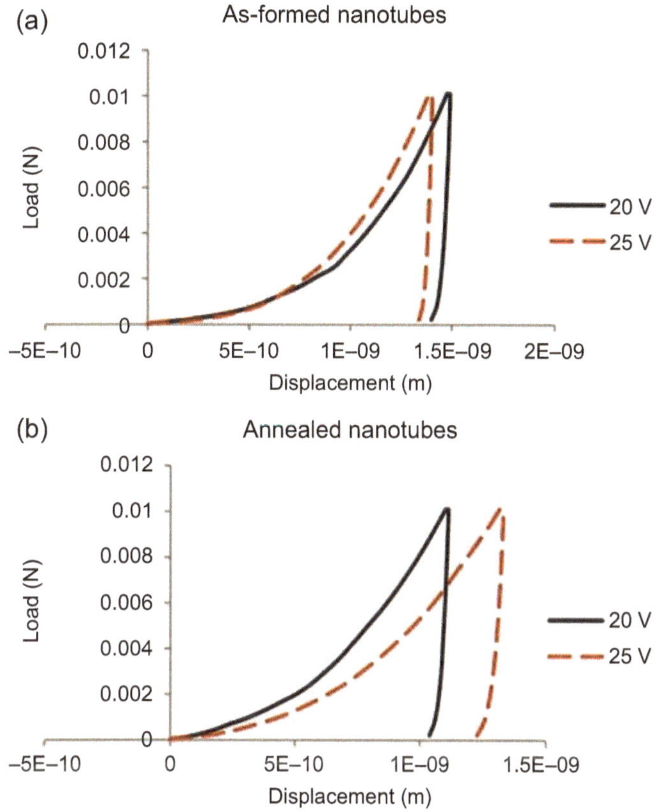

Figure 9.5 Loading–unloading force versus the nanoindentation depths of (a) as-formed $TiO_2-ZrO_2-ZrTiO_4$ and (b) annealed $TiO_2-ZrO_2-ZrTiO_4$ fabricated at the applied potential 20 and 25 V in aqueous electrolyte.

The nano Young's modulus and hardness were determined as a function of depth. The hardness and elastic modulus were calculated using the method described in Section 9.2.2 and are presented in Fig. 9.8.

The maximum hardness of the nanotubular layer of $TiO_2-ZrO_2-ZrTiO_4$ anodized in nonaqueous electrolyte was 330.2 and 4019.0 MPa before and after annealing, respectively, which was lower than the corresponding bare metal that was measured as 4.38 GPa. The maximum elastic modulus of the nanotubular layer of $TiO_2-ZrO_2-ZrTiO_4$ was 81.4 GPa before annealing and 84.4 GPa after annealing, which was lower than the corresponding bare metal at 102.9 GPa. It can be concluded that the nanotube porosity influenced the hardness, and the ceramic constituents of the nanotubular layer influenced the elasticity of the transformed metal surface. By increasing the applied potential and consequently the nanotube size, the hardness and elasticity of the as-formed nanotubes decreased, and the properties of the annealed nanotubes increased.

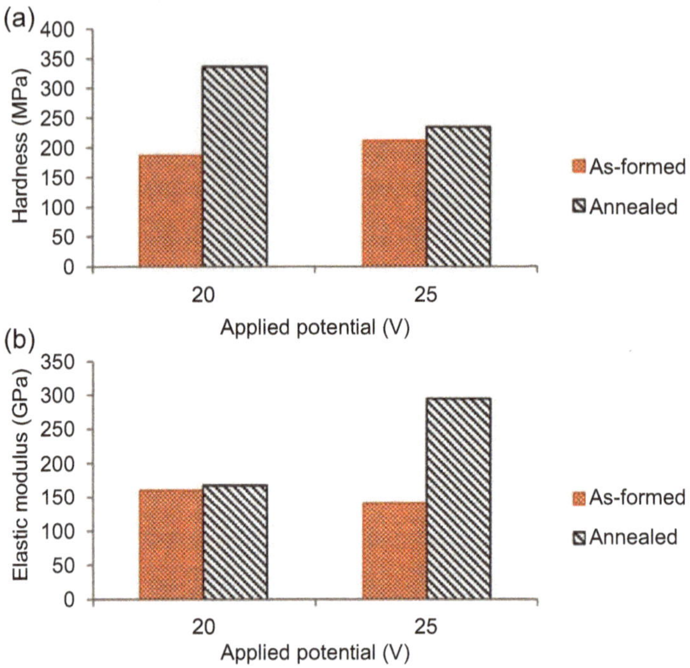

Figure 9.6 The nanomechanical properties of (a) hardness and (b) elastic modulus of TiO_2–ZrO_2–$ZrTiO_4$ nanotubes fabricated at different applied potentials in aqueous electrolyte.

The porosity of both nanotubular layers of TiO_2–ZrO_2–$ZrTiO_4$ fabricated in aqueous and nonaqueous electrolyte caused a decrease in the hardness of the Ti50Zr alloy surface. However, the ceramic properties of the metal oxide layer fabricated in aqueous electrolyte caused an increase in the elasticity of the alloy surface. The hard and brittle nanotubular layer fabricated in nonaqueous electrolyte exhibited a lower elastic modulus than the bare alloy. The nanohardness and elasticity were influenced by the values of the porosity, as reflected in the nanotube sizes, for both nanotubular layers.

9.3.4 Hydroxyapatite mineralization and bone cell attachment of TiO_2–ZrO_2–$ZrTiO_4$ nanotubes fabricated in aqueous and nonaqueous electrolyte

The bioactivity of TiO_2–ZrO_2–$ZrTiO_4$ nanotubes fabricated in aqueous and nonaqueous electrolyte was evaluated by immersing them in m-SBF. A dense and uniform layer of nanobristle spheres and nanoflakes of bone-like HA was formed on the surface of the nanotubular layers, as shown in Fig. 9.9(a–d). It has been reported that an anatase or a rutile structure of TiO_2 nanotubes was more favorable for HA formation than an amorphous structure [29,30]. Therefore samples of nanotubes fabricated in

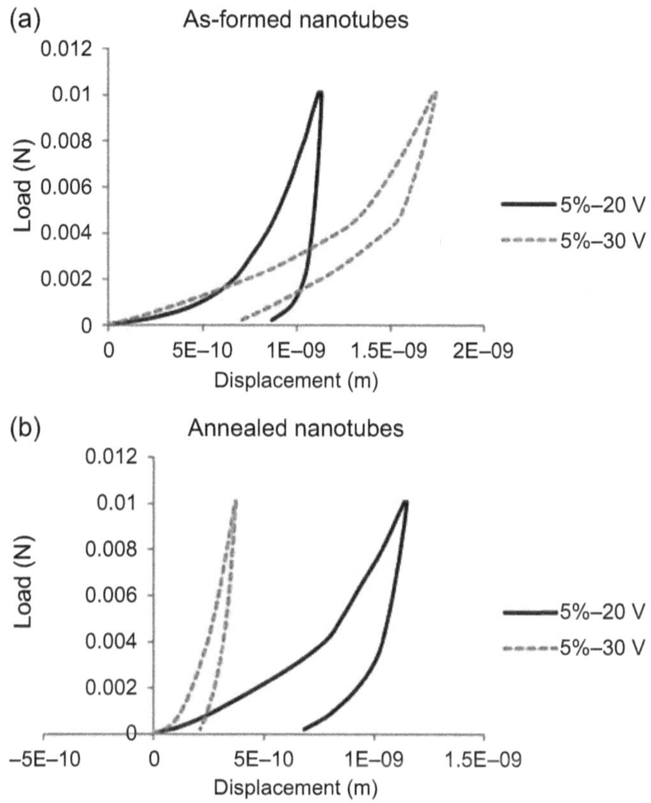

Figure 9.7 Loading–unloading forces versus the nanoindentation depths of (a) as-formed TiO_2–ZrO_2–$ZrTiO_4$ and (b) annealed TiO_2–ZrO_2–$ZrTiO_4$ fabricated at 5 wt% H_2O nonaqueous electrolyte at the applied potentials of 20 and 30 V.

aqueous electrolyte were annealed at 500°C for 3 h and (2) samples of nanotubes fabricated in nonaqueous electrolyte were annealed at 500°C for 2 h to obtain crystalline phases. The top layer of nanotubes fabricated in nonaqueous electrolyte was brittle and cracked after annealing. The brittle layer was removed, and the revealed dimpled surface of nanotubes was used for further investigation. Fig. 9.9(e–h) shows the SEM images after annealing.

The Ca/P ratio (in atomic percent) of the HA mineralized on the surface of nanotubular layers fabricated in aqueous and nonaqueous electrolyte is depicted in Fig. 9.10.

The mechanism of HA formation on nanotubes has been described in Chapter 7 of this book. The Ca/P ratio of HA precipitated on the nanotubular layer of TiO_2–ZrO_2–$ZrTiO_4$ increased with an increase of D_i (as a result of increasing applied potential) for both the as-formed and annealed nanotubes fabricated in aqueous electrolyte. On the other hand, for both the as-formed and annealed nanotubes fabricated in nonaqueous electrolyte, the Ca/P ratio of HA precipitated on the nanotubular layer of TiO_2–ZrO_2–$ZrTiO_4$ decreased with an increase of D_i (as a result of increasing applied potential).

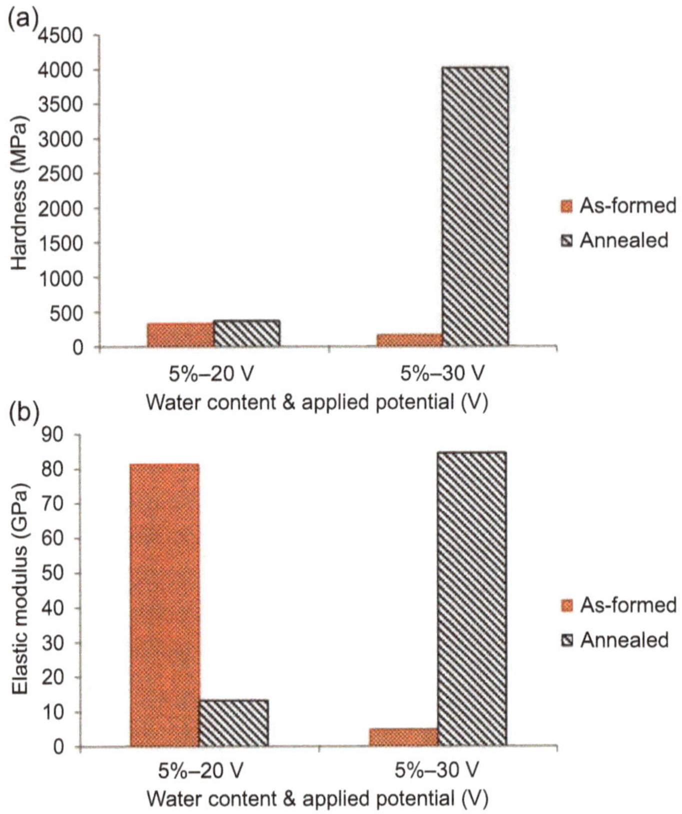

Figure 9.8 The nanomechanical properties of $TiO_2-ZrO_2-ZrTiO_4$ nanotubes fabricated in nonaqueous electrolyte with the same water content at different applied potentials: (a) hardness and (b) elastic modulus.

The nanotubular layers of $TiO_2-ZrO_2-ZrTiO_4$ fabricated in both aqueous and nonaqueous electrolytes with a range of nanotube sizes were bioactive. The size, shape, hydrophilic properties, and crystalline phase of the nanotubes influenced the Ca/P ratio of HA.

The cell behavior of osteoblasts (SaOS2) on the surface of $TiO_2-ZrO_2-ZrTiO_4$ nanotubes fabricated in aqueous and nonaqueous electrolyte with a variety of nanotube sizes and shapes with different physical and chemical properties was evaluated. Fig. 9.11 shows the SEM images of cell attachment on the nanotubular layers fabricated under two different conditions with similar distributions of D_i, and Fig. 9.12 shows the confocal microscopy images of the cells attached on the nanotubular layers.

The cell cluster with the highest percentage of attachment of 84.9% was on the surface of the nanotubular layer with $D_i = 25 \pm 5$ nm fabricated in nonaqueous electrolyte (Fig. 9.13). The percentage of cell attachment decreased when the D_i increased to 45 ± 6 nm. Also, the percentage of cell attachment on 40 ± 12 nm (fabricated in aqueous electrolyte) was 41%, which was higher than the percentage of cell attachment

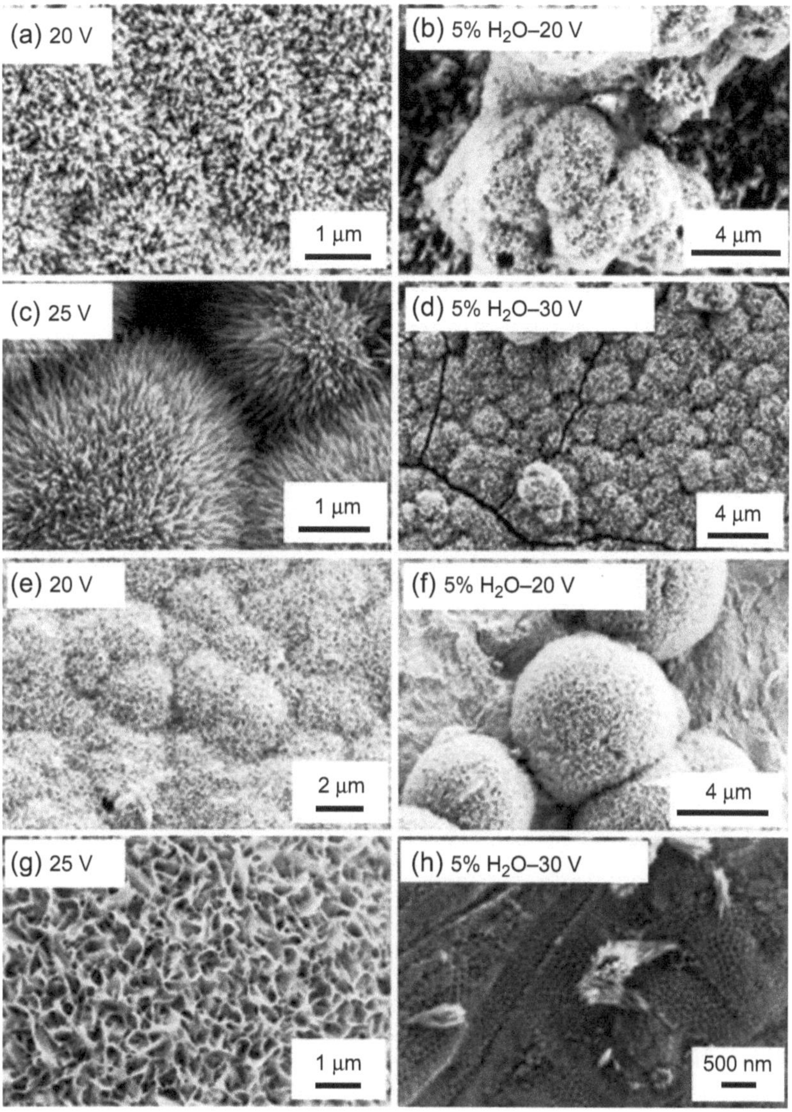

Figure 9.9 Scanning electron microscopy images of hydroxyapatite mineralization on the as-formed and annealed TiO_2–ZrO_2–$ZrTiO_4$ nanotubes: (a) as-formed at 20 V (aqueous); (b) as-formed 5 wt% H_2O at 20 V (nonaqueous); (c) as-formed at 25 V (aqueous); (d) as-formed 5 wt% H_2O at 30 V (nonaqueous); (e) annealed at 20 V (aqueous); (f) annealed 5 wt% H_2O at 20 V (nonaqueous); (g) annealed at 25 V (aqueous); and (h) annealed 5 wt% H_2O at 30 V (nonaqueous).

on nanotubes with higher D_i. The lowest percentage of cell attachment of 25.9% was on the nanotubular surface with $D_i = 59 \pm 17$ nm fabricated in an aqueous electrolyte.

The conditions for clustering of integrins on the surfaces with low roughness spacing parameters were not favorable, even though the nanospacing was optimal

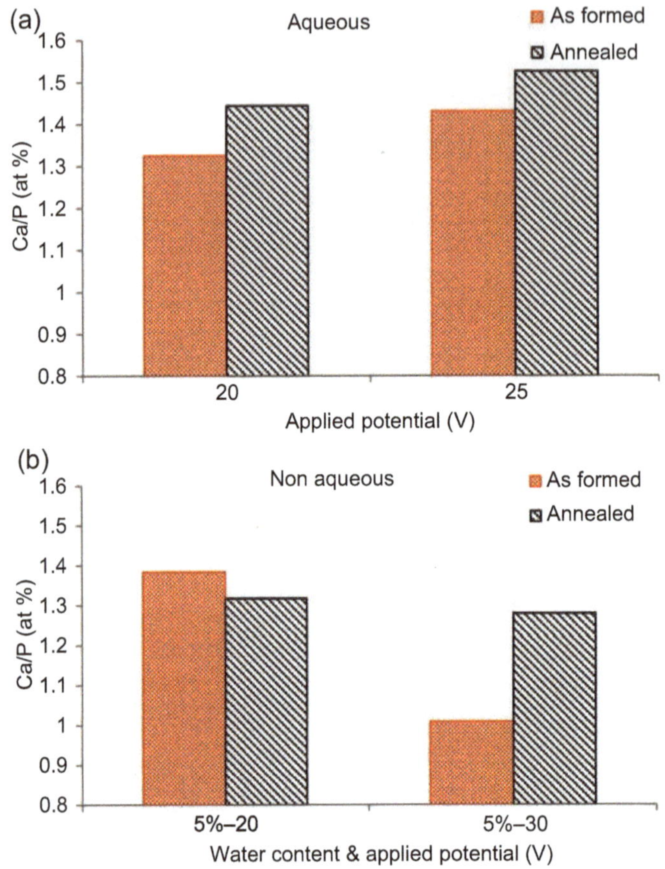

Figure 9.10 The atomic ratio, in percent, of Ca/P of mineralized hydroxyapatite on (a) as-formed and annealed TiO_2–ZrO_2–$ZrTiO_4$ nanotubes (aqueous) and (b) as-formed and dimpled TiO_2–ZrO_2–$ZrTiO_4$ nanotubes (nonaqueous).

since the surface geometry could potentially disrupt the formation of focal adhesion. It was reported that long-term adhesion is correlated to topography and the synthesis of extracellular matrix (ECM) proteins by the cells themselves, and cell–cell contacts are affected by the hybrid roughness parameters [17,18]. Table 9.2 summarizes the nanotubular surface parameters that influence cell attachment percentages. It can be determined that a high cell attachment was evident on the surface of nanotubes with either D_i or W_t in the range of the optimum nanospacing (<30 nm), and this was influenced by the roughness parameter of the surface.

Although the morphology and topography of the nanotubular layer fabricated in aqueous electrolyte are different from the nanotubular layer fabricated in nonaqueous electrolyte, they reveal almost the same surface energy. It can be concluded that the non-separate walled nanotubes fabricated in the nonaqueous electrolyte may adsorb more protein and serve as more suitable nanopattern surfaces for bone cell attachment. Besides

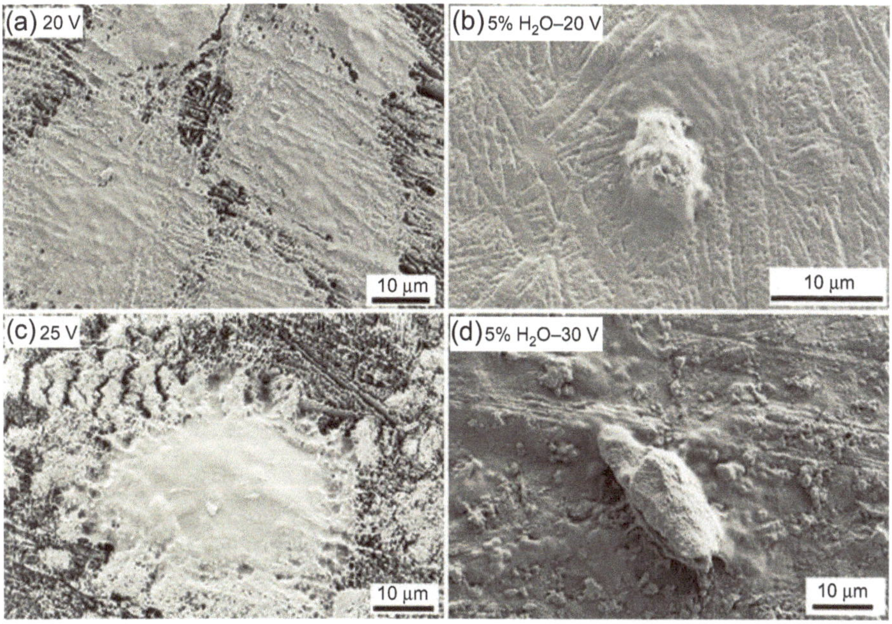

Figure 9.11 Scanning electron microscopy images of SaOS2 cells after culturing for 24 h on $TiO_2-ZrO_2-ZrTiO_4$ nanotubes fabricated at (a) 20 V, (b) 5 wt% H_2O at 20 V, (c) 25 V, and (d) 5 wt% H_2O at 30 V.

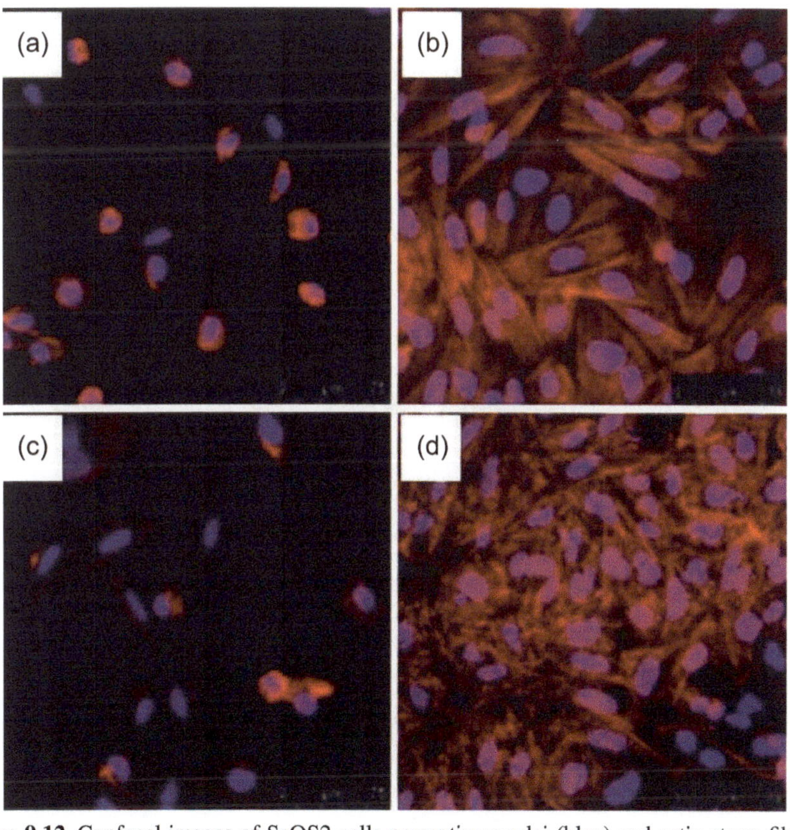

Figure 9.12 Confocal images of SaOS2 cells presenting nuclei (blue) and actin stress fibers (red) after culturing for 7 days on $TiO_2-ZrO_2-ZrTiO_4$ nanotubes fabricated at (a) 20 V, (b) 5 wt% H_2O at 20 V, (c) 25 V, and (d) 5 wt% H_2O at 30 V.

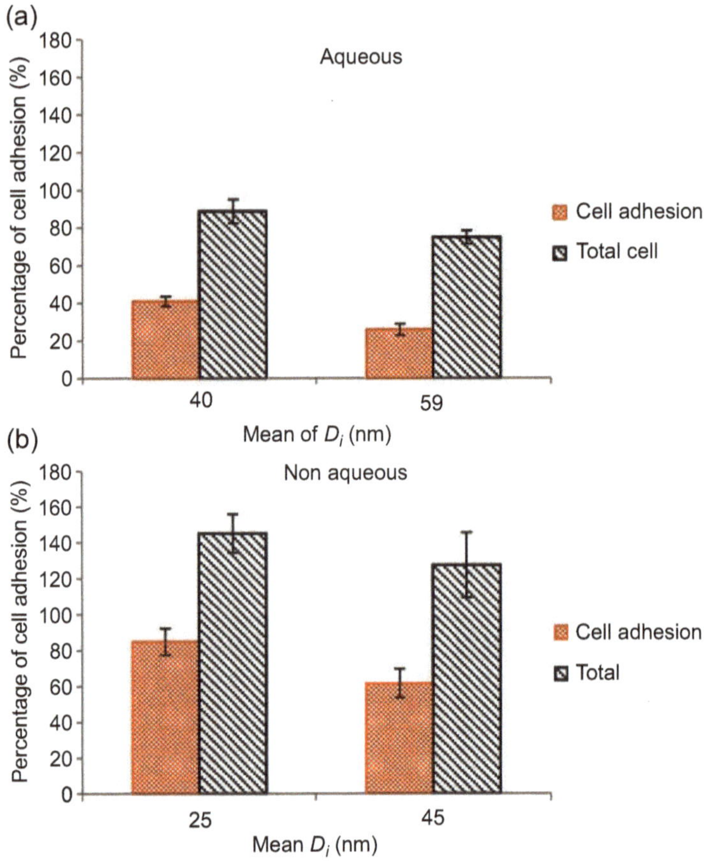

Figure 9.13 The percentage of cells attached to the nanotubular surface of TiO_2–ZrO_2–$ZrTiO_4$ fabricated in aqueous and nonaqueous electrolyte after culturing for 7 days.

the D_i of nanotubes, the topography of the nanotubular surface played an important role on the density of cell attachment when the hydrophilic properties were similar.

9.4 Conclusions

Two morphologies of TiO_2–ZrO_2–$ZrTiO_4$ nanotubes were fabricated using either an aqueous or nonaqueous electrolyte. The effect of an applied potential of 20 and 25 V in an aqueous electrolyte with 0.5 wt% NH_4F and the effect of an applied potential of 20 and 30 V in a nonaqueous electrolyte (ethylene glycol) that contained 0.5 wt% NH_4F and 5 wt% H_2O were investigated with regard to the fabrication of TiO_2–ZrO_2–$ZrTiO_4$ nanotubes. Regardless of the distribution of nanotube sizes of D_i, D_o, and W_t, nanotubes fabricated in a nonaqueous electrolyte exhibited a lower mean D_i, with nonseparated walls, within the range of applied potentials explored.

Table 9.2 The percentage of cells attached to the surfaces of different pore sizes and roughness parameters of $TiO_2-ZrO_2-ZrTiO_4$ nanotubes fabricated in aqueous and nonaqueous electrolyte after cell culturing for 7 days

		Nanotube sizes		Roughness parameters	
Anodization conditions	**Cell adhesion (%)**	**D_i (nm)**	**W_t (nm)**	**S_a (μm)**	**S_m (nm^3/nm^2)**
20 V	41.0 ± 2.6	40 ± 12	13 ± 4	0.64 ± 0.1	35 ± 9
25 V	25.9 ± 3.1	59 ± 17	17 ± 5	1.09 ± 0.14	43 ± 26
5 wt% H_2O, 20 V	84.9 ± 7.4	25 ± 5	27 ± 2	0.72 ± 0.12	62 ± 45
5 wt% H_2O, 30 V	61.5 ± 8.1	45 ± 6	24 ± 2	1.03 ± 0.28	57 ± 28

Sm, Surface material volume; Sc, Core void volume; Sv, Surface void volume.

The S_a and the RMS S_q of the $TiO_2-ZrO_2-ZrTiO_4$ nanotubular layers were evaluated using 3D profilometry. Because of the different oxidation and dissolution rates of the elements of the alloy, Ti and Zr, the nanotubes not only exhibited different nanotube sizes but also exhibited different lengths, resulting in different amplitude and space roughness parameters. The hardness and elastic modulus of both nanotubular layers of $TiO_2-ZrO_2-ZrTiO_4$ fabricated in aqueous and nonaqueous electrolyte were measured using nanoindentation. The porosity and ceramic properties of the nanotubular layers were reflected in a hardness decrease and an elastic modulus increase for layers fabricated in either aqueous or nonaqueous electrolytes.

The as-formed $TiO_2-ZrO_2-ZrTiO_4$ nanotubular layers on the surface of Ti50Zr fabricated in aqueous and nonaqueous electrolyte were amorphous. After annealing, crystalline phases formed, and their physical, chemical, and mechanical properties changed. The mean of the roughness parameter of S_a of the $TiO_2-ZrO_2-ZrTiO_4$ nanotubular layers decreased. The hydrophilic properties of the $TiO_2-ZrO_2-ZrTiO_4$ nanotubular layers represented by the water contact angle increased, and the calculated surface energy increased after annealing. After annealing, the hardness of the nanotubular layer of $TiO_2-ZrO_2-ZrTiO_4$ increased.

It can be concluded that the $TiO_2-ZrO_2-ZrTiO_4$ nanotubes on Ti50Zr alloy fabricated in a nonaqueous electrolyte with a variety of nanotube size distributions and morphologies possess higher bioactivity and bone cell attachment compared to those fabricated in an aqueous electrolyte.

Acknowledgments

This research is financially supported by the National Health and Medical Research Council through grant GNT1087290.

References

[1] Popat KC, Chalvanichkul KI, Barnes GL, Latempa Jr TJ, Grimes CA, Desai TA. Osteogenic differentiation of marrow stromal cells cultured on nanoporous alumina surfaces. J Biomed Mater Res – Part A 2007;80:955–64.

[2] Anselme K, Bigerelle M. Topography effects of pure titanium substrates on human osteoblast long-term adhesion. Acta Biomater 2005;1:211–22.

[3] Anselme K, Linez P, Bigerelle M, Le Maguer D, Le Maguer A, Hardouin P, et al. The relative influence of the topography and chemistry of TiAl6V4 surfaces on osteoblastic cell behaviour. Biomaterials 2000;21:1567–77.

[4] Anselme K, Ploux L, Ponche A. Cell/Material interfaces: influence of surface chemistry and surface topography on cell adhesion. J Adhes Sci Technol 2010;24:831–52.

[5] Anselme K, Ponche A, Bigerelle M. Relative influence of surface topography and surface chemistry on cell response to bone implant materials. Part 2: biological aspects. Proc Inst Mech Eng Part H: J Eng Med 2010;224:1487–507.

[6] Shin DH, Shokuhfar T, Choi CK, Lee SH, Friedrich C. Wettability changes of TiO_2 nanotube surfaces. Nanotechnology 2011;22:315704–11.

[7] Balaur E, Macak JM, Tsuchiya H, Schmuki P. Wetting behaviour of layers of TiO_2 nanotubes with different diameters. J Mater Chem 2005;15:4488.

[8] Minagar S, Berndt CC, Gengenbach T, Wen C. Fabrication and characterization of TiO_2-ZrO_2- $ZrTiO_4$ nanotubes on TiZr alloy manufactured via anodization. J Mater Chem B 2014;2:71–83.

[9] Park J, Bauer S, Von Der Mark K, Schmuki P. Nanosize and vitality: TiO_2 nanotube diameter directs cell fate. Nano Lett 2007;7:1686–91.

[10] Oh S, Brammer KS, Li YSJ, Teng D, Engler AJ, Chien S, et al. Stem cell fate dictated solely by altered nanotube dimension. Proc Natl Acad Sci USA 2009;106:2130–5.

[11] Brammer KS, Oh S, Cobb CJ, Bjursten LM, Heyde Hvd, Jin S. Improved bone-forming functionality on diameter-controlled TiO_2 nanotube surface. Acta Biomater 2009;5:3215–23.

[12] Chen X, Nouri A, Li Y, Lin J, Hodgson PD, Wen CE. Effect of surface roughness of Ti, Zr, and TiZr on apatite precipitation from simulated body fluid. Biotechnol Bioeng 2008;101: 378–87.

[13] Kim S, Lim J, Lee S, Nam S, Kang H, Choi J. Anodically nanostructured titanium oxides for implant applications. Electrochim Acta 2008;53:4846–51.

[14] Kim WG, Choe HC. Nanostructure and corrosion behaviors of nanotube formed Ti–Zr alloy. Trans Nonferrous Met Soc China (Engl Ed) 2009;19:1005–8.

[15] Jha H, Hahn R, Schmuki P. Ultrafast oxide nanotube formation on TiNb, TiZr and TiTa alloys by rapid breakdown anodization. Electrochim Acta 2010;55:8883–7.

[16] Grigorescu S, Pruna V, Titorencu I, Jinga VV, Mazare A, Schmuki P, et al. The two step nanotube formation on TiZr as scaffolds for cell growth. Bioelectrochemistry 2014;98: 39–45.

[17] Minagar S, Li Y, Berndt CC, Wen C. Cell response and bioactivity of titania-zirconia-zirconium titanate nanotubes with different nanoscale topographies fabricated in a non-aqueous electrolyte. Biomater Sci 2015;3:636–44.

[18] Minagar S, Li Y, Berndt CC, Wen C. The influence of titania–zirconia–zirconium titanate nanotube characteristics on osteoblast cell adhesion. Acta Biomater 2015;12:281–9.

[19] Oyane A, Onuma K, Ito A, Kim HM, Kokubo T, Nakamura T. Formation and growth of clusters in conventional and new kinds of simulated body fluids. J Biomed Mater Res - Part A 2003;64:339–48.

[20] Gadelmawla ES, Koura MM, Maksoud TMA, Elewa IM, Soliman HH. Roughness parameters. J Mater Process Technol 2002;123:133–45.
[21] Owens DK, Wendt RC. Estimation of the surface free energy of polymers. J Appl Polym Sci 1969;13:1741–7.
[22] Dann JR. Forces involved in the adhesive process. I. critical surface tensions of polymeric solids as determined with polar liquids. J Colloid Interf Sci 1970;32:302–20.
[23] Fischer-Cripps AC. Critical review of analysis and interpretation of nanoindentation test data. Surf Coat Technology 2006;200:4153–65.
[24] Oliver WC, Pharr GM. Measurement of hardness and elastic modulus by instrumented indentation: advances in understanding and refinements to methodology. J Mater Res 2004;19:3–20.
[25] Li H, Khor KA, Cheang P. Impact formation and microstructure characterization of thermal sprayed hydroxyapatite/titania composite coatings. Biomaterials 2003;24:949–57.
[26] Kokubo T, Takadama H. How useful is SBF in predicting in vivo bone bioactivity? Biomaterials 2006;27:2907–15.
[27] EL-010 SASNZC. Guidance on the measurement of wettability of insulator surfaces. GPO Box 5420, Sydney, NSW 2001. Australia: SAI Global; 2005. p. 15.
[28] Webb HK, Hasan J, Truong VK, Crawford RJ, Ivanova EP. Nature inspired structured surfaces for biomedical applications. Curr Med Chem 2011;18:3367–75.
[29] Tsuchiya H, Macak JM, Müller L, Kunze J, Müller F, Greil P, et al. Hydroxyapatite growth on anodic TiO_2 nanotubes. J Biomed Mater Res Part A 2006;77A:534–41.
[30] Kunze J, Muller L, Macak J, Greil P, Schmuki P, Muller F. Time-dependent growth of biomimetic apatite on anodic TiO_2 nanotubes. Electrochim Acta 2008;53:6995–7003.

Index

'*Note*: Page numbers followed by "f" indicate figures and "t" indicate tables.'

V

W